Progress in Inflammation Research

Series Editor

Prof. Dr. Michael J. Parnham
PLIVA
Research Institute
Prilaz baruna Filipovica 25
10000 Zagreb
Croatia

Published titles:
T Cells in Arthritis, P. Miossec, W. van den Berg, G. Firestein (Editors), 1998
Chemokines and Skin, E. Kownatzki, J. Norgauer (Editors), 1998
Medicinal Fatty Acids, J. Kremer (Editor), 1998
Inducible Enzymes in the Inflammatory Response, D.A. Willoughby, A. Tomlinson (Editors), 1999
Cytokines in Severe Sepsis and Septic Shock, H. Redl, G. Schlag (Editors), 1999
Fatty Acids and Inflammatory Skin Diseases, J.-M. Schröder (Editor), 1999
Immunomodulatory Agents from Plants, H. Wagner (Editor), 1999
Cytokines and Pain, L. Watkins, S. Maier (Editors), 1999
In Vivo *Models of Inflammation*, D. Morgan, L. Marshall (Editors), 1999
Pain and Neurogenic Inflammation, S.D. Brain, P. Moore (Editors), 1999
Anti-Inflammatory Drugs in Asthma, A.P. Sampson, M.K. Church (Editors), 1999
Novel Inhibitors of Leukotrienes, G. Folco, B. Samuelsson, R.C. Murphy (Editors), 1999
Vascular Adhesion Molecules and Inflammation, J.D. Pearson (Editor), 1999
Metalloproteinases as Targets for Anti-Inflammatory Drugs, K.M.K. Bottomley, D. Bradshaw, J.S. Nixon (Editors), 1999
Free Radicals and Inflammation, P.G. Winyard, D.R. Blake, C.H. Evans (Editors), 2000
Gene Therapy in Inflammatory Diseases, C.H. Evans, P. Robbins (Editors), 2000
New Cytokines as Potential Drugs, S. K. Narula, R. Coffmann (Editors), 2000

Forthcoming titles:
Immunology and Drug Therapy of Atopic Skin Diseases, C. Brujinzel-Koomen, E. Knol (Editors), 2000
Inflammatory Processes. Molecular Mechanisms and Therapeutic Opportunities, L. G. Letts, D. W. Morgan (Editors), 2000
Cellular Mechanisms in Airways Inflammation, C. Page, K. Banner, D. Spina (Editors), 2000
Novel Cytokine Inhibitors, G. Higgs, B. Henderson (Editors), 2000

High Throughput Screening
for Novel Anti-Inflammatories

Michael Kahn

Editor

Birkhäuser Verlag
Basel · Boston · Berlin

Editor

Dr. Michael Kahn
University of Washington
Department of Pathobiology, SC-38
Seattle, WA 98195
USA

Deutsche Bibliothek Cataloging-in-Publication Data

High throughput screening for novel anti-inflammatories /
Michael Kahn ed. - Basel ; Boston ; Berlin : Birkhäuser, 2000
  (Progress in inflammation research)
  ISBN 3-7643-5912-9

The publisher and editor can give no guarantee for the information on drug dosage and administration contained in this publication. The respective user must check its accuracy by consulting other sources of reference in each individual case.

The use of registered names, trademarks etc. in this publication, even if not identified as such, does not imply that they are exempt from the relevant protective laws and regulations or free for general use.

ISBN 3-7643-5912-9 Birkhäuser Verlag, Basel – Boston – Berlin

© 2000 Birkhäuser Verlag, P.O. Box 133, CH-4010 Basel, Switzerland
Printed on acid-free paper produced from chlorine-free pulp. TCF ∞
Cover design: Markus Etterich, Basel
Cover illustration: Automated Compound Distribution. With the friendly permission of Dr. Michael Kahn, Seattle, USA
Printed in Germany
ISBN 3-7643-5912-9

9 8 7 6 5 4 3 2 1

Contents

List of contributors

Mark A. Ator, Department of Biochemistry, Cephalon, Inc., 145 Brandywine Parkway, West Chester, PA 19380, USA; e-mail: mator@cephalon.com

J. David Becherer, Department of Molecular Biochemistry, Glaxo Wellcome Research and Development Inc., 5 Moore Drive, P.O. Box 13998, Research Triangle Park, NC 27709, USA; e-mail: jdb5617@glaxowellcome.com

D. Mark Bickett, Department of Molecular Biochemistry, Glaxo Wellcome Research and Development Inc., 5 Moore Drive, P.O. Box 13998, Research Triangle Park, NC 27709, USA; e-mail: dmbl4326@glaxowellcome.com

Terry L. Bowlin, BioChem Pharma, 275 Armand-Frappier Blvd., Laval, Quebec, Canada H7V 4A7; e-mail: bowlint@biochempharma.com

David T. Crowe, ICOS Corporation, 22021 20th Avenue SE, Bothell, WA 98021, USA

Sharon M. Dankwardt, Roche Bioscience, Inflammatory Disease Unit, Parallel Synthesis Group, 3401 Hillview Ave, R6E3, Palo Alto, CA 94303, USA;
e-mail: Sharon.Dankwardt@roche.com

Falguni Dasgupta, Bioorganic and Medicinal Chemistry, BioMarin Pharmaceuticals Inc., 11 Pimentel Ct., Novato, CA 94949, USA; e-mail: fdcarbo@hotmail.com

Kerry W. Fowler, ICOS Corporation, 22021 20th Avenue SE, Bothell, WA 98021, USA; e-mail: kfowler@icos.com

Tariq Ghayur, BASF Bioresearch Corporation, 100 Research Drive, Worcester, MA 01605, USA

Mark A. Giembycz, Thoracic Medicine, Imperial College School of Medicine at the National Heart and Lung Institute, Dovehouse Street, London SW3 6LY, UK; e-mail: m.giembycz@ic.ac.uk

Sheryl J. Hays, Parke-Davis Pharmaceutical Research, 2800 Plymouth Drive, Ann Arbor, MI 48105, USA

Mohamed A. Iqbal, Department of Chemistry, Cephalon, Inc., 145 Brandywine Parkway, West Chester, PA 19380, USA; e-mail: miqbal@cephalon.com

M. Anthony Leesnitzer, Department of Molecular Biochemistry, Glaxo Wellcome Research and Development Inc., 5 Moore Drive, P.O. Box 13998, Research Triangle Park, NC 27709, USA; e-mail: mtl4417@glaxowellcome.com

Anthony M. Manning, Signal Pharmaceuticals Inc., 5555 Oberlin Drive, San Diego, CA 92121, USA; e-mail: amanning@signalpharm.com

William A. Metz, Hoechst Marion Roussel, Inc., Route 202–206, P.O. Box 6800, Bridgewater, NJ 08807-0800, USA

William R. Moore, Department of Biology, Axys Pharmaceuticals Inc., 180 Kimball Way, South San Francisco, CA 94080, USA

Marcia L. Moss, Department of Molecular Biochemistry, Glaxo Wellcome Research and Development Inc., 5 Moore Drive, P.O. Box 13998, Research Triangle Park, NC 27709, USA

Brion W. Murray, Signal Pharmaceuticals Inc., 5555 Oberlin Drive, San Diego, CA 92121, USA; e-mail: bmurray@signalpharm.com

Norton P. Peet, Hoechst Marion Roussel, Inc., Route 202-206, P.O. Box 6800, Bridgewater, NJ 08807-0800, USA

Kenneth D. Rice, Department of Medicinal Chemistry, Axys Pharmaceuticals Inc., 180 Kimball Way, South San Francisco, CA 94080, USA; e-mail: ken_rice@axyspharm.com

Yoshitaka Satoh, Signal Pharmaceuticals Inc., 5555 Oberlin Drive, San Diego, CA 92121, USA; e-mail: ysatoh@signalpharm.com

Herman Schreuder, Hoechst Marion Roussel, D-65926 Frankfurt, Germany

Bernd Stein, Signal Pharmaceuticals Inc., 5555 Oberlin Drive, San Diego, CA 92121, USA; e-mail: bstein@signalpharm.com

Mark J. Suto, DuPont Pharmaceuticals Research Labs, 4570 Executive Drive, Suite 400, San Diego, CA 92121 USA; e-mail: msuto@combichem.com

Robert V. Talanian, BASF Bioresearch Corporation, 100 Research Drive, Worcester, MA 01605, USA

Stephen D. Yanofsky, Affymax Research Institute, Palo Alto, CA 94304, USA

Preface

Combinatorial chemistry, and in particular the ability to generate libraries of "drug-like" nonpeptide, nonnucleotide molecules is a valuable tool which has recently been added to the armamentarium utilized in drug discovery and development. It is, and will continue to play a critical role in both lead discovery and optimization. This volume outlines the incorporation of combinatorial chemistry and high throughput screening for the discovery of new anti-inflammatory agents. Dankwardt's chapter crisply reviews the use of solid phase chemistry for the creation of combinatorial libraries. Chapters by Iqbal and Ator (Proteasome), Ghayur, Hays and Talanian (Caspase), Metz and Peet (Elastase), Leesnitzer, Bicket, Moss and Becherer (TACE) and Rice and Moore (Tryptase) cover a group of proteolytic enzyme inhibitor discovery programs and the wide range of therapeutic indications in which they may have utility. Dasgupta (Selectins) and Fowler and Crowe (Integrins) discuss various aspects of programs directed at inhibition of cell adhesion and their pharmaceutical relevance. In the exciting fields of signal transduction and transcriptional regulation, Murray, Satoh, and Stein (MAPK) and Suto and Manning (NF-κB), respectively, describe ongoing efforts to discover and develop specific inhibitors of these pathways to both understand their roles in pathophysiological states and for therapeutic intervention. Bowlin, Yanofsky and Schreuder detail their efforts in the challenging arena of finding small molecule antagonists for protein/protein interaction in particular with regard to IL-1. Finally, Giembycz concludes with a detailed review of the field of phosphodiesterase inhibitors in regard to respiratory disease. Although just the tip of the iceberg, we hope that these chapters inspire further thought and innovation in the areas of combinatorial chemistry and the discovery of novel anti-inflammatory therapeutics.

Seattle, Washington   Michael Kahn, Ph.D.

Solid phase synthesis: Applications to combinatorial libraries

Sharon M. Dankwardt

Roche Bioscience, Inflammatory Disease Unit, Parallel Synthesis Group, 3401 Hillview Ave, R6E3, Palo Alto, CA 94303, USA

Introduction

Solid phase synthesis has expanded dramatically since the introduction of small molecule synthesis on solid support. Polymer-supported synthesis had previously been used primarily for peptide synthesis, but has recently become an indispensable tool for preparing large numbers of compounds due to the relative ease of manipulation and amenability to automation. Although this review will focus on applications to anti-inflammatory targets, there is widespread use of solid phase synthesis towards other disease areas and a large number of compound types can be prepared using this technology [1].

Structurally, there is a wide variety of compound classes and biological targets involved in anti-inflammatory research and solid phase synthesis of libraries is beginning to have an impact on drug research in these areas [2]. Currently the majority of the research published has been in terms of compound preparation of compounds on solid support which "may" be used towards a variety of biological targets without the corresponding details of screening or biological activity. Small molecule libraries that have been screened against targets dealing with anti-inflammatory processes and those prepared with the possibility of an application towards use as anti-inflammatory disease states will be discussed.

Libraries synthesized for specific biological targets associated with inflammation

Cyclooxygenase

Inhibitors of cyclooxygenase (COX) are important anti-inflammatory agents. The worldwide market is estimated to be about $ 5 billion [3]. The biological mode of action involves prostaglandin synthase or COX as a catalyst in the biosynthesis of prostaglandins (a primary class of mediators of inflammation) from arachidonic acid [4].

High Throughput Screening for Novel Anti-Inflammatories, edited by M. Kahn
© 2000 Birkhäuser Verlag Basel/Switzerland

4-Thiazolidinones

Researchers at Affymax have utilized solid phase synthesis to prepare libraries of 4-thiazolidinones to elaborate on a lead disclosed previously for COX-1 inhibition [5]. Using Tentagel S AC or Tentagel S RAM as their solid support, the chemistry elaborated in Scheme 1 was utilized to prepare 540 compounds using the split-pool combine technique. The amide, ester and carboxylic acid libraries were screened at ~10 µM with only the ester library showing any appreciable activity. Deconvolution of the other variables on the thiazolidinone system determined the best substituents for R', R and Y. For the α-thio acid, R' = Bu >> CH_2CO_2H, Pr, Me, H. For the aldehyde substituent, R = 3-PhOPh > 4-ClPhOPh >> 3-pyridyl, 3,5-$(MeO)_2$Ph, 2-naphthyl. Lastly Y is only active as p-Ph$(CH_2)_4$; L-Cys(Bn), D or L-Ser(OBn) or D/L-hPhe show no activity. Resynthesis of the most active compound confirmed the activity seen in the mixtures. The most active compound in the library has an IC_{50} 3.7 ± 1.5 µM towards COX-1.

Arylacetic acids

Ellman has prepared a library of arylacetic acid derivatives utilizing a safety catch linker on solid support as illustrated in Scheme 2 [6]. No biological data is presented to accompany these compounds, but this type of pharmacophore is very common

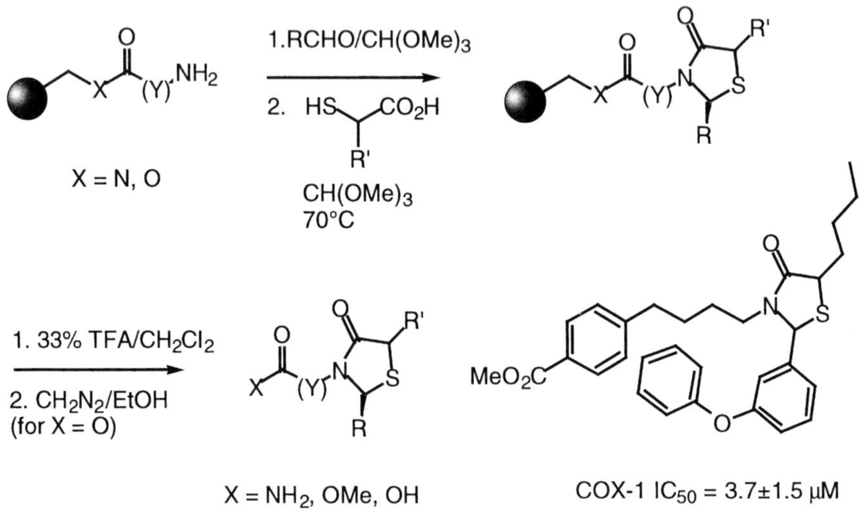

Scheme 1

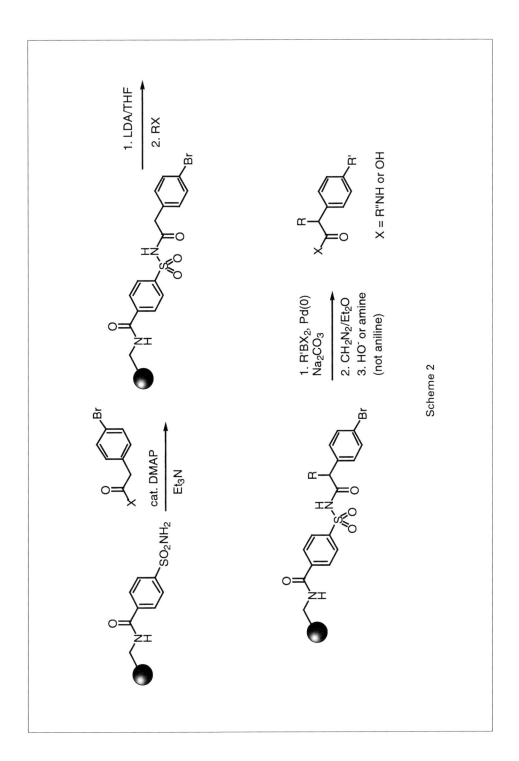

Scheme 2

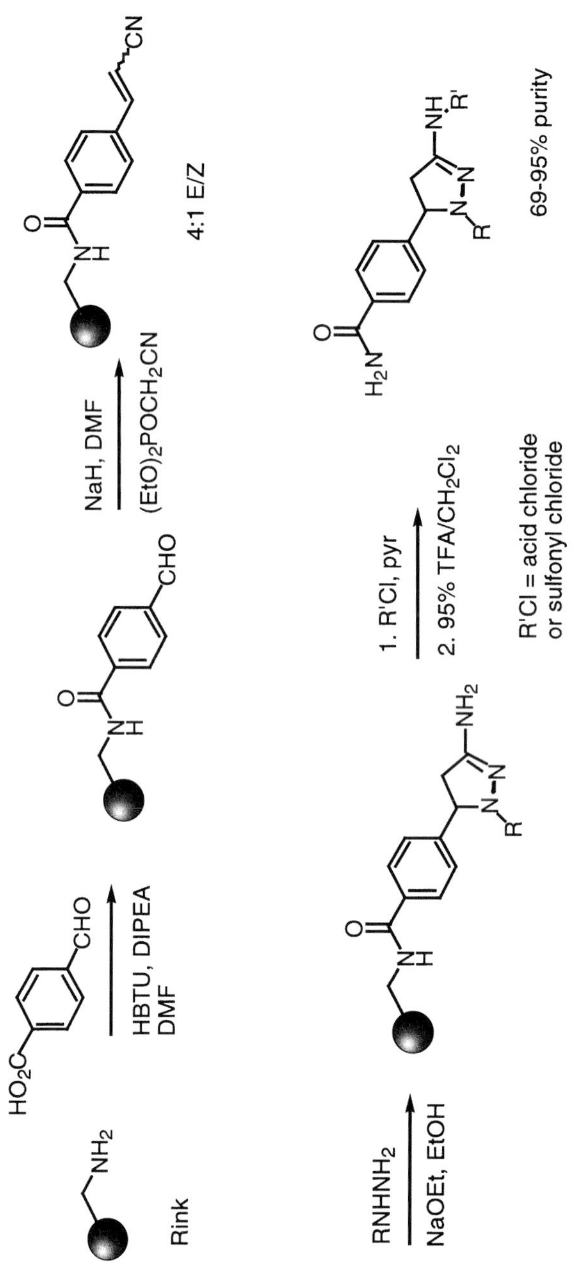
Rink
HBTU, DIPEA
DMF
NaH, DMF
(EtO)2POCH2CN
4:1 E/Z
RNHNH2
NaOEt, EtOH
1. R'Cl, pyr
2. 95% TFA/CH2Cl2
R'Cl = acid chloride
or sulfonyl chloride
69-95% purity

Scheme 3

among cyclooxygenase inhibitors. The key step in the construction of this library is the enolate alkylation of the acylsulfonamide. The yields for this synthesis is very good (87–100%) with the exception of the use of aniline as the final nucleophile which does not cleave the product from the resin.

3-Amino-2-pyrazolines

The pyrazolines synthesized as shown in Scheme 3 were selected as a combination of two known cyclooxygenase inhibitors with the desire to combine the attractive properties from each [7]. No biological data is shown to support their proposal although a library of twenty four compounds was presented using 6 different hydrazines and 4 different capping groups (R').

Matrix metalloproteinase

Matrix metalloproteinases (MMPs) are included in a family of zinc-dependent endopeptidases that are involved in extracellular matrix turnover and regulation. They have shown to be important for modulation of a variety of inflammatory and cell proliferative conditions [8]. Inhibition of these enzymes has currently been associated with diseases such as arthritis, cancer and multiple sclerosis [9].

Tripeptide hydroxamic acids

The methodology for the preparation of hydroxamic acids on solid support generally involves the use of either the nitrogen [10] or oxygen [11] of hydroxylamine as an attachment point to the support. In the case illustrated in Scheme 4, Floyd prepared a series of tripeptide hydroxamic acids on Wang resin modified through a two step procedure to afford an oxygen linked hydroxylamine [12]. The desired tripeptide was prepared using standard Fmoc peptide coupling protocols and was then cleaved from the resin with 70% TFA in dichloromethane containing ~2% water. After purification by flash chromatography (giving 25–88% isolated yields) the compounds were submitted for biological assay. Assay of the crude product gave similar results as the purified product. In a single illustrative example, a more acid labile resin, HMPA-MBHA was converted to the hydroxylamine linker in the same manner as the Wang resin and was converted into a tripeptide hydroxamic acid. Cleavage occurred with 1% TFA in dichloromethane in the presence of triisopropyl silane. This linker showed an increase from 71–90% in the purified yield. The compounds prepared were reported to give biological results in accord with those previously disclosed. The IC_{50}'s for CBz-Pro-Leu-Ala-NHOH were found for human recombinant collagenase, stromelysin and 72 kDa gelatinase as 8.0 μM, 3.5 μM and 8.0 μM respectively.

5

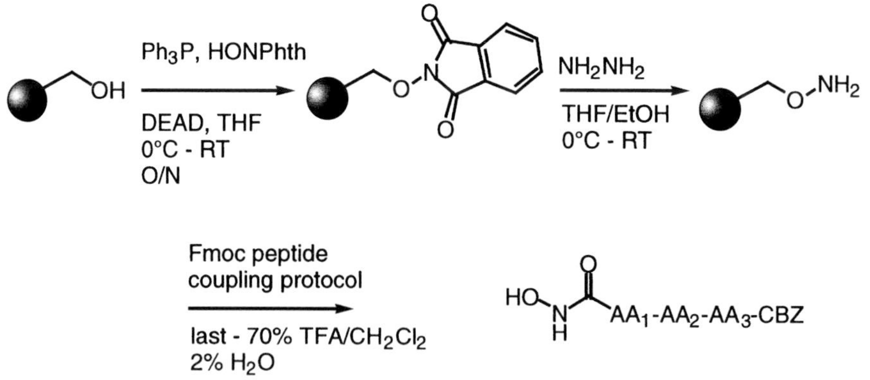

Scheme 4

Alternative approaches to the solid phase synthesis of hydroxamic acids include incorporation of hydroxylamine at a point remote to the linker [13] or using hydroxylamine as a nucleophile to directly displace the hydroxamic acid from the resin [14].

N-carboxyalkyl peptides

The N-carboxyalkyl peptides were prepared as inhibitors of human stromelysin (MMP-3) and human neutrophil collagenase (MMP-8) [15]. The synthesis outlined in Scheme 5 gives a 1:1 mixture of epimers with purities of > 50%. Since previous studies have shown that R = Me and R' = phenethyl have good potency against MMP-3, these substituents were kept constant. A library with > 100 different amines (R"NH$_2$) was prepared and screened, without purification, for inhibition of MMP-3 at 200 µM. (±)-1-Phenethylamine was found to be weakly active (10% MMP-3 inhibition at 100 µM), and the corresponding (R) isomer gave 6% inhibition and the (S) gave 33% inhibition at 100 µM. The resultant SAR data was then applied to a series of succinate derivatives and eventually led to the preparation of an inhibitor with a K$_i$ of 9 nM.

Thiols

Foley et al. have utilized thiols as a zinc binding ligand for collagenase and gelatinase inhibitors [16]. They have also prepared carboxylic acid and imidazole containing compounds as alternative zinc binding ligands (replacement of cysteine for

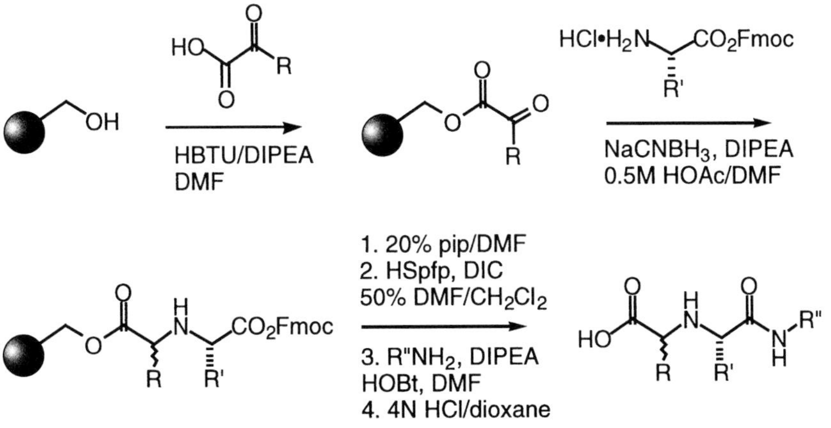

Scheme 5

aspartic acid, glutamic acid and histidine in Scheme 6). The first library prepared included 50 natural and unnatural amino acids varying R, with acetyl as the capping group. This was screened against human fibroblast collagenase (MMP-1). From this library it was deduced that heteroaromatic and aliphatic side chains from L amino acids were preferred. The IC_{50}'s reported for variation of Fmoc–AA–OH were: Phe > 100 µM, Leu = 7 µM, Trp = 5 µM, 2-thienylalanine = 4 µM, 3-pyridyl-alanine = 4 µM. A second library was prepared with about 150 different capping reagents keeping the first amino acid constant with L-Phe. These were screened against MMP-1 and 92 kD gelatinase (MMP-9). Inhibition of MMP-1 is seen most effectively with R' = CF_3 or heteroaromatics (benzotriazole or pyrazole derived). MMP-9 inhibition, on the other hand, is seen with large lipophilic groups, with the best selectivity seen with phenethyl. A matrix was then prepared that incorporated the best substituents at each position, with the most potent illustrated below. Replacement of cysteine in one analog with Asp, Glu or His resulted in less active compounds.

Diketopiperazines

Diketopiperazines were synthesized as shown in Scheme 7 and were screened against collagenase-1, stromelysin-1 and gelatinase-B [17]. The zinc ligand for these compounds is a thiol and is kept constant by using cysteine as the first amino acid (R = CH_2SH) in the first library (DKP-I) or with cysteine as the second amino acid (R" = CH_2SH) for the second library (DKP-II). There were 684 compounds prepared in DKP-I, which utilized D and L Cys (R = CH_2SH), 19 R'CHO and 18 amino

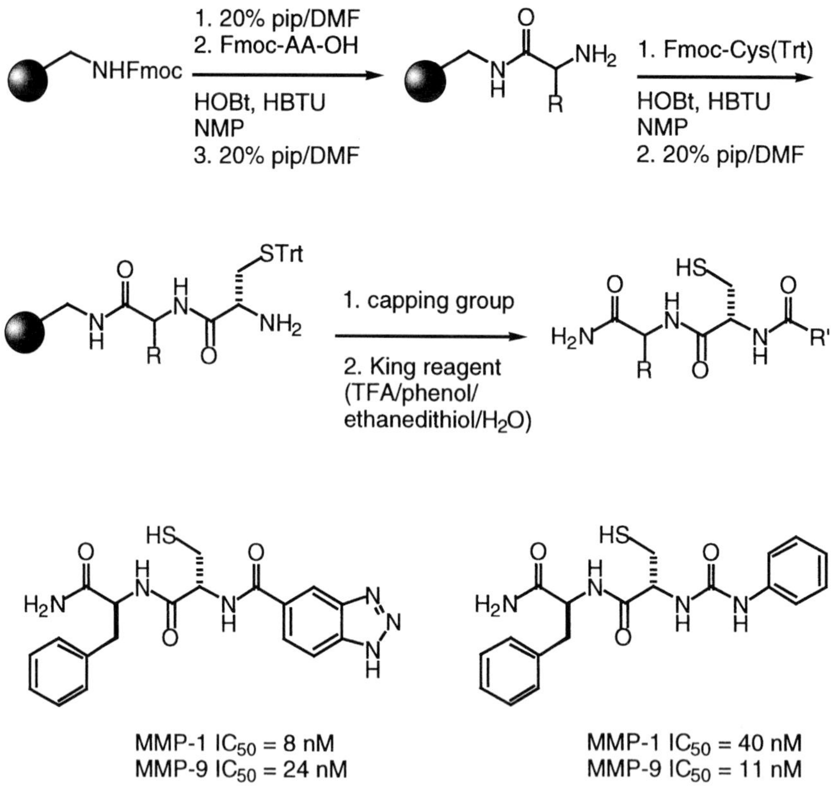

Scheme 6

acids (R"). DKP-II also contained 684 compounds with 19 amino acids (R), 18 R'CHO and D and L Cys (R"). The most active in DKP-I was low micromolar and was not investigated further. DKP-II consisted of 36 pools of 19 of which a number showed submicromolar activities for Col-1 and Gel-B. None of the pools however showed appreciable activity towards matrilysin or strom-1. R'CHO with large, non-flexible groups showed decreased activity, L-Cys was only slightly more active than D-Cys (due to partial racemization during coupling). The coupling agent was changed to dimethyl-2-fluoropyridinium 4-toluenesulfonate (DMFP) to alleviate this problem. The first deconvolution was with R" as L-Cys and R'CHO as 4-MeOBn. This led to the following observations about R on the first amino acid: (1) L configuration is preferred, (2) polar groups are not well tolerated and (3) extended R groups show a preference for Gel-B compared with Col-1 and α-branching shows a loss in activity. The best amino acid incorporating R is L-cyclohexylalanine,

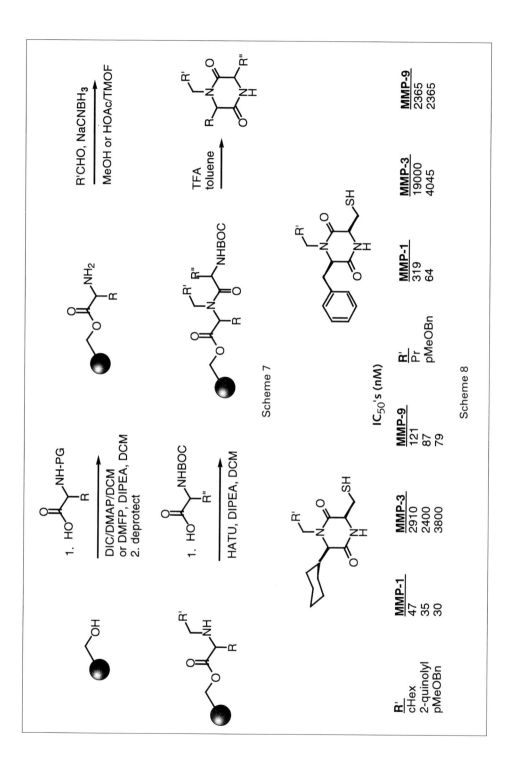

Scheme 7

Scheme 8

IC$_{50}$'s (nM)

R'	MMP-1	MMP-3	MMP-9
cHex	47	2910	121
2-quinolyl	35	2400	87
pMeOBn	30	3800	79

R'	MMP-1	MMP-3	MMP-9
Pr	319	19000	2365
pMeOBn	64	4045	2365

for both Col-1 and Gel-B. Some of the most active compounds were resynthesized and accurate IC_{50}'s were obtained. These are illustrated in Scheme 8.

Bradykinin

Bradykinin, a nonapeptide, is a known inflammatory mediator that is produced by tissue and plasma kallikreins. Although a number of potent peptide antagonists have been prepared that effectively block the action of bradykinin, there has not yet been a successful small molecule antagonist prepared [18].

Substituted piperazines

Goodfellow et al. have synthesized a small molecule library synthesis towards the preparation of antagonists of bradykinin [19]. Their design of substituted piperazines was based on a molecular modeling approach. The compounds were prepared as shown in Scheme 9 and screened as mixtures. They selected ten amino acids (with variable R) (5-D/L mixtures). These were combined and split into 12 lots. Ten of these were treated with one of ten different aldehydes or ketones (R'). The other two lots were taken on without the reductive amination step (R' = H). Each of these groups was further divided into 12 portions and treated with 1 of 12 different amines. Each of these were then divided in half. CBz side chain protecting groups on R' or R" were then removed and some were guanidated. The other half also had CBz side chains removed and were then reduced to a substituted piperazine followed by guanidation. From the initial screening against human B2 receptor binding a compound CP-2458 (structure not provided) had IC_{50} = 4.1 μM. They state that further modification has led to much more potent antagonists (IC_{50} = 130–500 nM, human receptor clone).

$\alpha_4\beta_1$ integrin

The leukocyte $\alpha_4\beta_1$ integrin is a receptor for fibronectin (an adhesive protein). This integrin has many roles including invasion of inflammed tissues. It mediates chromic inflammatory diseases such as rheumatoid arthritis, asthma and others [20].

β turn mimics

Scheme 10 illustrates the chemistry to prepare β-turn mimics that were used to mimic a cyclic hexapeptide antagonist of the α_4 integrins [21]. A library of over 5500 individual compounds was prepared using 12 R/S α-bromoacids (R"), 14 D/L Fmoc-amino acids (R') and 9 primary amines (R). From all of these structures, 2304

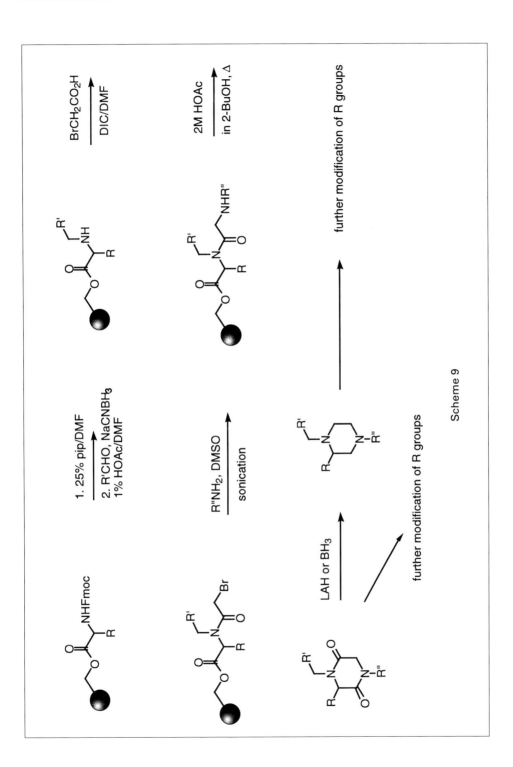

Scheme 9

11

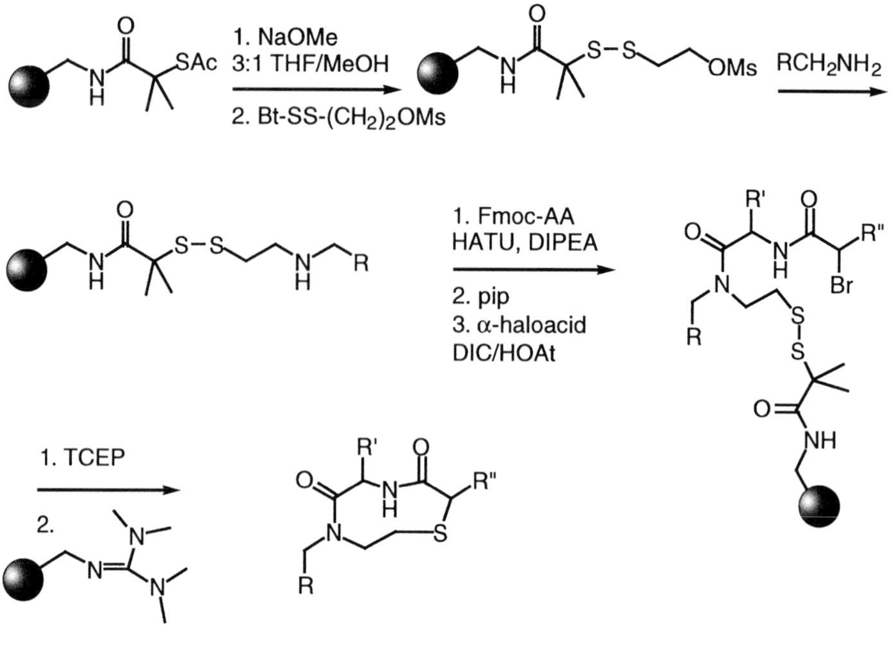

Scheme 10

were selected which had a crucial aspartic acid residue at least one site, with the other positions being varied. The library was assayed at 1 µM for inhibitory effect on the binding of fluorescently labeled Ramos cells in immobilized CS1 peptide. Nearly all of the active compounds had R" = CH_2CO_2H and R' = a hydrophobic residue, whereas R showed both hydrophobic and hydrophilic residues as having activity. Four of the most active compounds were resynthesized on larger scale and reassayed and their structures and activity are shown in Scheme 11.

Prostaglandins

Prostaglandins are the products of the arachidonic acid cascade and are a primary class of mediators of inflammation [4].

Prostaglandins

Illustrated in Scheme 12 is an approach on solid support toward the synthesis of prostaglandins [22]. This method has been applied to the preparation of a number

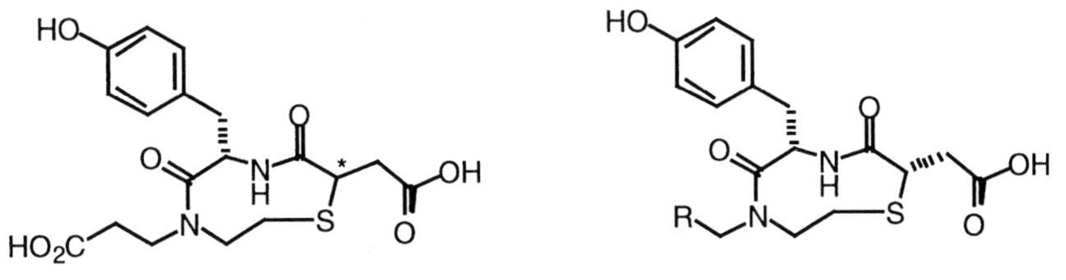

	IC$_{50}$
S- isomer	8 ± 2 μM
R- isomer	5 ± 1 μM

R	IC$_{50}$
$CH_3(CH_2)_2$	>100 μM
$(CH_3)_2CHCH_2$	>>100 μM

Scheme 11

of prostaglandins in the E and F series. There have also been reported synthesis of PGE$_2$ and PGF$_{2\alpha}$ on soluble polymer support as single compounds [23]. The compounds prepared had no biological results presented, but the synthesis illustrates some examples of complex chemical reactions that can be carried out on solid support.

Aminohydantoins
BW68C has been identified as a prostaglandin D receptor agonist and as a result the following solid phase approach (Scheme 13) could be applied towards elaboration of this series [24]. This synthesis utilizes a traceless cyclization-cleavage strategy to obtain the desired aminohydantoin by heating with bis(trimethylsilyl)trifluoroacetamide (BSTFA). The resin linked hydrazino acid used as the starting material was obtained either by coupling the desired bromoacetic acid to the resin followed by treatment with t-butylcarbazate or direct coupling of the preformed hydrazino acid using Mitsunobu esterification conditions. The urea formation was determined to give the best results using triphosgene followed by treatment with the desired amine (especially for anilines).

Conclusion

This chapter serves to illustrate some of the chemistries involved in the preparation of compounds involved in anti-inflammatory research. The number of reactions applicable to solid support is rapidly increasing and more technically demanding reaction conditions are continually being incorporated into solid phase chemistry.

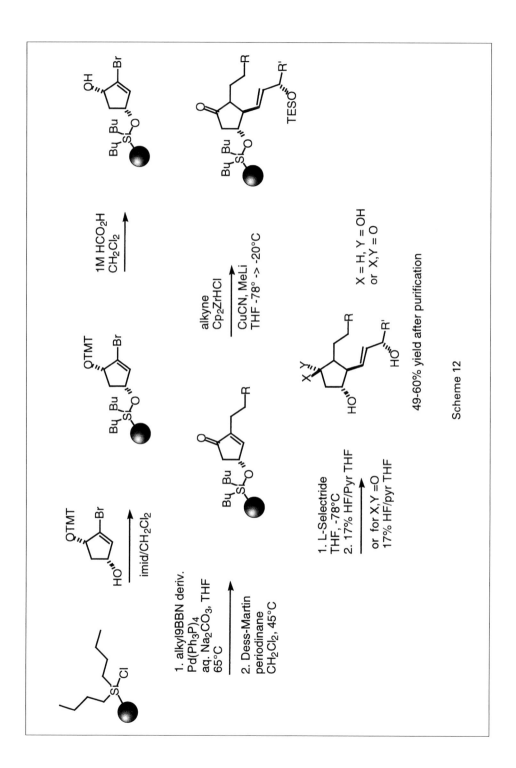

Scheme 12

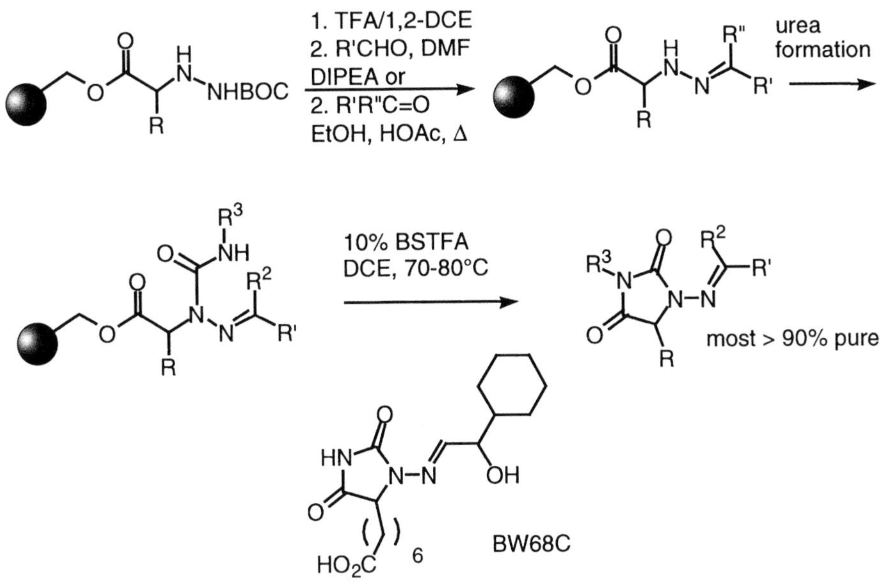

Scheme 13

The number of published libraries that have been screened is increasing and it will certainly increase as more active drug candidates are discovered using both solid phase synthesis and high throughput screening.

References

1   Fecik RA, Frank KE, Gentry EJ, Menon SR, Mitscher LA, Telikepalli H (1998) The search for orally active medications through combinatorial chemistry. *Med Res Rev* 18: 149–185
Cowley PM, Rees DC (1997) Applications of solid-phase synthesis to drug discovery. *Curr Med Chem* 4: 211–227
Felder ER, Poppinger D (1997) Combinatorial compound libraries for enhanced drug discovery approaches. *Adv Drug Res* 30: 111–199
Dolle RE (1997) Discovery of enzyme inhibitors through combinatorial chemistry. *Mol Diversity* 2: 223–236
2   Campbell DA (1997) The application of combinatorial and parallel diversity libraries to the discovery of antiinflammatory agents. *Curr Pharm Design* 3: 503–513

3 Carter JS (1997) Recently reported inhibitors of cyclooxygenase-2. *Exp Opin Ther Patents* 8: 21–29

4 Vane JR, Bakhle YS, Botting RM (1998) Cyclooxygenases 1 and 2. *Annu Rev Pharmacol Toxicol* 38: 97–120

5 Look GC, Schullek JR, Holmes CP, Chinn JP, Gordon EM, Gallop MA (1996) The identification of cyclooxygenase-1 inhibitors from 4-thiazolidinone combinatorial libraries. *Bioorg Med Chem Lett* 6: 707–712

6 Ellman JA (1996) Design, synthesis, and evaluation of small-molecule libraries. *Acc Chem Res* 29: 132–143

7 Lyngsø LO, Nielsen J (1998) Solid phase synthesis of 3-amino-2-pyrazolines. *Tetrahedron Lett* 39: 5845–5858

8 Trocmé C, Gaudin P, Berthier S, Barro C, Zaoui P, Morel F (1998) Human B lymphocytes synthesize the 92-kDa gelatinase, matrix metalloproteinase-9. *J Biol Chem* 273: 20677–20684

9 Beckett RP, Davidson AH, Drummond AH, Huxley P, Whittaker M (1996) Recent advances in matrix metalloproteinase inhibitor research. *Drug Disc Today* 1: 16–26

10 Ngu K, Patel DV (1997) A new and efficient solid phase synthesis of hydroxamic acids. *J Org Chem* 62: 7088–7089

11 Bauer U, Ho W-B, Koskinen AMP (1997) A novel linkage for the solid-phase synthesis of hydroxamic acids. *Tetrahedron Lett* 38: 7233–7236
Mellor SL, McGuire C, Chan WC (1997) N-Fmoc-aminooxy-2-chlorotrityl polystyrene resin: A facile solid-phase methodology for the synthesis of hydroxamic acids. *Tetrahedron Lett* 38: 3311–3314
Richter LS, Desai MC (1997) A TFA-cleavable linkage for solid-phase synthesis of hydroxamic acids. *Tetrahedron Lett* 38: 321–322
Mellor SL, Chan WC (1997) 4-[2,4- Dimethoxy(N-fluoren-9-ylmethoxycarbonyl-N-alkylaminooxy)-methyl]phenoxymethyl polystyrene: A multiple solid-phase approach to N-alkylhydroxamic acids. *J Chem Soc Chem Commun* 2005–2006

12 Floyd CD, Lewis CN, Patel SR, Whittaker M (1996) A method for the synthesis of hydroxamic acids on solid phase. *Tetrahedron Lett* 37: 8045–8048

13 Chen JJ, Spatola AF (1997) Solid phase synthesis of peptide hydroxamic Acids. *Tetrahedron Lett* 38: 1511–1514

14 Dankwardt SM (1998) Solid phase synthesis of hydroxamic acids. *Synlett* 761

15 Rockwell A, Melden M, Copeland RA, Hardman K, Decicco SP, DeGrado WF (1996) Complementarity of combinatorial chemistry and structure-based ligand design: Application to the discovery of novel inhibitors of matrix metalloproteinases. *J Am Chem Soc* 118: 10337–10338

16 Foley MA, Hassman AS, Drewry DH, Greer DG, Wagner CD, Feldman PL, Berman J, Bickett DM, McGeehan GM, Lambert MH, Green M (1996) Rapid synthesis of novel dipeptide inhibitors of human collagenase and gelatinase using solid phase chemistry. *Bioorg Med Chem Lett* 6: 1905–1910

17 Szardenings AK, Harris D, Lam S, Shi L, Tien D, Wang Y, Patel DV, Navre M, Camp-

bell DA (1998) Rational design and combinatorial evaluation of enzyme inhibitor scaffolds: Identification of novel inhibitors of matrix metalloproteinases. *J Med Chem* 41: 2194–2200

18 Abe Y, Kayakiri H, Satoh S, Inoue T, Sawada Y, Imai K, Inamura N, Asano M, Hatori, C, Katayama A et al (1998) A novel class of orally active non-peptide bradykinin B$_2$ receptor antagonists. 1. Construction of the basic framework. *J Med Chem* 41: 564–578 and references therein

19 Goodfellow VS, Laudeman CP, Gerrity JI, Burkard M, Strobel E, Zuzack JS, McLeod DA (1996) Rationally designed non-peptides: Variously substituted piperazine libraries for the discovery of bradykinin antagonist and other G-protein-coupled receptor ligands. *Mol Div* 2: 97–102

20 Mousa SA (1998) Cell adhesion molecules and extracellular matrix proteins; potential therapeutic applications. *Exp Opin Invest Drugs* 7: 1159–1171

21 Souers AJ, Virgilio AA, Schürer SS, Ellman JA, Kogan TP, West HE, Ankener W, Vanderslice P (1998) Novel inhibitors of $\alpha_4\beta_1$ integrin receptor interactions through library synthesis and screening. *Bioorg Med Chem Lett* 8: 2297–2302

22 Thompson LA, Moore FL, Moon Y-C, Ellman JA (1998) Solid-phase synthesis of diverse E- and F-series prostaglandins. *J Org Chem* 63: 2066–2067

23 Chen S, Janda KD (1997) Synthesis of prostaglandin E$_2$ methyl ester on a soluble-polymer support for the construction of prostanoid libraries. *J Am Chem Soc* 119: 8724–8725

Chen S, Janda KD (1998) Total synthesis of naturally occurring prostaglandin F$_{2\alpha}$ on a non-cross-linked polystyrene support. *Tetrahedron Lett* 39: 3943–3946

24 Wilson LJ, Li M, Portlock DE (1998) Solid phase synthesis of 1-aminohydantoin libraries. *Tetrahedron Lett* 39: 5135–5138

Proteasome inhibitors

Mohamed A. Iqbal[1] and Mark A. Ator[2]

Department of [1]Chemistry and [2]Biochemistry, Cephalon, Inc., 145 Brandywine Parkway, West Chester, PA 19380, USA

Introduction

The proteasome is a large multifunctional proteolytic complex responsible for non-lysosomal protein degradation [1–3]. The form of the enzyme most frequently studied is the 20S proteasome, a 700 kDa complex which catalyzes at least five proteolytic activities. The 20S proteasome is the catalytic core of the 26S proteasome, a larger particle (2000 kDa) which also contains two copies of a 19S regulatory complex. The 26S form of the proteasome catalyzes ATP-dependent hydrolysis of ubiquitinated proteins, while the 20S proteasome is not ATP-dependent. The enzyme is conserved from archaebacteria and eubacteria, which contain only the 20S proteasome, through eukaryotes, which express both 20S and 26S forms of the enzyme [4]. The proteasome is located in both the cytosol and nucleus of eukaryotic cells and is a predominant cellular component, comprising up to 1% of the total protein in most cells. The enzyme plays a major role in the degradation of misfolded, damaged or abnormal proteins, as well as in the modulation of levels of key cell signaling regulators [5]. The activity of the proteasome is highly regulated, and any deregulation has the potential to lead to pathological conditions.

The complex nature of the proteasome with its multiple proteolytic activities has hampered the process of inhibitor design and potential drug development for this important enzyme. Despite the absence of specific substrates and the only recently emerging understanding of the mechanism of action for this new class of threonine proteases, many research groups are attempting to develop inhibitors for this enzyme. Here, we summarize the status of such efforts. The reader is encouraged to refer to excellent reviews on the proteasome in the areas of biology [6–8], structure-function [9–11], and inhibitor design [12].

High Throughput Screening for Novel Anti-Inflammatories, edited by M. Kahn
© 2000 Birkhäuser Verlag Basel/Switzerland

Proteasome

Biochemistry

The proteasome has been reported to exhibit at least five distinct proteolytic activities, as defined by the cleavage preference at the P1, or carboxyl terminal, residue [13]. The major catalytic activities include the chymotrypsin-like (Ch-like), trypsin-like, peptidylglutamyl-peptide hydrolyzing activity (PGPH), branched-chain amino acid preferring (BrAAP), and small neutral amino acid preferring (SNAAP) activities. Most inhibitor design to date has focused on the Ch-like activity. The substrate requirements for different activities and their kinetic and mechanistic differences have been discussed in detail [13, 14]. However, other investigators have suggested fewer catalytic activities of the enzyme. Studies employing monoclonal antibodies and mutation of the β subunits validate the presence of only three major proteolytic activities [15]. Consistent with this hypothesis is the kinetic argument that the BrAAP activity is actually a combination of the chymotrypsin-like and PGPH activities [16]. It is possible that the variable subunit composition of the proteasome may contribute to minor proteolytic reactions and to the overlap of these activities.

Measurement of the catalytic activity of proteasomes is typically accomplished with small fluorogenic peptide substrates, which display some selectivity for particular catalytic activities of the complex. Typical substrates employed for measurement of the Ch-like, trypsin-like and PGPH activities are Suc-Leu-Leu-Val-Tyr-AMC, Z-Leu-Leu-Arg-AMC, and Z-Leu-Leu-Glu-2NA, respectively (AMC = 7-amino-4-methyl coumarin; 2NA = 2-naphthylamine) [16]. Rigorous evaluation of the kinetics of substrate hydrolysis by the 20S proteasome revealed a complex, cooperative mechanism consistent with the presence of multiple active sites [17].

Structure of the 20S proteasome

The 20S proteasome consists of two classes of subunits, α and β, which are similar in sequence to each other, but unrelated to any other family of proteins [3]. Based on the evidence summarized below, the β subunits appear to be responsible for the catalytic activity of the enzyme. The primitive proteasome from the archaebacterium *Thermoplasma acidophilum* contains only one type of α and of β subunit, while eukaryotic proteasomes are comprised of seven representatives of each class which are encoded by distinct genes. The α subunits contain a highly conserved 35 amino acid helical extension, which appears to be important in the assembly and recognition process. Most β subunits contain a prosequence that is cleaved off during maturation of the particle, liberating the essential N-terminal threonine residue in the case of those subunits that have catalytic activity.

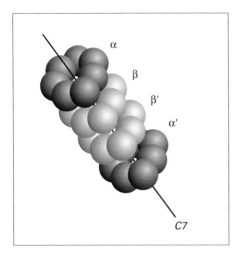

Figure 1
Drawing of the C7-symmetrical arrangement of α and β subunits of the 20S proteasome [3].

The subunit composition of the eukaryotic proteasome can vary depending on conditions. For example, interferon γ (IFNγ) stimulates the substitution of three constitutive β subunits by inducible subunits encoded by the major histocompatability complex (MHC), resulting in alteration of the substrate specificity of the particle to better suit antigen presentation [18]. The subunit composition in proteasomes isolated from different tissues of the same species can vary, resulting in differential expression of catalytic activities [19].

The complex architecture of the proteasome has been the subject of intense interest for many years. Electron microscopy and related antibody-tagging experiments suggested that the prokaryotic and eukaryotic proteasomes share a cylindrical $\alpha_7\beta_7\beta_7\alpha_7$ quaternary structure (Fig. 1) [4]. This conclusion was confirmed through determination of the crystal structure of the *Thermoplasma* 20S proteasome [20]. The enzyme is barrel-shaped, containing three large cavities within the cylinder and narrow constrictions defined by the α subunits at the ends (Fig. 2). The structure of the proteasome complexed with Ac-Leu-Leu-norleucinal demonstrated binding of inhibitors within the central cavity to Thr_1 of all 14 β subunits. The localization of the active sites within the particle and the tight packing of the α/α and α/β rings therefore mandates that substrates pass through the narrow channels at the ends of the barrel, requiring that they be unfolded and in an extended conformation. In spite of the limited sequence homology of the α and β subunits, they display very similar three-dimensional structures.

The crystal structure of the 20S proteasome from the yeast *Saccharomyces cerevisiae* was recently determined, revealing a quaternary structure identical to that of

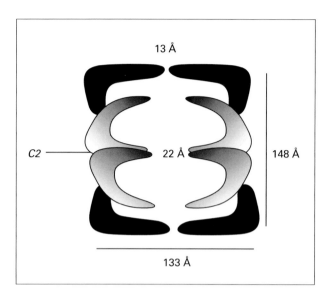

Figure 2
Cross-section view showing C2 symmetrical arrangement of the α and β subunits and the overall dimension of the proteasome [4, 21].

the prokaryotic enzyme and a unique position in the complex for each of the seven α and seven β submits [21]. The prosequences of three of the seven β subunits (β_1, β_2 and β_5) are cleaved to produce an N-terminal threonine residue; only these subunits are catalytically active and capable of reacting covalently with Ac-Leu-Leu-norleucinal. Based on these results and mutagenesis experiments, the three major catalytic activities of the proteasome can be assigned to specific subunits [21].

Mechanism of action

The mechanistic classification of the proteasome has long been controversial due to its lack of homology to other proteases and its ambiguous reactivity with class-specific protease inhibitors. Several lines of evidence indicate that Thr_1 of the β subunit is the nucleophile required for amide bond hydrolysis by the proteasome, making the enzyme a member of the N-terminal nucleophile (Ntn) hydrolase family [22]. Site-directed mutagenesis of Thr_1 of the *Thermoplasma* proteasome demonstrated the essential nature of that residue, with catalytic activity abolished by its deletion or replacement with alanine [23]. The demonstration by crystallography that inhibitors such as Ac-Leu-Leu-norleucinal [20, 21] and lactacystin [21] bind to the N-terminal threonine further supports this conclusion.

A general base is required to enhance the nucleophilicity of the threonine hydroxyl, similar to the role played by histidine in serine or cysteine proteases. The crystal structure of the *Thermoplasma* proteasome suggests that this function is fulfilled by either the side chain of Lys_{33} or the α-amino group of Thr_1 [20]. Mutation of Lys_{33} to either Ala or Arg results in a properly folded and assembled, but catalytically inactive proteasome [23]. However, it is not clear whether the lysine side chain is required for proton transfer or polarization of the threonine hydroxyl. Based on considerations of pK_a and geometry, the α-amino group of Thr_1 was favored as the general base [23].

26S proteasome

The 26S proteasome catalyzes the ATP-dependent hydrolysis of proteins marked for destruction by ubiquitination on lysine residues [24]. The additional machinery required for recognition and hydrolysis of ubiquitinated proteins is found in the 19S regulatory particles, which appear in electron micrographs as asymmetric caps on both ends of the typical 26S proteasome structure [10]. Among the approximately 15 subunits of the 19S complex are several ATPases as well as subunits that appear to bind ubiquitin and an isopeptidase, which releases it from the protein. The overall function of the 19S complex is proposed to involve unfolding of target proteins and transport of the substrates into the 20S proteolytic core. However, the mechanism by which these events might occur remains elusive.

Biological functions of the proteasome

In addition to its role in protein degradation, the proteasome participates in many specific proteolytic reactions which regulate critical cellular functions [5, 25]. As described above, the proteasome is involved in the processing of intracellular antigens, which are presented via the MHC-1 complex [18]. Among the important proteasome substrates are IκB, the inhibitor of the transcription factor NF-κB [26], the cyclin-dependent kinase inhibitors p21 [27] and p27 [28], and the cell cycle regulator p53 [29]. The ability to intervene in these processes with a proteasome inhibitor could have important therapeutic implications for treatment of inflammatory disease, cancer, and a variety of other conditions.

Inhibitors

Enzyme inhibitors are broadly divided into two main classes, reversible and irreversible, depending upon their mode of interaction with the enzyme [30].

23

Reversible inhibitors bind with the enzyme through hydrogen-bonding, hydrophobic and electrostatic interactions, as well as with rapidly reversible covalent linkages. Irreversible inhibitors bind to the enzyme and form a permanent covalent bond to a functional group of the enzyme. Examples of the reversible inhibitors of the proteasome include the peptide-based aldehydes, boronic acids and boronic esters. Irreversible inhibitors include ketoepoxides, vinyl sulfones and lactacystin. Inhibitors whose design is based on substrates have a recognition sequence and an active functional group known as an enzyme-reactive group (ERG). Early studies focussed on peptide aldehydes in which the aldehyde group serves as the ERG. The types of proteasome inhibitors reported in the literature are summarized in Table 1.

Table 1 - Structures of proteasome inhibitors

Aldehydes [14, 32, 35, 37]

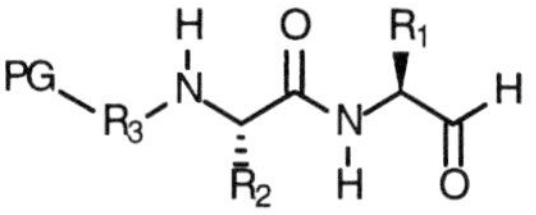

PG = Protecting group, acyl group (alkyl and aryl)
R1 = Alkyl, aryl, biaryl, substituted aryl group
R2 = Alkyl, aryl, polar group masked alkyl groups
R3 = PG, hydrophobic amino acid or absent

Ketocompounds

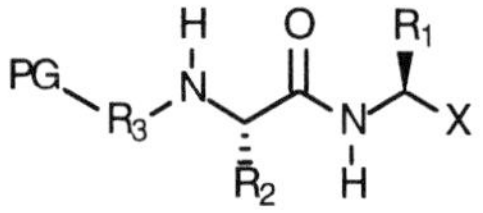

X = –COCHO   Ketoaldehyde [43]
    –CONHEt..   Ketoamide [44]
    –COCOCOOEt   Diketoester [50]
    –COCH₂Cl   Chloromethyl ketone [44]

Keto epoxide and keto benzoxazole [12, 42, 50]

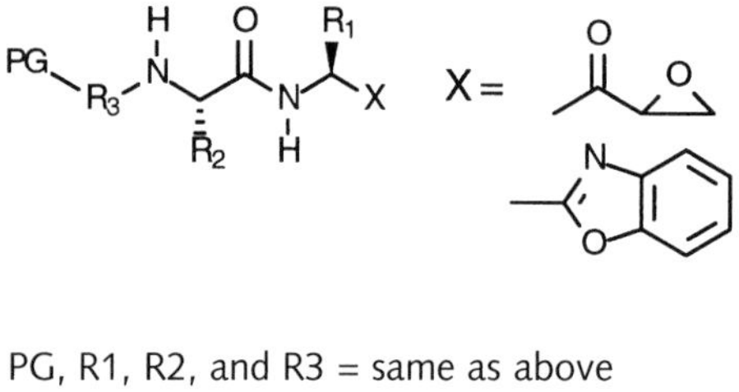

PG, R1, R2, and R3 = same as above

24

Table 1 (continued)

Boronic acid and ester [44, 47, 49]

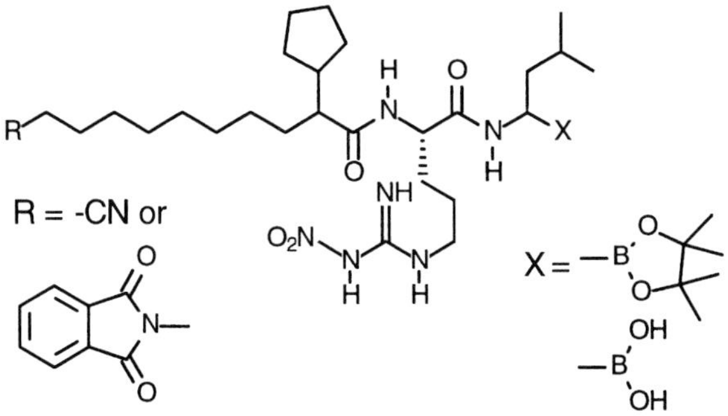

R = -CN or

X =

Boronic acid [12, 50]

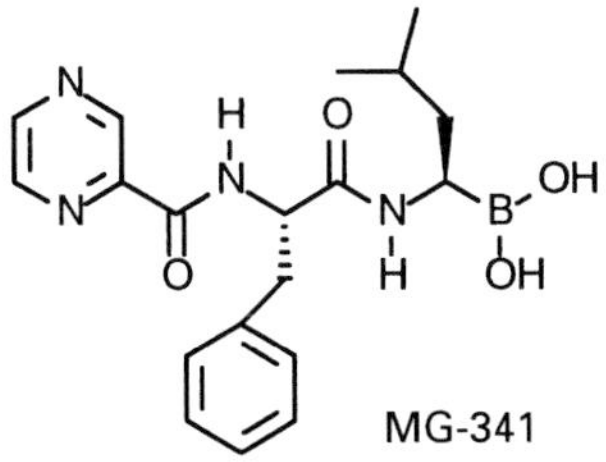

MG-341

Preferred
P1 = Leu, naphthyl-Ala, or any hydrophobic group
P2 = Leu, Phe, or hydrophobic amino acid

Vinyl sulfones [53]

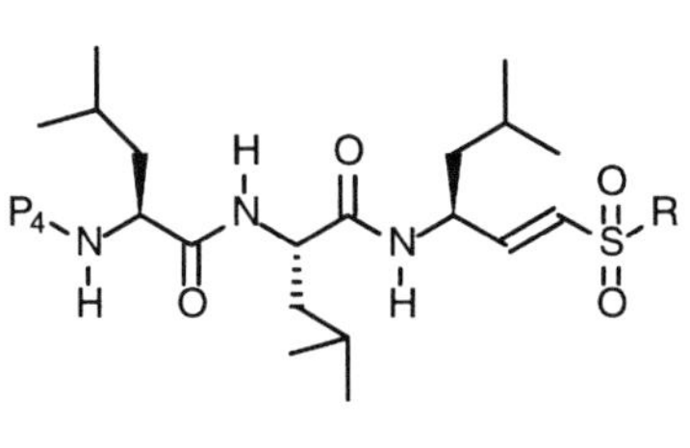

P4 = H, Gly, Leu, Tyr, or benzophenylalanine
  R = Methyl or phenyl group

Table 1 (continued)

Indanone derivative [54]

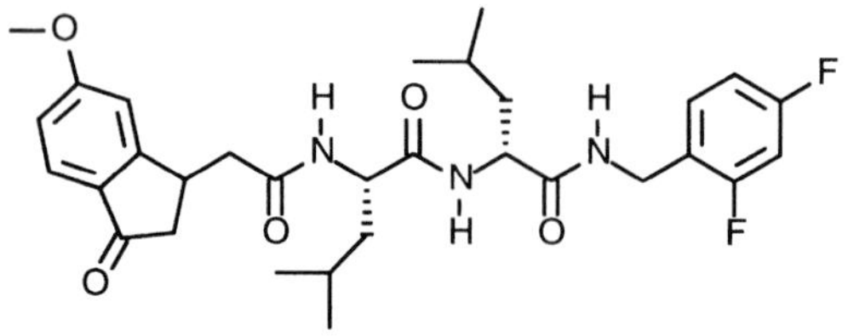

Lactacystin and clasto-lactacystin [55, 56]

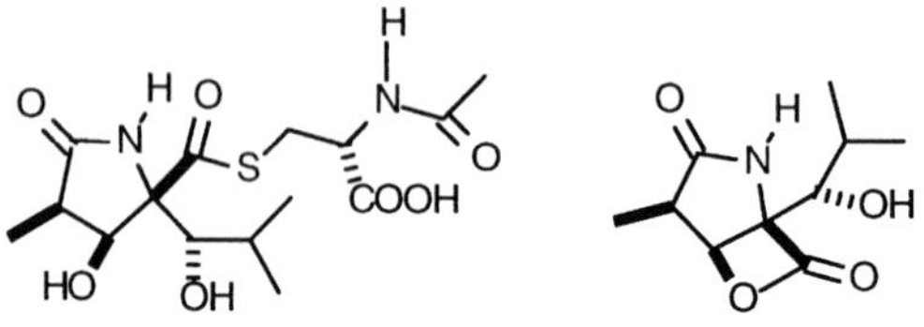

LC

cLC

Aclacinomycin A

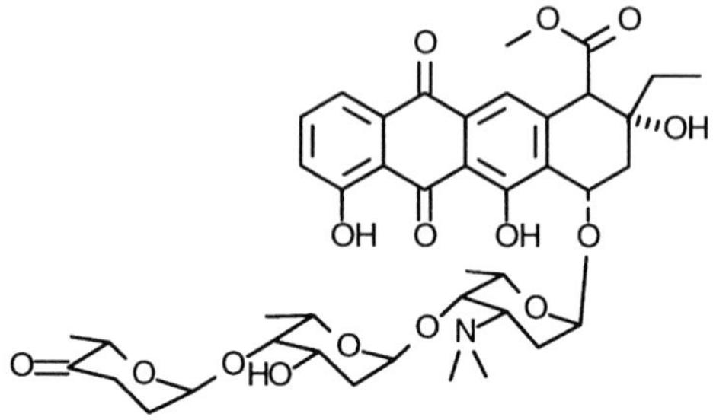

Ritonavir [58]

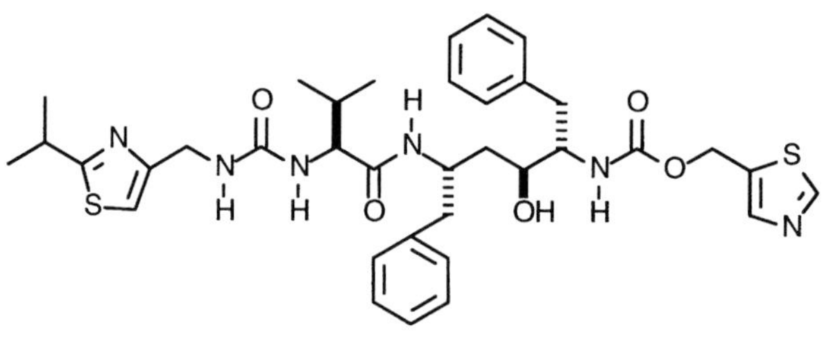

Peptide aldehydes

Peptide aldehydes are known reversible inhibitors of serine, cysteine, and aspartyl proteases [31]. Initially, peptide-based inhibitors were used to study the chymotrypsin-like activity of the proteasome [14]. Sets of hydrophobic acylated peptide aldehydes were reported as inhibitors from extensive SAR studies [14, 32]. A branched aliphatic or aromatic residue at the P1 site was tested extensively [33, 34]. Various modifications at P1, P2, and in some cases P3 were carried out. An impressive investigation was reported by Goldberg and his group describing potent aldehyde inhibitors [35]. According to their studies, the preferred amino acids at the P1 and P2 positions are Leu, naphthylalanine and other hydrophobic amino acids. The preferred N-terminal capping groups are aromatic urethane benzoyl groups. Another study reported inhibitors in which the hydrophobic property of the preferred amino acid at the P1 and P2 position was derived from a protected polar amino acid residue [36]. In our laboratory, a systematic search was carried out to identify aldehyde-based inhibitors of the proteasome. The preferred residues are Phe or Leu at the P1 site, a side-chain protected Arg residue at the P2 site, and a long chain hydrophobic acyl group at P3. The (S)-chirality at the P1 and P2 sites is critical, but the P3-chirality was not as sensitive [37, 38]. One of these dipeptide inhibitors has been shown to selectively induce apoptosis in multiple human solid tumor cell lines, but not in normal cells [39].

The two-fold symmetry of the two heptameric β subunits was observed in the crystal structure of bacterial proteasome. Based on these studies, bivalent inhibitors were synthesized by joining two peptide aldehydes (at the amino terminal) through a polyethylene glycol chain [40]. The bivalent inhibitor demonstrated, as the authors anticipated, higher potency (> 100 fold) than the simple aldehyde. It was suggested that these inhibitors may enhance binding affinity and bioavailability and may lead to an effective *in vivo* inhibitor of the proteasome.

Non-aldehyde inhibitors

In recent studies, peptide-based irreversible inhibitors have been designed using epoxide and chloromethyl ketone ERGs. Reversible inhibitors incorporating α-ketoamides, α-ketoaldehydes, boronic esters, boronic acids, indanone derivatives, and vinyl sulfones have been identified using both *in vivo* and *in vitro* assays.

α-keto epoxides

Epoxides are known irreversible inhibitors of the cysteine proteases [41]. The ketoepoxide molecule can act both as a reversible (using an activated carbonyl ERG) and an irreversible (forming a covalent bond using the active epoxide ERG) inhibitor. A preliminary report indicated that a tripeptide epoxyketone is an effective inhibitor of the proteasome (IC_{50} = 5 nM) [42]. One epoxide diastereomer was 50-fold more active and kinetic results indicate that the epoxide acted as a covalent, irreversible inhibitor of the proteasome [12].

Keto compounds

A set of ketoaldehydes (or glyoxals) was reported as inhibitors of Ch-like activity of the proteasome [43]. Dipeptide ketoaldehydes containing branched aliphatic and aromatic P1 residues showed moderate activities. However, potency of the tripeptide keto aldehyde is comparable to the known tripeptide aldehyde inhibitors (K_i values of 3–4 nM). We have tested α-ketoamide and chloromethylketone-containing proteasome inhibitors and found the α-ketoamides to be moderately active inhibitors. The chloromethylketones were less effective [44]. Similarly, a keto benzoxazole-containing peptide was shown to be a weak proteasome inhibitor [50].

Boronic acids and boronic esters

Peptide boronic acids and the corresponding esters are known serine protease inhibitors [45, 46]. In addition, it has been demonstrated that boronic acid is the active species, which is produced as a result of hydrolysis of the ester by the assay buffer [47]. Our group [44, 48, 49] and Stein's group [12, 50] undertook a systematic study to identify potent boronic acid-containing proteasome inhibitors. Stein and co-workers derived a peptide backbone using aldehyde as the ERG, and subsequently converted the aldehyde to a boronic acid to achieve very effective boronic acid inhibitors. Interestingly, bulky aromatic substituents at the P1 position increased activity. One of the potent inhibitors, MG-341 (PS-341), has been shown to be active in both cell culture and *in vivo* studies [12, 51]. It is also claimed that these compounds show antitumor and anti-inflammatory activity in various animal models.

In our group, potent aldehyde inhibitors were converted to the corresponding boronic acid and its pinacol ester [48, 49]. The boronic acid derivatives are somewhat more active (IC_{50} = 2–3 nM) than the corresponding pinacol esters (IC_{50} = 6–8 nM). Because of the presence of epimers at the P1 and P3 sites in these initial compounds, they are a mixture of four diastereomeric compounds. One can expect that an enantiomerically pure boronic acid inhibitor might be more potent.

Vinyl sulfones

Vinyl sulfones have been demonstrated to be irreversible inhibitors of cysteine proteases [52]. A series of tri- and tetrapeptide-containing vinyl sulfones were synthesized and tested for inhibitory activity [53]. P1 side-chain modification (methyl vs phenyl) modified the substrate specificity. The authors clearly demonstrated the influence of hydrophobic groups at the P3 and P4 sites. Moreover, variations at the P4 residue modulated the activity to fine-tune the subunit selectivity. It was proposed that selective inhibition for a specific proteolytic activity on the catalytic subunit could be achieved.

Other compounds

Indanone-containing peptide carboxamides are reported as inhibitors of 20S and 26S proteasomes [54]. This new class of hydrophobic peptide derivatives contain D-amino acids and no ERGs. The preferred compounds have L-Leu and D-Leu as first and second residues after the indanone group, and a simple or substituted aromatic residue as the third residue. In addition, a strict requirement for a methoxyl group on indanone is reported. Five representative compounds were shown to inhibit with moderate potency the Ch-like activity of the 20S proteasome, as well as lipopolysaccharide induced TNFα production in RAW cells (IC_{50} = 0.14 to 17.7 μM).

Lactacystin

The most widely studied irreversible inhibitor of the proteasome is lactacystin (LC), a microbial metabolite from *Streptomyces*. Initially, this compound and its analogs were reported as neurotrophic agents and inhibitors of cell cycle progression in cancer cell lines [55]. LC and its analogs were compared for inhibitory activity of the proteasome, and the specificity of these analogs was established. Mechanistic studies on the inactivation of the proteasome by LC indicate that the active species is clasto-lactocystin (cLC) derived from LC. Also, the activity of cLC is 50 times more potent than the LC [34, 56]. The electrophilic carbonyl group of LC or cLC reacts covalently with the nucleophilic Thr on the proteasome. It is interesting to note that LC binds predominantly to a single catalytically active subunit of the proteasome in contrast to tripeptide aldehyde inhibitors, which bind to all three active sites [21].

Aclacinomycin A

Aclacinomycin A (also known as aclarubicin, Ac), an antitumor drug, is an anthracyclic antibiotic consisting of an aglycone group linked to a trisaccharide moiety (see Tab. 1). It is the first non-peptide molecule shown to inhibit the 20S proteasome in a reversible non-competitive manner [57]. Similar to LC, Ac also inhibits only the Ch-like activity. The authors suggest an allosteric binding of Ac leading to favorable exposure of the chymotrypsin-like active site and blocking the other proteolytic sites. Deletion of any one of the sugar residues from Ac, or substitution of other sugar residues, attenuated inhibitory activity. The β5-β5' subunits of the proteasome responsible for the Ch-like activity, and the β1-β1' and β2-β2' units, which harbor the PGPH and trypsin-like activity, respectively, are located on opposite sides of the heptameric ring. The binding of Ac on or near the β5-β5' subunits may alter the conformation of the subunits, thus masking the other two active subunits.

An inhibitor of HIV protease, ritonavir, was reported to inhibit the Ch-like activity of the 20S proteasome as potent as the aldehyde, Ac-Leu-Leu-norLeu-H, and was shown to impair cytotoxic T lymphocyte activity [58].

Conclusion

Despite the importance of the proteasome, little work has been done on the design and development of small molecule inhibitors. Except for lactacystin analogs, few small organic molecules have been reported. Peptide-based aldehyde and boronic acid-containing inhibitors developed in our group and in Stein's show considerable potency both in *in vivo* and *in vitro* assay systems.

Successful design of synthetic inhibitors requires a thorough understanding of the catalytic mechanism and the substrate specificity of the proteasome. Because of the absence of structural similarity between lactacystin analogs and the peptide-based inhibitors, it is possible that different inactivation mechanisms are involved. We are beginning to understand the specific interaction of hydrophobic molecules with the enzyme resulting in modulation of proteasome activity. With the available structural information on the proteasome and inhibitor molecules, it is now possible to design inhibitors targeting the specific catalytic sites.

Acknowledgements
We thank Dr. John P. Mallamo and Dr. James C. Kauer for helpful comments and review of this manuscript.

References

1   Orlowski M (1990) The multicatalytic proteinase complex, a major extralysosomal proteolytic system. *Biochemistry* 29: 10289–10297

2   Goldberg AL, Rock KL (1992) Proteolysis, proteasomes and antigen presentation. *Nature* 357: 375–379

3   Coux O, Tanaka K, and Goldberg, AL (1996) Structure and functions of the 20S and 26S proteasomes. *Annu Rev Biochem* 65: 801–847

4   Baumeister W, Lupas A (1997) The proteasome. *Curr Opin Stru Biol* 7: 273–278

5   Goldberg AL, Stein RL, Adams J (1995) New insight into proteasome function: from archaebacteria to drug development. *Chem Biol* 2: 503–508

6   Pickart CM (1997) Targeting of substrates to the 26S proteasome. *FASEB J* 11: 1055–1066

7   Smith SE, Koegl M, Jentsch S (1996) Role of the ubiquitin/proteasome system in regulated protein degradation in *Saccharomyces cerevisiae*. *Biol Chem* 377: 437–446

8   Goldberg AL, Akopian TN, Kisselev AF, Lee DH, Rohrwild M (1997) New insights into the mechanism and importance of the proteasome in intracellular protein degradation. *Biol Chem* 378: 131–140

9   Lupas A, Zwickl P, Wenzel T, Seemuller E, Baumeister W (1995) Structure and function of the 20S proteasome and of its regulatory complexes. *Cold Spring Harbor Symp Quant Biol* LX: 515–524

10   Tanaka K (1998) Proteasomes: structure and biology. *J Biochem* 123: 195–204

11   Hilt W, Wolf DH (1995) Proteasomes of the yeast *S. cerevisiae*: genes, structure and function. *Mol Biol Repor* 21: 3–10

12   Adams J, Stein R (1996) Novel inhibitors of the proteasome and their therapeutic use in inflammation. *Annu Rep Med Chem* 31: 279–288

13   Orlowski M, Cardozo C, Michaud C (1993) Evidence for the presence of five distinct proteolytic components in the pituitary multicatalytic proteinase complex. Properties of two components cleaving bonds on the carboxyl side of branched chain and small neutral amino acids. *Biochemistry* 32: 1563–1572

14   Vinitsky A, Cardozo C, Sepp-Lorenzino L, Michaud C, Orlowski M (1994) Inhibition of the proteolytic activity of the multicatalytic proteinase complex (proteasome) by substrate-related peptidyl aldehydes. *J Biol Chem* 269: 29860–29866

15   Arendt CS, Hochstrasser M (1997) Identification of the yeast 20S proteasome catalytic centers and subunit interactions required for active-site formation. *Proc Natl Acad Sci USA* 94: 7156–7161

16   McCormack TA, Cruikshank AA, Grenier L, Melandri FD, Nunes SL, Plamondon L, Stein RL, Dick, LR (1998) Kinetic studies of the branched chain amino acid preferring peptidase activity of the 20S proteasome: development of a continuous assay and inhibition by tripeptide aldehydes and *clasto*-lactacystin β-lactone. *Biochemistry* 37: 7792–7800

17   Stein RL, Melandri F, Dick LR (1996) Kinetic characterization of the chymotryptic activity of the 20S proteasome. *Biochemistry* 35: 3899–3908

18   Groettrup M, Soza A, Kuckelkorn U, Kloetzel P-M (1996) Peptide antigen production by the proteasome: complexity provides efficiency. *Immunol Today* 17: 429–435

19   Cardozo C, Eleuteri AM, Orlowski M (1995) Differences in catalytic activities and subunit pattern of multicatalytic proteinase complexes (proteasomes) isolated from bovine pituitary, lung, and liver. *J Biol Chem* 270: 22645–22651

20   Löwe J, Stock D, Jap B, Swickl P, Baumeister W, Huber R (1995) Crystal structure of the 20S proteasome from the archaeon *T. acidophilum* at 3.4 A resolution. *Science* 268: 533–539

21   Groll M, Ditzel L, Lowe J, Stock D, Bochtler M, Bartunik HD, Huber R (1997) Structure of 20S proteasome from yeast at 2.4 A resolution. *Nature* 386: 463–471

22   Brannigan JA, Dodson G, Duggleby HJ, Moody PCE, Smith JL, Tomchick DR, Murzin AG (1995) A protein catalytic framework with an N-terminal nucleophile is capable of self-activation. *Nature* 378: 416–419

23   Seemüller E, Lupas A, Stock D, Löwe J, Huber R, Baumeister W (1995) Proteasome from *Thermoplasma acidophilum*: a threonine protease. *Science* 268: 579–582

24   Ciechanover A (1994) The ubiquitin-proteasome proteolytic pathway. *Cell* 79:13–21

25   Hilt W, Wolf DH (1996) Proteasomes: destruction as a programme. *Trends Biochem Sci* 21: 96–102

26   Ghosh S, May MJ, Kopp EB (1998) NF-κB and Rel proteins: evolutionarily conserved mediators of immune responses. *Annu Rev Immunol* 16: 225–260

27   Blagosklonny MV, Wu GS, Omura S, El-Deiry WS (1996) Proteasome-dependent regulation of p21$^{WAF1/CIP1}$ expression. *Biochem Biophys Res Comm* 227: 564–569

28   Pagano M, Tam SW, Theodoras AM, Beer-Romero P, Del Sal G, Chau V, Yew PR, Draetta GF, Rolfe M (1995) Role of the ubiquitin-proteasome pathway in regulating abundance of the cyclin-dependent kinase inhibitor p27. *Science* 269: 682–685

29   Scheffner M, Huibregtse JM, Vierstra RD, Howley PM (1993) The HPV-16 EG and E6-AP complex functions as an ubiquitin-protein ligase in the ubiquitination of p53. *Cell* 75: 495–505

30   Knight CG (1986) The characterization of enzyme inhibition. In: AJ Barrett, G Salvesen (eds): *Proteinase inhibitors*. Elsevier, New York, 23–51

31   Sandler M, Smith HJ (eds) (1989) *Design of enzyme inhibitiors as drug*. Oxford University Press, New York

32   Vinitsky A, Michaud C, Powers JC, Orlowski M (1992) Inhibition of the chymotrypsin-like activity of the pituitary multicatalytic proteinase complex. *Biochemistry* 31: 9421–9428

33   Tsubuki S, Kawasaki H, Saito Y, Miyashita N, Inomata M, Kawashima S (1993) Purification and characterization of a Z-Leu-Leu-Leu-MCA degrading protease expected to regulate neurite formation: a novel catalytic activity in proteasome. *Biochem Biophys Res Commun* 196: 1195–1201

34   Dick LR, Cruikshank A, Grenier L, Melandri F, Plamondon L, Stein R (1996) Mechanistic studies on the inactivation of the proteasome by lactacystin: a central role for clasto-lactacystin beta-lactone. *J Biol Chem* 271: 7273–7276

35   Stein RL, Ma Y-T, Brand S (1997) Inhibitors of the 26S proteasome complex and the 20S proteasome contained therein. Patent US 5693617

36   Figueiredo-Pereira ME, Wu-E C, Yuan H-M, Wilk S (1995) A novel chymotrypsin-like component of the multicatalytic proteinase complex optimally active at acidic pH. *Arch Biochem Biophys* 317: 69–78

37   Iqbal M, Diebold J, Siman R, Chatterjee S, Kauer JC (1995) Multicatalytic protease inhibitors. Patent US 5550262

38   Iqbal M, Chatterjee S, Kauer JC, Das M, Messina PA, Freed B, Biazzo W, Siman R (1995) Potent inhibitors of proteasome. *J Med Chem* 38: 2276–2277

39   An B, Goldfarb RH, Siman R, Dou QP (1999) Novel dipeptidyl proteasome inhibitors

overcome Bcl-2 protective function and selectively accumulate the cyclin-dependent kinase inhibitor p27 and induce apoptosis in transformed, but not normal, human fibroblasts. *Cell Death Differ* 5: 1062–1075

40 Loidl G, Musiol H-J, Groll M, Ditzel, Huber R, Moroder L (1998) Bivalent inhibitors of the yeast proteasome. *J Pep Sci* (Special issue) 4: 122

41 Hanada K, Tamai M, Yamagishi M, Ohmura S, Sawada J, Tanaka I (1978) Studies on thiol protease inhibitors. Part I. Isolation and characterization of E-64, a new thiol protease inhibitor. *Agric Biol Chem* 42: 523–528

42 Spaltenstein A, Leban JJ, Huang JJ, Reinhardt KR, Viveros H, Sigafoos J, Crouch R (1996) Design and synthesis of novel protease inhibitors. Tripeptide α',β'-epoxyketones as nanomolar inactivators of the proteasome. *Tetrahedron Lett* 37: 1343–1346

43 Lynas JF, Harriott P, Healy A, McKervey MA, Walker B (1998) Inhibitors of the chymotrypsin-like activity of proteasome based on di- and tri-peptidyl α-ketoaldehyde (glyoxals). *Bioorg Med Chem Lett* 8: 373–378

44 Iqbal M, Chatterjee S, Kauer JC, Mallamo JP, Messina PA, Reiboldt A, Siman R (1996) Potent a-ketocarbonyl and boronic ester derived inhibitors of proteasome. *Bioorg Med Chem Lett* 6: 287–290

45 Shenvi AB (1986) Alpha-Aminoboronic acid derivatives: effective inhibitors of aminopeptidases. *Biochemistry* 25: 1286–1291

46 Kettner C, Mersinger L, Knabb R (1990) The selective inhibition of thrombin by peptides of boroarginine. *J Biol Chem* 259: 18289–18297

47 Kettner CA, Shenvi AB (1984) Inhibition of the serine proteases leukocyte elastase, pancreatic elastase, cathepsin G, and chymotrypsin by peptide boronic acids. *J Biol Chem* 259: 15106–15114

48 Iqbal M, Diebold J, Siman R, Chatterjee S, Kauer JC (1995) Multicatalytic protease inhibitors. Patent US 5614649

49 Iqbal M, Diebold J, Siman R, Chatterjee S, Kauer JC (1995) Multicatalytic protease inhibitors. Patent WO 96/14857

50 Adams J, Behnke M, Chen S, Cruickshank AA, Dick LR, Grenier L, Klunder JM, Ma Y-T, Plamondon L, Stein RL (1998) Potent and selective inhibitors of the proteasome: dipeptidyl boronic acids. *Bioorg Med Chem Lett* 8: 333–338

51 Adams J, Ma Y-T, Stein R, Baevsky M, Grenier L, Plamondon L (1996) Boronic ester and acid compounds, synthesis and uses. Patent WO 96/13266

52 Sok DE, Choi DS, Kim YB, Lee YH, Cha SH (1993) Selective inactivation of glyceraldehyde-3-phosphate dehydrogenase by vinyl sulfones. *Biochem Biophys Res Commun* 195: 1224–1229

53 Bogyo M, Shin S, McMaster JS, Ploegh HL (1998) Substrate binding and sequence preference of the proteasome revealed by active-site-directed affinity probes. *Chem Biol* 5: 307–320

54 Lum R, Schow S, Joly A, Kerwar S, Nelson M, Wick M (1998) Indanone derivatives that inhibits 26S and 20S proteasome-useful for the treatment of e.g. rheumatoid arthritis, lupus, diabetes, multiple sclerosis, cancer and restenosis. Patent WO 98/13061–A1

55 Fenteany G, Standaert RF, Lane WS, Reichard GA, Corey EJ, Schreiber SL (1994) A b-lactone related to lactacystin induces neurite outgrowth in a neuroblastoma cell line and inhibits cell cycle progression in an osteosarcoma cell line. *Proc Natl Acad Sci USA* 91: 3358–3362

56 Fenteany G, Standaert RF, Lane WS, Choi S, Corey EJ, Schreiber SL (1995) Inhibition of proteasome activities and subunit-specific amino-terminal threonine modification by lactacystin. *Science* 268: 726–729

57 Figueiredo-Pereira ME, Chen WE, Li J, Johdo O (1996) The antitumor drug aclacino-mycin A, which inhibits the degradation of ubiquitinated proteins, shows selectivity for the chymotrypsin-like activity of the bovine pituitary 20S proteasome. *J Biol Chem* 271: 16455–16459

58 Andre P, Groettrup M, Klenerman P, de Giuli R, Booth BL, Cerundolo V, Bonneville M, Jotereau F, Zinkernagel RM, Lotteau V (1998) An inhibitor of HIV-1 protease modulates proteasome activity, antigen presentation, and T cell responses. *Proc Natl Acad Sci USA* 95: 13120–13124

Caspase-1 (ICE) and other caspases as drug discovery targets: Opportunities and progress

Tariq Ghayur[1], Sheryl J. Hays[2] and Robert V. Talanian[1]

[1]BASF Bioresearch Corporation, 100 Research Drive, Worcester, MA 01605, USA, and
[2]Parke-Davis Pharmaceutical Research, 2800 Plymouth Drive, Ann Arbor, MI 48105, USA

Introduction

The caspases are a family of intracellular cysteine proteases that have critical roles in cytokine maturation and apoptosis. Pharmacologic modulation of caspase activity *in vivo* may be effective in inflammatory diseases such as rheumatoid arthritis and septic shock, or, more speculatively, in conditions where inappropriate apoptosis contributes to pathology, such as neurodegenerative diseases and ischemia-related cell death. The caspases have thus attracted a great deal of attention as drug discovery targets. Here we review our understanding of the biological roles and properties of the caspases, particularly caspase-1 (or interleukin-1β converting enzyme, ICE), and progress in the discovery of caspase-specific inhibitory drugs.

Biological roles of caspases

Background

Interleukin-1β (IL-1β) has been implicated as a key mediator of a variety of inflammatory diseases. IL-1β is activated intracellularly by proteolysis. Caspase-1, which catalyzes this cleavage, was described in 1989 [1, 2]. The unusual substrate specificity of caspase-1 suggested that the design of selective inhibitors might be achieveable. The cDNA and predicted amino acid sequences of human caspase-1 were reported in 1992 [3]. This enabled the production of recombinant caspase-1 in sufficient quantities for mass screening and inhibitor/enzymatic studies, as well as structure determination.

A landmark publication in 1993 suggested by sequence homology that caspase-1 is a mammalian ortholog of ced-3, one of two *C. elegans* genes required for developmental cell death [4]. This raised concerns that inhibition of caspase-1 might interfere with normal apoptosis. Currently, 12 human caspase-1/ced-3 homologs have been reported [5–7]. These were renamed "caspases" (for cysteine aspartate-specific proteases), numbered by the order of their discovery [5]. As described below, a picture of specialized caspase function is emerging, in which the primary role of caspase-1 and probably that of its closest homologs is cytokine maturation, and that of the remaining caspases is apoptosis. This has diminished the concern that selective caspase inhibition might globally block apoptosis.

Roles in cytokine maturation

Caspase-1 was identified by its ability to activate IL-1β, but it was unknown whether it had additional functions or whether other enzymes could also produce mature IL-1β. To address these questions, we and others have utilized biochemical approaches, cell-based assays, and caspase-1 knockout (caspase-1$^{-/-}$) mice [8, 9]. Caspase-1 activates IL-1β *in vitro* most efficiently among the caspases. Similarly, in COS cell co-transfection assays, only caspase-1 generated biologically active IL-1β. Caspase-1$^{-/-}$ mice were severely deficient in generation of mature IL-1β. Surprisingly, caspase-1$^{-/-}$ mice were also defective in generation of mature IL-1α, even though IL-1α is not a caspase-1 substrate [8]. Caspase-1 processes *in vitro* calpastatin [10], a cellular inhibitor of calpain, which itself cleaves IL-1α. The defect in LPS-induced mature IL-1α in caspase-1$^{-/-}$ mice might therefore be due to calpain degradation of IL-1α. Similarly, the caspase-1 inhibitor Ac-YVAD-cho [3] can block LPS-induced production of mature IL-1α from human PBMCs, although with about 10-fold higher IC_{50} values than that of IL-1β inhibition.

We and others recently demonstrated that interleukin-18 (IL-18, or IGIF for interferon-γ inducing factor) is a natural caspase-1 substrate [11, 12]. IL-18 is a potent inducer of interferon-γ (IFNγ) production by T-helper type-1 (TH1) and natural killer (NK) cells [13], and is therefore pro-inflammatory. Caspase-1 cleaved pro-IL-1β and pro-IL-18 *in vitro* with similar catalytic efficiencies, and in COS cells, Ac-YVAD-cho inhibited both LPS-induced IL-1β and IFNγ with similar IC_{50} values [11]. Caspase-1$^{-/-}$ mice are also deficient in the LPS-induced production of IFNγ, which is dependent on IL-18 production [11]. Thus, caspase-1 directly and indirectly regulates production of IL-1β, IL-18, IL-1α, and IFNγ. These results strengthen the idea that caspase-1 inhibitors might be effective as anti-inflammatory drugs.

Roles in apoptosis

With few exceptions, the actions of caspases are required for apoptosis. Many studies show that blocking caspase activation or activity can inhibit apoptosis. There is a large and growing list of known caspase substrates. These include (i) cytokines, (ii) other caspases, (iii) enzymes that function in signal transduction (e.g. PKC-δ, PLC-γ, and c-PLA2), (iv) structural proteins (e.g. actin, fodrin, lamins), and (v) factors involved in DNA metabolism (e.g. PARP, DNA-PK, and p45). Some are activated by caspase cleavage, and others are inactivated. Caspase action on DNA-metabolizing enzymes, such as p40 nuclease activation by cleavage of its inhibitor p45 (the murine orthologs are called CAD and ICAD, respectively), and inactivation of the DNA repair factor PARP, clearly contribute to the DNA cleavage that is a hallmark of apoptosis. Likewise, cleavage of structural proteins contributes to common apoptotic morphology, such as membrane blebbing and cell shrinkage. The roles of the caspase substrates that function in signal transduction, many of which are kinases that are activated by caspase cleavage, are less clear. While our current understanding allows prediction that caspase inhibitors would be effective apoptosis-modulating drugs, many important details remain unclear.

Physical and biochemical properties of caspases

Caspase activation

The caspases are synthesized as inactive precursors. Activation occurs by proteolysis, releasing a pro-domain of a few to more than 150 residues, and separating the large (ca. 20 kDa) and small (ca. 10 kDa) subunits that comprise the active enzyme. These cleavages occur at aspartic acid residues and are primarily autoproteolytic or conducted by other caspases. The pro-domains have roles in subcellular localization [14, 15], dimerization [16] and autocatalytic activation [17].

Caspase three-dimensional structures

The crystal structures of caspase-1 [18, 19] and -3 [20, 21] have yielded insights into the assembly, stability, substrate recognition, and catalytic properties of the caspase family. In its active form, each enzyme is a noncovalently associated homodimer of heterodimeric large and small subunits. The two catalytic sites in the homodimer are distant from one another, with no significant allosteric interaction between them. Substrate recognition and catalytic residues are derived from both subunits of each heterodimer.

Biochemical evidence identified Cys285 as the active site nucleophile of caspase-1 [3], and this was confirmed by the crystal structure. A catalytic role was also suggested for His237 due to its proximity to Cys285. The catalytic residues and geometry of the caspase-3 active site were similar to those of caspase-1, suggesting conservation of those features as well as the catalytic mechanism throughout the caspase family [20, 21].

Mutation complementation studies showed that the large and small subunits of an active caspase can derive from separate translation products, which might be different gene products [22, 23]. Also, homodimeric pairs can exist in a simple equilibrium [24, 25], suggesting the formation of active oligomeric species containing portions of up to four separate gene products. Such species might vary in their specificity or susceptibility to regulation. Other factors that may influence caspase properties in cells include association with other proteins and splice variation.

Caspase substrate specificity

Compared to many proteases, the caspases display remarkable substrate specificity. Understanding this specificity helps predict the biological roles of these enzymes, and offers opportunities for the design of inhibitors that distinguish caspases from other enzymes and one another. Caspase specificity toward peptide substrates has been studied by defined-substrate and combinatorial methods [26, 27], and is summarized in Table 1.

All caspases require Asp in P1. This specificity is shared with granzyme B, a serine protease that also has proapoptotic activity [28]. In addition, all caspases prefer Glu in P3. The x-ray structures of caspase-1 [18, 19] and -3 [20, 21] bound with peptidic inhibitors show that P1 and P3 specificity is determined at least partially by contact with conserved caspase residues. These include interaction of the acidic side-chains of P3 and P1 with the guanidinium of a conserved Arg. Similar interactions have been inferred from a modeling study of caspase-8 [29].

P4 specificity distinguishes the caspases from one another. The caspase-1 and -3 structures reveal substantial differences in the identities of the residues in the P4 region as well as the steric features of the pocket that they form. Differences in the

Table 1 - Caspase specificity and roles

Caspase	Peptide specificity	Probable physiologic roles
1, 4, 5, 13*	W-E-x-D	Cytokine maturation
2	V-D-V-x-D	Apoptosis signalling
8, 9, 10, 14*	L-E-x-D	
6	V-E-x-D	Apoptosis effectors
3,7	D-E-x-D	

*Caspase-13 and -14 specificity have not been studied in detail, and are presumed to be similar to those of caspase-1, -4 and -5, and caspase-2 and -9, respectively, because of sequence similarity.

breadth of P4 specificity between the caspases suggests that they vary in their P4 flexibility as well.

P1' specificity has been studied in detail only for caspase-1 and -4 [26]. Both prefer Gly in this position, but also efficiently recognise aromatic and hydroxyl/thiol-containing amino acids.

The caspases also make contacts with the backbones of peptidic inhibitors. For efficient recognition, caspase-2 requires that peptidic inhibitors contain at least 5 residues; all other caspases require four. The importance of each contact to favorable recognition varies along the chain. For caspase-1, substantial differences in the effects on inhibitor potency were observed when peptidic inhibitors were methylated at each of their amides, with P1 and P3 being most important [30]. Attempts to deduce the cellular roles of the caspases from their specificity toward peptidic substrates have been hampered by the fact that the enzymes efficiently recognise substrate and inhibitor peptides of sub-optimal sequence.

Caspase-1 inhibitor discovery

Mass screening

A common means to generate inhibitor leads is to screen a diverse chemical library. This has been applied to caspase-1, but with little success. The only reported nonpeptide lead from a proprietary compound collection was an arylpyridazine 1 with an IC_{50} of 3 μM [31]. While this compound and its analogs are selective for caspase-1 compared to other cysteine proteases, such reactive compounds are typically not useful leads [32]. Other reactive as well as redox-active compounds have inhibitory activity for caspase-1, but these also act by undesirable mechanisms.

Peptidic inhibitors

Another method of caspase-1 inhibitor design is the use of peptide substrates. Some success in inhibitor optimization based on caspase specificity studies has been realized. A peptidic aldehyde inhibitor incorporating the preferred residue Trp in P4 (Ac-WEVD-cho) displayed a K_i for caspase-1 of 56 pM [27]. Several reviews have comprehensively discussed peptidic caspase inhibitors [33, 34]. These electrophilic peptides include aldehydes [35, 36] and ketones [37, 38] that bind the active site cysteine reversibly and acyloxymethylketones [39, 40], aryloxymethylketones [41], phosphinyloxymethylketones [42] and heteroaryloxymethylketones [43, 44] that contain leaving groups a to the carbonyl moiety at S1, resulting in a covalent, irreversible linkage with the active site cysteine.

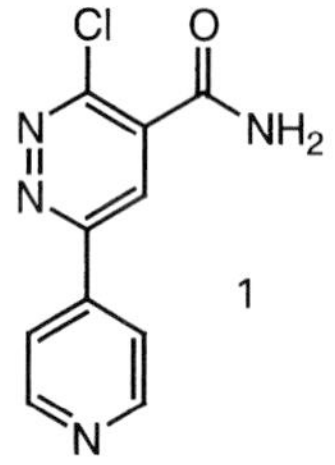

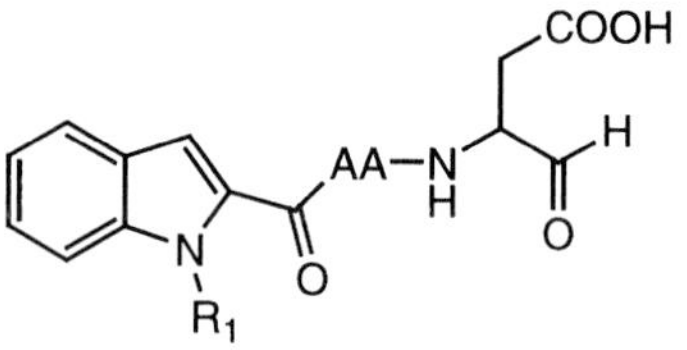

Compound #	R1	AA	IC$_{50}$ (µM)
2	-CH$_3$	alanine	0.177
3	-(CH$_2$)$_2$COOH	alanine	0.198
4	-(CH$_2$)$_3$PH	valine	0.133
	Cbz-Val-Ala-Asp-H		0.064

Recent patents show continuing progress in new caspase-1 peptidic inhibitors. One exemplifies a series of N-substituted indoles that interact at P3 (compounds 2–4). These are 2–3 times less potent than the reference compound Cbz-VAD-cho. This is a modest loss in activity, considering that these analogs lack functionality to interact with caspase-1 at P4 [45, 46].

Other new peptides show that an interaction on the "primeside" of the enzyme can increase potency. Peptides exemplified by compounds 5 and 6 have primeside moieties that are not leaving groups [47, 48]. The naphthylacetic acid moiety of analog 7 may be a leaving group depending upon the interactions on the P-side of the inhibitor [49]. Such bimodal inhibitors have been discussed in detail [50]. Primeside functionality can interact with a lipophilic pocket of caspase-1 to produce substantial increases in potency. While this is demonstrated by peptides 5–7, such primeside groups may also contribute to potency in nonpeptidic compounds.

Peptidomimetics

While peptidic caspase-1 inhibitors contribute to SAR understanding and permit key "proof-of-concept" studies, they suffer from undesirable properties such as inadequate oral absorption and rapid metabolism. Caspase-1/inhibitor cocrystal structures along with conventional drug design strategies have resulted in new peptidomimetic inhibitors. A starting point for peptidomimetic design was identification of a surrogate for the S$_3$–S$_2$ dipeptide of peptidic inhibitors [51]. All such compounds retain the S$_1$ aspartic acid residue and the critical hydrogen-bonding functionality (S$_1$ and S$_3$ NH, S3 C=O) that are required for potent inhibition by peptidic inhibitors (Fig. 1). An initial study examined pyridone and pyrmidone-based mimet-

$$R_1 \overset{O}{\underset{}{\parallel}}\!\!-NH\text{-Val-Ala-Asp}\overset{O}{\underset{}{\parallel}}\!\!-X$$

Compound	R_1	X	IC50 (μM)	Reference
5	Ph-(CH$_2$)$_2$-		0.03	47
6	Ph-CH$_2$-O-		0.015	48
7	Ph-CH$_2$-O-		0.02	49
Reference Compound	Ph-CH$_2$-O-	H	0.064	46

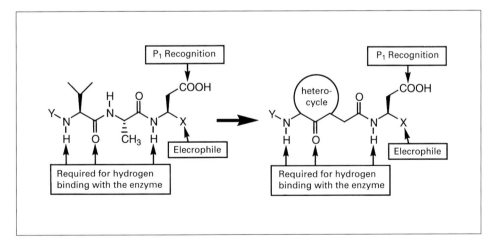

Figure 1
Design features for a peptidomimetic strategy.

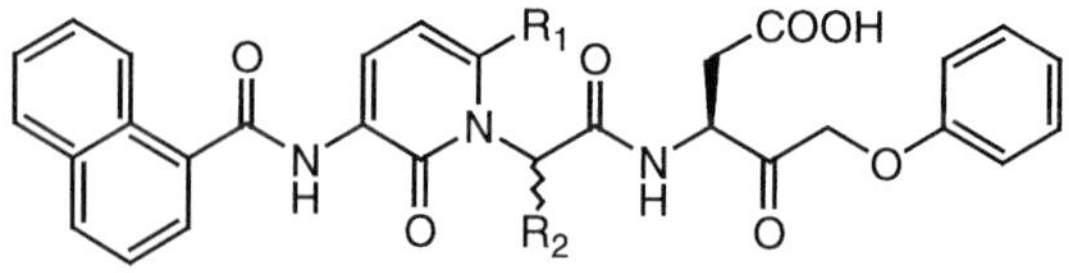

Compound #	R$_1$	R$_2$	Ki (µM)
8	-CH$_2$Ph	H	0.010
9	H	-n-Pr	0.0018
10	-CH$_3$	-n-Pr	2.2

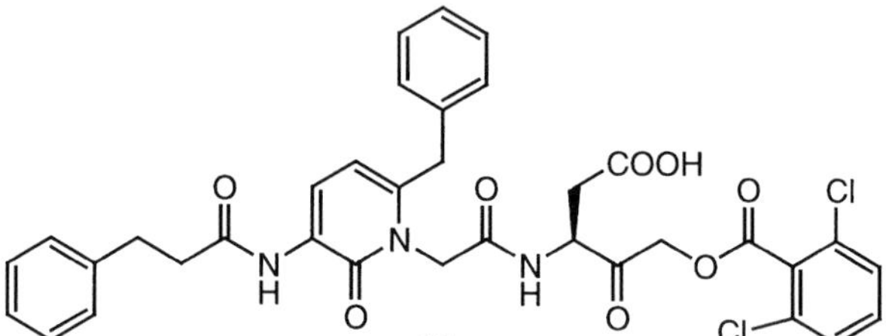

ics to replace the Val-Pro motif at S$_3$–S$_2$ [52]. This suggested that alkyl substitution at R$_1$ or R$_2$ improved activity (compounds 8 and 9), but when both groups were alkyl (compound 10), potency was reduced 100- to 1000-fold, suggesting that both groups compete for one binding site. The caspase-1 cocrystal structure with the irreversible analog 11 suggested that a benzyl group off the 6-position of the pyridone ring could access a lipophilic pocket near P$_2$ [53]. Molecular modeling and x-ray studies supported the idea that the steric interactions between a P$_2$ methyl (R$_2$ = CH$_3$) and the 6-benzyl substituent hinder adoption of the requisite binding conformation, reducing potency [53].

Other peptidomimetic heterocycles have been used as scaffolds in the design of caspase-1 inhibitors (compounds 12–15) [46, 54, 55]. Although several patents claimed improved *in vivo* activity and enhanced pharmacokinetic properties compared to peptide inhibitors, only compound 15 has data supporting these claims. The N-benzoyl compound inhibited IL-1β production by > 95% in a mouse model of biochemical efficacy at 100 mg/kg i.p. The compound exhibited stablity in *ex vivo* liver and intestinal slice assays, had a plasma clearance rate of 7 mL/min/kg, and demonstrated oral bioavailability of 12 and 16% in two dogs [54].

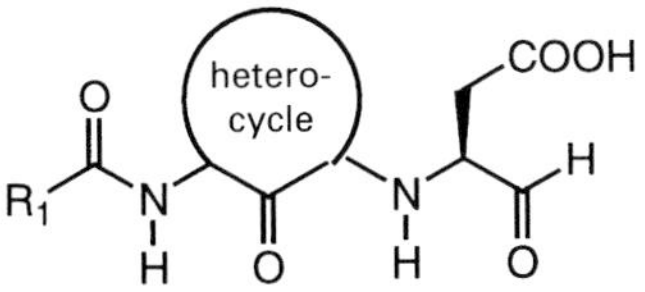

compound #	R₁	Heterocycle	Ki (μM)	Reference
12	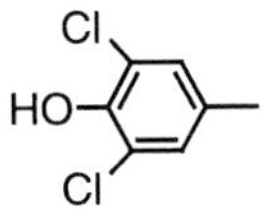	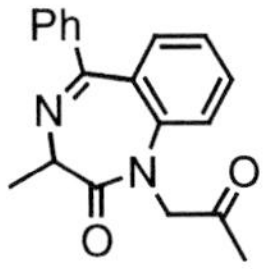	0.0025	55
13	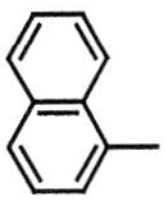	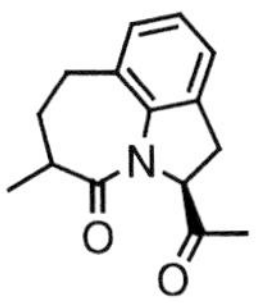	0.010	46
14	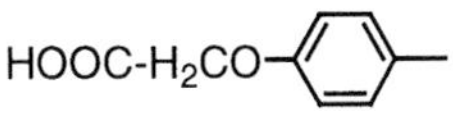 HOOC-H₂CO-	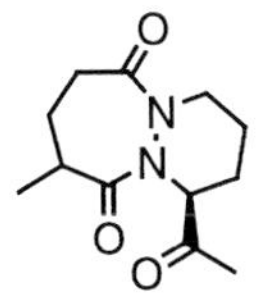	0.001	54
15	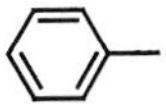	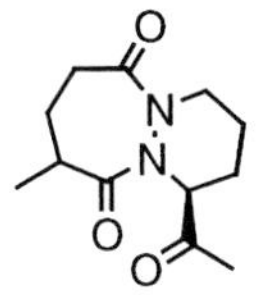	0.005	54

Gold salts and the regulation of IL-1β production

In monocytic/macrophage cells and cell lines caspase-1 plays a critical role not only in the processing of pro-IL-1β, but also in the release of mature IL-1β from cells. Gold salts (aurothiomalate and auranofin) inhibited IL-1β release from human peripheral blood mononuclear cells. The co-crystal structure of caspase-1 and gold-thiomalate showed that these compounds bind to Cys364 and Cys397, located near the 2-fold axis of the crystal [19], possibly disrupting the oligomeric structure of the enzyme.

Conclusions and prospects

At this stage, the promise of caspase inhibitors as anti-inflammatory drugs seems clear, while their application to diseases of inappropriate apoptosis remains somewhat speculative. Nevertheless, the wide range of important clinical indications that have been proposed as targets for caspase inhibitors supports a continued high level of interest in elucidating the biological roles of these enzymes in health and disease. While mass screening has been largely unsuccessful, progress in the design of caspase-1 inhibitors has been made based on understanding of the catalytic and structural properties of the enzyme as well as a great deal of creativity. Similar progress can be expected for other caspases. With further work, caspase inhibitors efficacious in a variety of clinical indications will certainly be produced.

References

1   Black RA, Kronheim SA, Sleath PR (1989) Activation of interleukin-1β by a co-induced protease. *FEBS Lett* 247: 386–390
2   Kostura MJ, Tocci MJ, Limjuco G, Chin J, Cameron P, Hillman AG, Chartrain NA, Schmidt JA (1989) Identification of a monocyte specific pre-interleukin 1β convertase activity. *Proc Natl Acad Sci USA* 86: 5227–5231
3   Thornberry NA, Bull HG, Calaycay JR, Chapman KT, Howard AD, Kostura MJ, Miller DK, Molineaux SM, Weidner JR, Aunins J et al (1992) A novel heterodimeric cysteine protease is required for interleukin-1β processing in monocytes. *Nature* 356: 768–774
4   Yuan J, Shaham S, Ledoux S, Ellis HM, Horvitz HR (1993) The *C. elegans* cell death gene ced-3 encodes a protein similar to mammalian interleukin-1β-converting enzyme. *Cell* 75: 641–652
5   Alnemri ES, Livingston DJ, Nicholson DW, Salvesen G, Thornberry NA, Wong WW, Yuan J (1996) Human ICE/CED-3 protease nomenclature. *Cell* 87: 171
6   Humke EW, Ni J, Dixit VM (1998) ERICE, a novel FLICE-activatable caspase. *J Biol Chem* 273: 15702–15707
7   Hu S, Snipas SJ, Vincenz C, Salvesen G, Dixit VM (1998) Caspase-14 is a novel developmentally regulated protease. *J Biol Chem* 273: 29648–29653
8   Li P, Allen H, Banerjee S, Franklin S, Herzog L, Johnston C, McDowell J, Paskind M, Rodman L, Salfeld J et al (1995) Mice deficient in IL-1β-converting enzyme are defective in production of mature IL-1β and resistant to endotoxic shock. *Cell* 80: 401–411
9   Kuida K, Lippke JA, Ku G, Harding MW, Livingston DJ, Su MS-S, Flavell RA (1995) Altered cytokine export and apoptosis in mice deficient in interleukin-1β converting enzyme. *Science* 267: 2000–2003
10   Wang KKW, Posmantur R, Nadimpalli R, Nath R, Mohan P, Nixon RA, Talanian RV, Keegan M, Herzog L, Allen H (1998) Caspase-mediated fragmentation of calpain inhibitor protein calpastatin during apoptosis. *Arch Biochem Biophys* 356: 187–196

11   Ghayur T, Banerjee S, Hugunin M, Butler D, Herzog L, Carter A, Quintal L, Sekut L, Talanian R, Paskind M, et al (1997) Caspase-1 processes IFN-γ-inducing factor and regulates LPS-induced IFN-γ production. *Nature* 386: 619–623

12   Gu Y, Kuida K, Tsutsui H, Ku G, Hsiao K, Fleming MA, Hayashi N, Higashino K, Okamura H, Nakanishi K et al (1997) Activation of interferon-γ inducing factor mediated by interleukin-1β converting enzyme. *Science* 275: 206–209

13   Takeda K, Tsutsui H, Yoshimoto T, Adachi O, Yoshida N, Kishimoto T, Okamura H, Nakanishi K, Akira S (1998) Defective NK cell activity and Th1 response in IL-18-deficient mice. *Immunity* 8: 383–390

14   Ashkenazi A, Dixit VM (1998) Death receptors: Signaling and modulation. *Science* 281: 1305–1308

15   Mao PL, Jiang Y, Wee BY, Porter AG (1998) Activation of caspase-1 in the nucleus requires nuclear translocation of pro-caspase-1 mediated by its prodomain. *J Biol Chem* 273: 23621–23624

16   Butt AJ, Harvey NL, Parasivam G, Kumar S (1998) Dimerization and autoprocessing of the Nedd2 (caspase-2) precursor requires both the prodomain and the carboxyl-terminal regions. *J Biol Chem* 273: 6763–6768

17   Colussi PA, Harvey NL, Shearwin-Whyatt LM, Kumar S (1998) Conversion of procaspase-3 to an autoactivating caspase by fusion to the caspase-2 prodomain. *J Biol Chem* 273: 26566–26570

18   Walker NPC, Talanian RV, Brady KD, Dang LC, Bump NJ, Ferenz CR, Franklin S, Ghayur T, Hackett MC, Hammill LD et al (1994) Crystal structure of the cysteine protease interleukin-1β-converting enzyme: A (p20/p10)2 homodimer. *Cell* 78: 343–352

19   Wilson KP, Black J-AF, Thomson JA, Kim EE, Griffith JP, Navia MA, Murcko MA, Chambers SP, Aldape RA, Raybuck SA et al (1994) Structure and mechanism of interleukin-1β converting enzyme. *Nature* 370: 270–275

20   Rotonda J, Nicholson DW, Fazil KM, Gallant M, Gareau Y, Labelle M, Peterson EP, Rasper DM, Ruel R, Vaillancourt JP et al (1996) The three-dimensional structure of apopain/CPP32, a key mediator of apoptosis. *Nature Struct Biol* 3: 619–625

21   Mittl PRE, Di Marco S, Krebs JF, Bai X, Karanewsky DS, Priestle JP, Tomaselli KJ, Grütter MG (1997) Structure of recombinant human CPP32 in complex with the tetrapeptide acetyl-Asp-Val-Ala-Asp fluoromethyl ketone. *J Biol Chem* 272: 6539–6547

22   Gu Y, Wu J, Faucheu C, Lalanne J-L, Diu A, Livingston DJ, Su MS-S (1995) Interleukin-1β converting enzyme requires oligomerization for activity of processed forms *in vivo*. *EMBO J* 14: 1923–1931

23   Fernandes-Alnemri T, Takahashi A, Armstrong R, Krebs J, Fritz L, Tomaselli KJ, Wang L, Yu Z, Croce CM, Salveson G et al (1995) Mch3, a novel human apoptotic cysteine protease highly related to CPP32. *Cancer Res* 55: 6045–6052

24   Dang LC, Talanian RV, Banach D, Hackett MC, Gilmore JL, Hays SJ, Mankovich JA, Brady KD (1996) Preparation of an autolysis-resistant interleukin-1β converting enzyme mutant. *Biochemistry* 35: 14910–14916

25   Talanian RV, Dang LC, Ferenz CR, Hackett MC, Mankovich JA, Welch JP, Wong WW,

Brady KD (1996) Stability and oligomeric equilibria of refolded interleukin-1β converting enzyme. *J Biol Chem* 271: 21853–21858

26 Talanian RV, Quinlan C, Trautz S, Hackett MC, Mankovich JA, Banach D, Ghayur T, Brady KD, Wong WW (1997) Substrate specificities of caspase family proteases. *J Biol Chem* 272: 9677–9682

27 Thornberry NA, Rano TA, Peterson EP, Rasper DM, Timkey T, Garcia-Calvo M, Houtzager VM, Nordstrom PA, Roy S, Vaillancourt JP et al (1997) A combinatorial approach defines specificities of members of the caspase family and granzyme B. *J Biol Chem* 272: 17907–17911

28 Talanian RV, Yang X, Turbov J, Seth P, Ghayur T, Casiano CA, Orth K, Froelich CJ (1997) Granule-mediated cell killing: Pathways for granzyme B-initiated apoptosis. *J Exp Med* 186: 1323–1331

29 Chou K-C, Jones D, Heinrikson RL (1997) Prediction of the tertiary structure and substrate binding site of caspase-8. *FEBS Lett* 419: 49–54

30 Mullican MD, Lauffer DJ, Gillespie RJ, Matharu SS, Kay D, Porritt GM, Evans PL, Golec JMC, Murcko MA, Luong YP et al (1994) The synthesis and evaluation of peptidyl aspartyl aldehydes as inhibitors of ICE. *Bioorgan Med Chem Lett* 4: 2359–2364

31 Dolle RE, Hoyer D, Rinker JM, Ross TM, Schmidt SJ, Helaszek C, Ator MA (1997) 3-Chloro-4-carboxamido-6-arylpyridazines as a non-peptide class of interleukin-1β converting enzyme inhibitor. *Bioorg Med Chem Lett* 7: 1003–1006

32 Rishton RM (1997) Reactive compounds and *in vitro* false positives in HTS. *Drug Disc Today* 2: 382–384

33 Ator MA, Dolle RE (1995) Interleukin-1β converting enzyme: Biology and the chemistry of inhibitors. *Curr Pharm Des* 1: 191–210

34 Livingston DJ (1997) *In vitro* and *in vivo* studies of ICE inhibitors. *J Cell Biochem* 64: 19–26

35 Chapman KT (1992) Synthesis of a potent, reversible inhibitor of interleukin-1β converting enzyme. *Bioorg Med Chem Lett* 2: 613–618

36 Graybill TL, Dolle RE, Helaszek CT, Miller RE, Ator MA (1994) Preparation and evaluation of peptidic aspartyl hemiacetals as reversible inhibitors of interleukin-1β converting enzyme (ICE). *Int J Pept Protein Res* 44: 173–182

37 Mjalli AMM, Chapman KT, MacCoss M, Thornberry NA (1993) Phenylalkyl ketones as potent reversible inhibitors of interleukin-1β converting enzyme. *Bioorg Med Chem Lett* 3: 2689–2692

38 Mjalli AMM, Chapman KT, MacCoss M, Thornberry NA, Peterson EP (1994) Activated ketones as potent reversible inhibitors of interleukin-1β converting enzyme. *Bioorg Med Chem Lett* 4: 1965–1968

39 Dolle RE, Hoyer D, Prasad CVC, Schmidt SJ, Helaszek CT, Miller RE, Ator MA (1994) P1 aspartate-based peptide α-((2,6-dichlorobenzoyl)oxy)methyl ketones as potent time-dependent inhibitors of interleukin-1β-converting enzyme. *J Med Chem* 37: 563–564

40 Prasad CVC, Prouty CP, Hoyer D, Ross TM, Salvino JM, Awad M, Graybill TL, Schmidt SJ, Osifo IK, Dolle RE et al (1995) Structural and stereochemical requirements

of time-dependent inactivators of the interleukin-1β converting enzyme. *Bioorg Med Chem Lett* 5: 315–318

41   Mjalli AMM, Zhao JJ, Chapman KT, Thornberry NA, Peterson EP, MacCoss M, Kagmann WK (1995) Inhibition of interleukin-1β converting enzyme by N-acyl-aspartyl aryloxymethyl ketones. *Bioorg Med Chem Lett* 5: 1409–1414

42   Dolle RE, Singh J, Whipple D, Osifo IK, Speier G, Graybill TL, Gregory JS, Harris AL, Helaszek CT, Miller RE et al (1995) Aspartyl α-((diphenylphosphinyl)oxy)methyl ketones as novel inhibitors of interleukin-1β converting enzyme. Utility of the diphenylphosphinic acid leaving group for the inhibition of cysteine proteases. *J Med Chem* 38: 220–222

43   Graybill TL, Prouty CP, Speier GJ, Hoyer D, Dolle RE, Helaszek CT, Ator MA, Uhl J, Strasters J (1997) α-((Tetronoyl)oxy)- and α-((tetramoyl)oxy)methyl ketone inhibitors of the interleukin-1β converting enzyme (ICE). *Bioorg Med Chem Lett* 7: 41–46

44   Dolle RE, Singh J, Rinker J, Hoyer D, Prasad CV, Graybill TL, Salvino JM, Helaszek CT, Miller RE, Ator MA (1994) Aspartyl α-((1-phenyl-3-(trifluoromethyl)-pyrazol-5-yl)oxy)methyl ketones as interleukin-1β converting enzyme inhibitors. Significance of the P1 and P3 amido nitrogens for enzyme-peptide inhibitor binding. *J Med Chem* 37: 3863–3866

45   Karanewsky D, Bai X (1998) C-terminal modified (N-substituted)-2-indolyl dipeptides as inhibitors of the ICE/ced-3 family of cysteine proteases. Patent WO9811129

46   Fritz L, Tomaselli K (1998) Inhibition of apoptosis using interleukin-1β converting enzyme (ICE)/CED-3 family inhibitors. Patent WO9810778

47   Kazuyuki O, Makoto T, Tohru M, Hiroyuki O (1997) Peptidic tetrazole compounds having interleukin-1β converting enzyme inhibitory activity. Patent EP761680

48   Albrecht HP, Allen HJ, Brady KD, Harter WG, Kostlan CR, Roth BD, Walker N (1998) Sulfonamide interleukin-1β converting enzyme inhibitors. Patent WO9816505

49   Albrecht HP, Allen HJ, Brady KD, Caprathe BW, Gilmore JL, Harter WG, Hays SJ, Kostlan CR, Lunney EA, Para KS et al (1998) Preparation of aspartate ester inhibitors of interleukin-1β converting enzyme. Patent WO9816502

50   Brady KD (1998) Bimodal inhibition of caspase-1 by aryloxymethyl and acyloxymethyl ketones. *Biochemistry* 37: 8508–8515

51   Dolle RE, Prouty CP, Prasad CV, Cook E, Saha A, Ross TM, Salvino JM, Helaszek CT, Ator MA (1996) First examples of peptidomimetic inhibitors of interleukin-1β converting enzyme. *J Med Chem* 39: 2438–2440

52   Semple G, Ashworth DM, Baker GR, Batt AR, Baxter AJ, Benzies DWM, Elliot LH, Evans DM, Franklin RJ, Hudson P et al (1997) Pyridone-based peptidomimetic inhibitors of interleukin-1β-converting enzyme (ICE). *Bioorg Med Chem Lett* 7: 1337–1342

53   Golec JMC, Mullican MD, Murcko MA, Wilson KP, Kay DP, Jones SD, Murdoch R, Bemis GW, Raybuck SA, Luong Y-P et al (1997) Structure-based design of non-peptidic pyridone aldehydes as inhibitors of interleukin-1β converting enzyme. *Bioorgan Med Chem Lett* 7: 2181–2186

54 Dolle RE, Prasad CVC, Prouty CP, Salvino JM, Awad MMA, Schmidt SJ, Hoyer D, Ross TM, Graybill TL, Speier GJ et al (1997) Pyridazinodiazepines as a high-affinity, P_2–P_3 peptidomimetic class of interleukin-1β-converting enzyme inhibitor. *J Med Chem* 40: 1941–1946

55 Golec JMC, Lauffer DJ, Livingston DJ, Mullican MD, Murcko MA, Nyce PL, Robidoux ALC, Wannamaker MW (1998) Inhibitors of interleukin-1β converting enzyme. Patent WO9824805

Elastase inhibitors

William A. Metz and Norton P. Peet

Hoechst Marion Roussel, Inc., Route 202–206, P.O. Box 6800, Bridgewater, NJ 08807-0800, USA

Introduction

Polymorphonuclear leukocyte elastase or neutrophil elastase (EC 3.4.21.37), herein referred to as elastase, is the name collectively given to endogenous proteinases which are capable of hydrolyzing and thus degrading a variety of structural matrix proteins, among them elastin. Elastin is an insoluble protein responsible for the elastic properties of mammalian connective tissue and organs. Elastin is an extremely hydrophobic protein which is not a substrate for most other proteinases. In mammalian physiology, elastase is necessary to provide homeostasis for tissue repair and normal degradation of damaged tissue. It is regulated by endogenous inhibitors or antiproteinases. When the balance of elastase and endogenous inhibitor is upset, as during an acute inflammatory response, the balance must be restored by the endogenous inhibitors or excess elastase will perpetuate the destruction of healthy elastic fibers. This unopposed excess is believed to play a major role in the development of many inflammatory diseases and contributes to the progression through the chronic obstructive pulmonary disease (COPD) continuum.

Most research to this end is based on the hypothesis that supplementation of the endogenous elastase inhibitor with an exogenous inhibitor would help restore the normal balance between endogenous inhibitor and elastase and thus serve as a therapy for such chronic diseases. Although it is now known that the elastase-antielastase hypothesis is oversimplified, it has still spurred a flurry of research activity in this area over the last decade. There are many factors involved in tissue degradation and it is still unclear which cells and proteinases are actually involved in the pathogenesis of tissue destruction in inflammatory diseases such as emphysema. Nevertheless, the design and development of elastase inhibitors as therapeutic agents, whether broad spectrum or selective inhibitors, is a formidable challenge in drug discovery and has shown promise for the treatment of inflammatory diseases in the COPD continuum.

On this note it is the authors' intent to provide a recent survey of the research which has been reported over the last several years with regard to elastase inhib-

High Throughput Screening for Novel Anti-Inflammatories, edited by M. Kahn
© 2000 Birkhäuser Verlag Basel/Switzerland

49

itors. It is not within the scope of this review to be all-inclusive or to go into specific detail on the biological aspects of various diseases and numerous proteinases suspected to be involved. Since both human neutrophils and macrophages contain a large number of proteolytic enzymes which aid in the defense mechanism during an inflammatory response, these enzymes will only be mentioned relative to elastase. A vast amount of research has been directed toward the synthesis of small molecule inhibitors of elastase. Therefore, this chapter will reflect mostly on that work with mention of some of the work reported on natural or recombinant proteinaceous inhibitors. Included is a survey of the recent literature on the relatively new areas of combinatorial chemistry and matrix metalloproteinases and the effect this pioneering research may have on the direction of future research for new designs and targets of elastase inhibitors.

Elastase and inflammatory diseases

Elastase is one of the most abundant destructive enzymes in the body and is a key component of the inflammatory response system. Stored in the azurophil granules of the neutrophil, it is one of many proteolytic enzymes that is released to combat invading foreign bodies during inflammation [1, 3]. Elastase is most commonly associated with inflammatory diseases of the lung, since neutrophils are immediately recruited to the lung in an immune response to bacterial and viral infections. Elastase assists neutrophils in their migration to the site of inflammation, and participates in the degradation of invading microorganisms [2] and the digestion of bacterial proteins [3] in a process called phagocytosis. In addition, extracellular elastase is involved in tissue remodeling which initiates the wound healing process [4]. This process, call elastolysis, appears to target elastin [5] which is the primary elastic component of the lungs, blood vessels and other organs [6].

During chronic inflammation the balance between human neutrophil elastase (HNE) and the endogenous inhibitor α_1-proteinase inhibitor (α_1-PI) can be shifted in favor of HNE and lead to the uncontrolled destruction of connective tissue [7]. This indiscriminant destruction of extracellular matrix proteins [8] has been observed mostly in chronic inflammatory diseases of the lung [9], although elastase is believed to play a role in the pathogenesis of acute and chronic diseases of the skin [10] and joints [11] (rheumatoid arthritis). Neutrophil elastase has been shown to degrade fibronectin [12], laminin [13], collagen [14] and proteoglycans [15].

Over 30 years have past since experimental and clinical evidence revealed that the causative factor in emphysema was the destruction of elastic fibers by elastase [16, 17]. Since then it has been determined that a mutation in the α_1-PI gene impairs the secretion and circulation of endogenous proteinase inhibitor, which allows neutrophil elastase to act unopposed and cause tissue destruction and emphysema [18].

Currently, one treatment for this type of emphysema is infusion with partially puri-fied human plasma α_1-PI on a routine basis. Maintenance of the serum level of this endogenous elastase inhibitor within normal limits has been shown to protect the lung tissue from HNE infiltration [19]. More common cases of emphysema are non-genetic and are induced by pulmonary inflammation as the result of smoking. Although a direct link between HNE and the pathogenesis of this more common form of emphysema is still uncertain, it is still hypothesized that HNE is involved. Smokers demonstrate normal levels of α_1-PI but it is believed that cigarette smoke decreases the protective effect of α_1-PI and also secretory leukocyte proteinase (SLPI), which protects the upper respiratory airways, by oxidative inactivation of these endogenous inhibitors. Oxidative damage combined with an increased num-ber of neutrophils, which delivers elastase to the lung recruited by cigarette smoke, may promote protein degradation.

Matrix metalloelastase (MME), which exists in macrophages, has recently been implicated in emphysema since most smokers have a ten-fold increase in the num-ber of macrophages. Since macrophages are the most abundant defense cell in the lung, both under normal conditions and especially during chronic inflammation, it is plausible that macrophages have the capacity to degrade elastin and contribute to the pathogenesis of emphysema. Although this conclusion is still somewhat contro-versial, research is being reported that suggests a causative role for macrophage matrix metalloproteinase (MME) in COPD.

Elevated levels of elastase in the lung have also been attributed to lung destruc-tion associated with cystic fibrosis (CF) [20], acute respiratory distress syndrome (ARDS) [21], and bronchitis [22]. Cystic fibrosis is derived from a mutated gene which results in dysfunction of a chloride channel membrane in the exocrine glands [23]. Bacterial infection usually ensues, which promotes neutrophil infiltration into the lung as the inflammatory response. A vast amount of HNE is released into the extracellular matrix protein which leads to progressive tissue damage. Treatment of CF presently involves a combination of antibiotics and aerosol application of α_1-PI to counter excess HNE infiltration. These diseases demonstrate the destructive nature of elastase that has made inhibitors of elastase attractive therapeutic targets.

Neutrophil elastase

Human neutrophils contain many proteolytic enyzmes that respond to inflamma-tion. HNE has received the most attention in the literature due to its abundance in the cell and its broad specificity. HNE, sometimes referred to as human leukocyte elastase (HLE), is a serine proteinase whose primary role appears to be the hydrol-ysis of proteins that are taken up by the neutrophil during phagocytosis. Its ability to digest bacterial proteins and its broad specificity make it a popular target for the design of synthetic inhibitors. Elastase may also have an extracellular function in

Table 1 - Human proteinases that possess elastinolytic activity

Proteinase (pH 7.5)	Cell source	Catalytic class	Elastolytic capacity
Elastase	Neutrophil	Serine	100%
Cathepsin G	Neutrophil	Serine	20%
Proteinase 3	Neutrophil	Serine	40%
Collagenase	Neutrophil	Metalloproteinase	30%
Gelatinase (92 kDa)	Neutrophil, Macrophage	Metalloproteinase	30%
Metalloelastase	Macrophage	Metalloproteinase	35%
Cathepsin B, L, S	Macrophage	Cysteine	80%
			(L inactive at pH 7.5)

neutrophil migration that may be regulated by circulating plasma and tissue local-ized endogenous inhibitors. Both neutrophils and macrophages contain a variety of proteinases that are capable of degrading elastin (see Tab. 1).

Catalytic mechanism of neutrophil elastase

Neutrophil elastase, as with all mammalian serine proteinases, interacts with the scissile amide bond of a protein substrate by a charge transfer mechanism to form a tetrahedral intermediate. This intermediate is formed with the catalytic triad residues of histidine 57, aspartic acid 102 and serine 195 (Scheme 1) and as a result, cleavage of the substrate occurs in a reversible manner. Initiation of hydrolysis begins when the hydroxyl group of the serine 195 residue of the enzyme is close enough to the carbonyl functionality of the peptide bond of the substrate to be cleaved. This is followed by migration of the hydroxyl proton to the histidine 57 residue. The resulting oxyanion attacks the carbonyl functionality of the substrate to form a tetrahedral intermediate and the new oxyanion is stabilized by interaction with the amide groups of serine 195 and glycine 193. The tetrahedral intermediate then decays to give an amine product, leaving behind the acylated enzyme. Hydra-tion of the acyl enzyme then forms a second tetrahedral intermediate that decom-poses to regenerate active enzyme.

Interaction of the amino acid residues on the substrate (e.g. P2, P1, P1', P2') with specific subsites of the enzyme (S2, S1, S1', S2') make up the extended binding region. The amino acids extending toward the N-terminus of the substrate are P1, P2, P3, etc., and those extending to the C-terminus, from the scissile amide bond, are P1', P2', P3', etc. The substrate sidechains interact with specific subsites of the

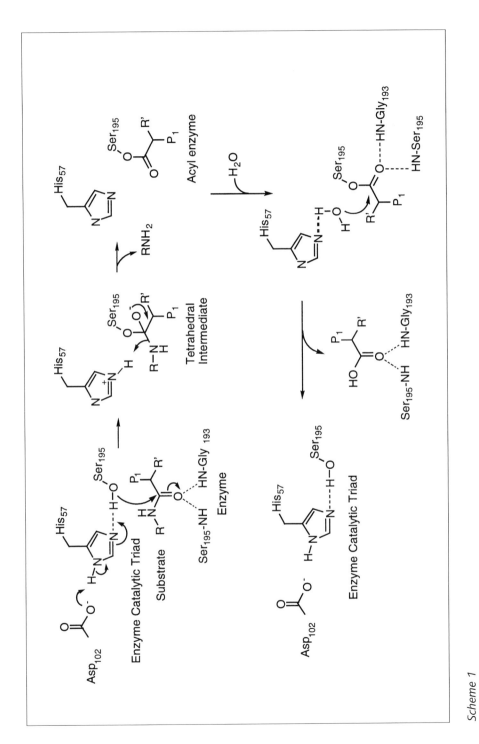

Scheme 1
Mechanism of hydrolysis by serine proteinases.

Table 2 - Natural inhibitors of elastase

Inhibitor	Source	Mol. Wt. (kDa)	P1-P1' (active site)
α_1-PI	Human	52	methionine-serine
SLPI	Human	12	leucine-methionine
Elafin	Human	6	alanine-methionine
Eglin c	Leech	8	leucine-aspartic acid
EIM	Human	42	cysteine-methionine

proteinase [24]. These subsites generally consist of several amino acid residues. In most cases, this model is used in the design of many small molecule peptide [25–27] and non-peptide inhibitors [28–31].

Proteinaceous inhibitors of elastase

An intense research effort over the last two decades has been directed towards developing inhibitors to supplement the natural ability to inhibit elastase, e.g. to provide a balance between the proteinase and the endogenous proteinase inhibitors. One approach has been to administer endogenous inhibitors with high molecular weight polypeptide inhibitors isolated from plant or animals, although the most clinically successful inhibitors have been isolated from human plasma or are recombinant human proteins [32]. Proteinaceous inhibitors such as α_1-pro-teinase inhibitor (α_1-PI) [33], eglin c [34], secretory leukocyte proteinase inhibitor (SLPI) [35] or elafin [36] are natural inhibitors that have site-specific inhibitory activity (see Tab. 2). Some of these inhibitors have been isolated or prepared by recombinant technology and have been formulated into drugs for aerosol or intra-venous administration [37].

α_1-Proteinase inhibitor (α_1-PI)

The best known of the natural inhibitors is α_1-proteinase inhibitor (α_1-PI). α_1-PI, also known as α_1-antitrypsin (α_1-AT), is a 52 kDa glycopeptide made up of 394 amino acid residues. The bulk of α_1-PI is produced in the liver and its major physi-ological target is HNE. It is one of many serine proteinase inhibitors that provides most of the antielastinolytic protection in the lower respiratory airways. It infiltrates tissue, complexes with HNE and is cleared through the circulatory system. α_1-PI deficient patients, whether through an inherited deficiency [38] or as a consequence of smoking [39], were found to develop emphysema. The inactivation of α_1-PI, the main plasma inhibitor of HNE [40], by cigarette smoke is a major cause of emphysema and has been implicated in other respiratory tract diseases [41]. Cigarette smoke is believed to oxidize the methionine residue at position P1 of α_1-PI which decreases the rate of inhibition of HNE. It is known that α_1-PI binds tightly to HNE and the inhibitor is cleaved at the methionine-serine scissile amide bond to give inactive inhibitor.

α_1-PI has been cloned and the recombinant protein [42] is one of several marketed endogenous inhibitors of HNE (prolastin; Miles Pharmaceuticals) for patients with α_1-PI genetic deficiency. Although the recombinant protein differs from the native protein in that it is nonglycosylated [43], elastase inhibitory properties are not impaired. Therapy using partially purified plasma α_1-PI has also been shown to be effective for genetically deficient patients and provides protection from HNE infiltration into the lungs [44].

Secretory leukocyte proteinase inhibitor (SLPI)

Secretory leukocyte proteinase inhibitor (SLPI) is a single polypeptide, 12 kDa endogenous reversible inhibitor of HNE, cathepsin G, trypsin and α-chymotrypsin [45]. It is a 107-amino acid residue peptide with N-terminal and C-terminal domains stabilized with four disulfide bonds. The disulfide bridges render the molecule resistant to denaturation. SLPI is found in all mucous secretions, it inhibits a broad range of serine proteinases and is a major endogenous inhibitor of HNE. It forms a reversible complex with HNE by which the inhibitor dissociates uncleaved. It is less tightly bound to HNE and therefore less effective than α_1-PI in inhibiting HNE. The cleavage site (P1-P1') is leucine-methionine and is located in the C-terminal domain [46]. As with α_1-PI, the methionine residue at P1' is easily oxidized to render the inhibitor inactive.

SLPI is suspected to play a role in attenuating elastase activity in upper respiratory tract diseases [41] and could be useful for supplemental treatment in patients with these disorders. The recombinant form of SLPI is identical to the native form and provides an abundant source of inhibitor for therapy. Tests in animal models have shown significant protection against HNE-induced emphysema [47] and aerosol application of recombinant SLPI in sufficient amounts reduces HNE levels significantly in the lungs of cystic fibrosis patients [48]. SLPI (Synergen) is in Phase II clinical trials for cystic fibrosis.

Elafin

Elafin is a low molecular weight (6 kDa) inhibitor of elastase that is isolated from human skin of psoriasis patients [49] and has also been found in human sputum [50]. It is a polypeptide composed of 57 amino acids and is a substrate-like reversible inhibitor of HNE [51]. It appears to be specific for elastases. Elafin has a 38% homology to the key amino acids of SLPI in the region of P1' to P6' of the cleavage site. The positions of all eight cysteines are identical to the C-terminal domain of SLPI and form analogous disulfide bridges, suggesting similar tertiary structure. The cleavage site is alanine-methionine and the methionine residue is prone to oxidation, which leads to loss of inhibitory activity. Elafin is the only human protein to have a relationship to SLPI. Although the precise biological function of elafin is uncertain, it appears to have a role in the regulation of neutrophil-dependent tissue destruction in cutaneous inflammation [52].

Eglin c

Eglin c, which is isolated from leeches (*Hirudo medicinalis*), is a potent, reversible inhibitor of HNE. Consisting of a single polypeptide chain of 70 amino acids [34] and having a molecular weight of 8 kDa, eglin c is unlike elafin and SLPI in that it has no sulfur-containing amino acids and is resistant to denaturation. The cleavage site is leucine-aspartic acid [53]. Eglin c complexes with HNE in a noncovalent manner and is a reversible inhibitor [54]. Recombinant eglin c is identical to the native inhibitor and is effective in preventing HNE-induced lung damage in pretreated hamsters [55]. However, in dogs eglin c elicited a severe allergic response which culminated in anaphylaxis. This clearly precludes its use as a clinical agent for humans and demonstrates the disadvantage of using protein inhibitors isolated from a non-human source for therapy.

Enzyme inhibitor of monocytes (EIM)

Enzyme inhibitor of monocytes (EIM) is a 42 kDa endogenous inhibitor of HNE that is found in human monocytes, neutrophils and macrophages [56]. It is composed of a single polypeptide chain of 379 amino acid residues [57] and has a 30% homology with α_1-PI. The cleavage site is cysteine-methionine that leaves it susceptible to oxidation and nucleophilic cleavage. Therefore, it is presumed to have the same mechanism of action as α_1-PI.

Factors regulating the activity, properties, and selectivity of the proteinase inhibitors have recently been reviewed [58].

Synthetic inhibitors of elastase

Small molecule synthetic inhibitors of elastase are an alternative to naturally occurring polypeptide, proteinaceous inhibitors for attenuating the effects of elastase. Synthetic inhibitors can be designed to provide better selectivity and bioavailability. Many potent synthetic inhibitors have been reported that have K_i values in the nanomolar range and have demonstrated oral activity. For this discussion we will focus on mechanism-based inhibitors of elastase. These inhibitors will be classified

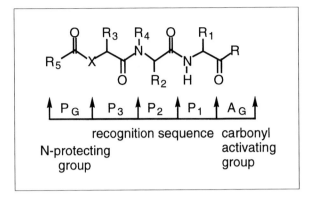

Figure 1
Recognition sequence of substrate-based inhibitors.

as either reversible or irreversible inhibitors. They belong to several chemical classes of compounds that will be briefly described with representative examples. These include peptidic electrophilic ketones, acylating and alkylating agents, heterocyclic and nonheterocyclic inhibitors and those of unknown mechanism.

Reversible inhibitors

There is a fine distinction between inhibitors that are reversible and those that are irreversible. Sometimes a class of inhibitor may be described as reversible but the covalent adduct is so stable that the inhibitor is functionally irreversible. Therefore, for this discussion when an inhibitor is described as reversible, both active inhibitor and enzyme can be regenerated.

Substrate-based electrophilic ketones are comprised mostly of short peptide sequences that contain an electrophilic carbonyl functionality. The design is centered around a known recognition sequence, as shown in Figure 1, which interacts with the N-terminal extended binding region of HNE. Initial studies focused on small substrate inhibitors of porcine pancreatic elastase (PPE) and HNE [59].

For the most part, substrate-based electrophilic ketone inhibitors are reversible inhibitors. Although the peptide sequence is necessary for affinity, the mechanistic basis for inhibition is usually due to the predisposition of the inhibitor to interact with the catalytic functionality of the enzyme (Fig. 2). Computer generated models of enzyme-inhibitor complexes have been built using X-ray crystal structure coordinates of HNE or PPE, which has a 40% homology with HNE. These models have been used successfully to predict structure-activity relationships based on the enzyme recognition sequence. One of the earliest crystal structures reported for a peptide inhibitor-enzyme complex was that of methoxysuccinyl-Ala-Ala-Pro-Val-

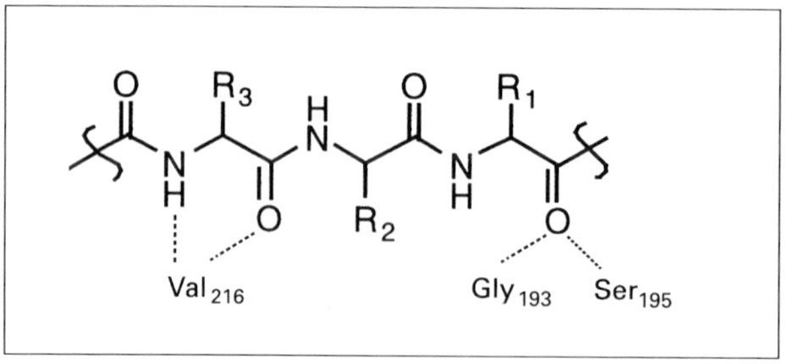

Figure 2
Hydrogen bonding between substrate-based inhibitor and HNE.

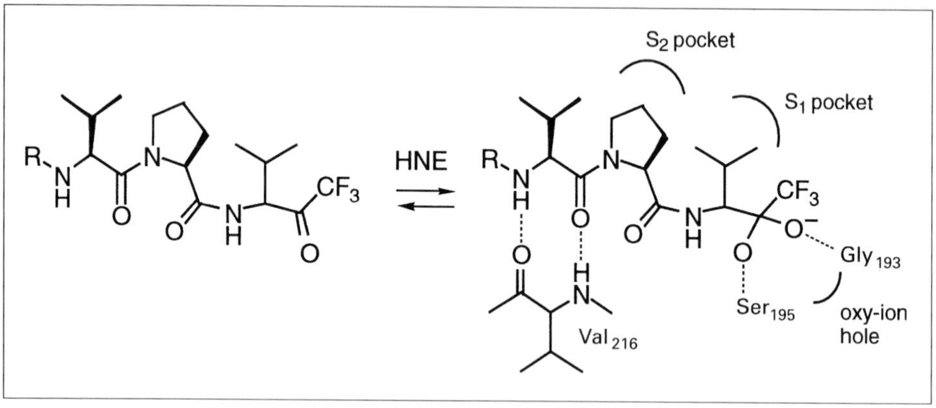

Scheme 2
Mechanism of enzyme inactivation by substrate-based electrophilic ketones.

CH_2Cl and HNE [60, 61]. This structure complex has served as a model for structure-based design of many other inhibitors.

The electrophilic ketones described below are perfluoro ketone inhibitors of HNE. They form a stable, non-hydrolyzable covalent adduct at the electrophilic carbonyl with the serine 195 hydroxyl group in the active site of the enzyme which is a tetrahedral intermediate. Other binding interactions, based on PPE X-ray crystal structure data and modeling experiments, suggest that these inhibitors may also hydrogen bond with valine 216, and the inhibitor alkoxide oxygen is hydrogen bound in the oxy-anion hole to the NH groups of glycine 193 and serine 195. The key design feature is incorporation of a ketone-activating group that can withdraw electron density from the ketone. This allows for formation of a tetrahedral intermediate with the enzyme and stablizes the hemiketal intermediate (Scheme 2).

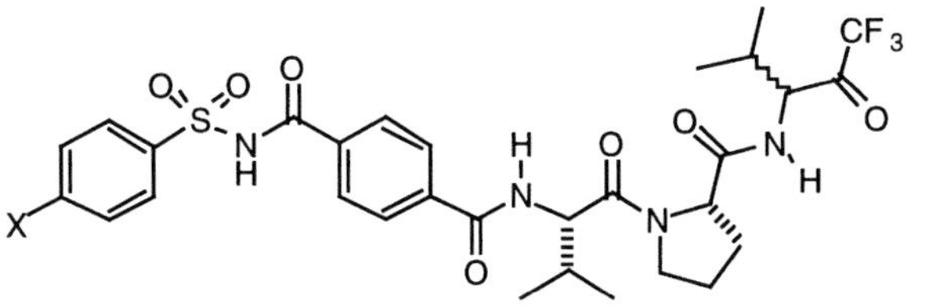

1 X = Cl, K_i = 0.5 nM
X = Br, K_i = 0.6 nM

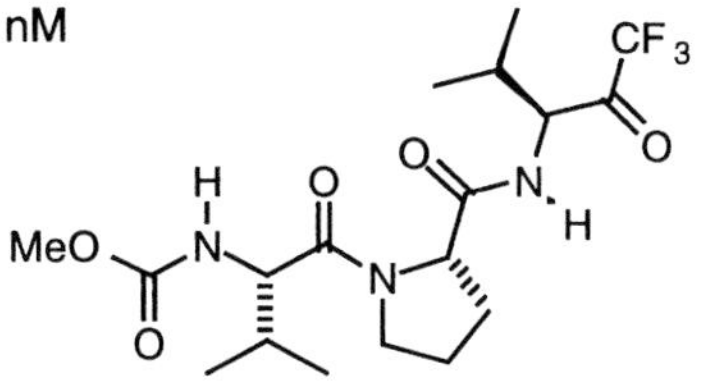

2 K_i = 13 nM

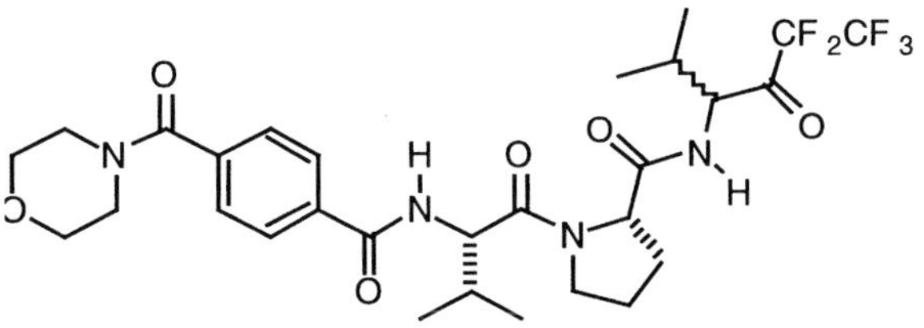

3a K_i = 20 nM

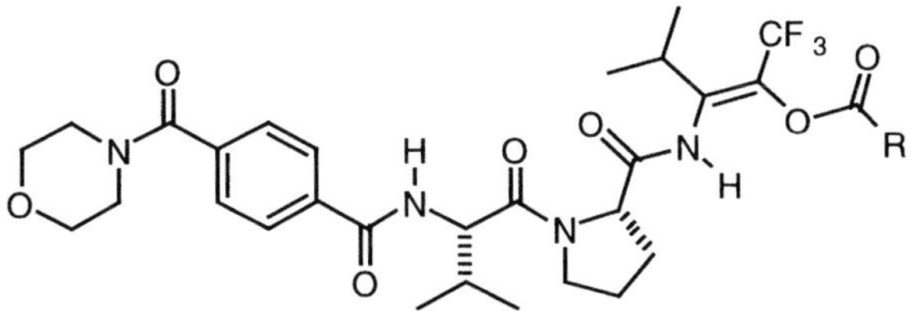

3b R = CH$_3$, CH$_2$CH$_3$, CH(CH$_3$)$_2$

Mechanistically, this is reversible inhibition, since retro-addition provides the inhibitor and the active enzyme. Inhibitors **1–6** fall into this chemical class.

Inhibitors **1** and **2** are compounds designed by Zeneca researchers [62]. Compound **1** is the Zeneca prototype (K_i = 0.5 nM) which possesses an N-terminal protecting group designed specifically to provide a longer half-life but was found not to be orally active. Compound **2** was synthesized in stereochemically pure form, demonstrates good binding activity (K_i = 13 nM) and has good oral availability

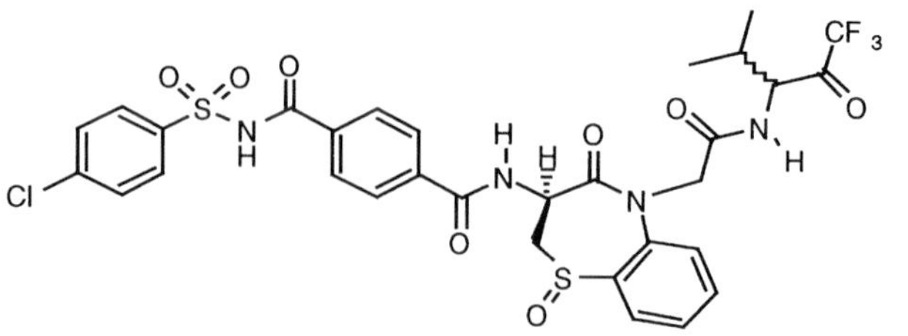

4 $K_i = 6.8$ nM

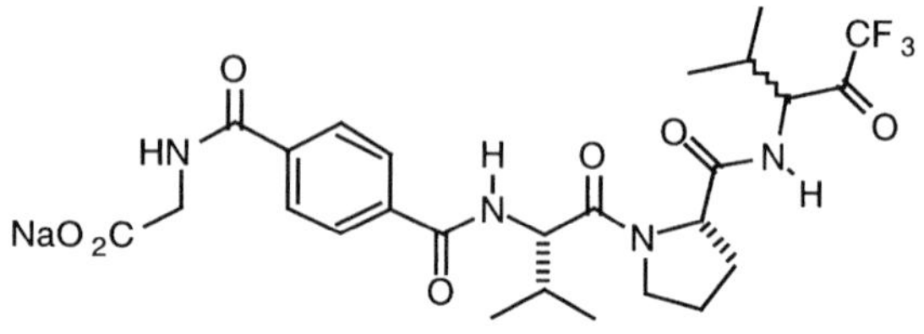

5 $K_i = 4.2$ nM

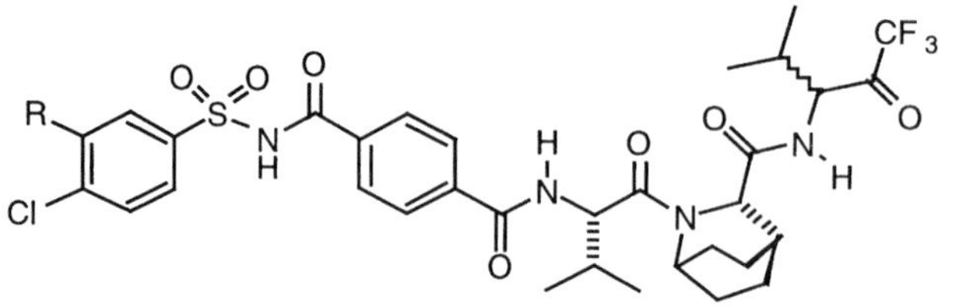

6a R = H, $K_i = 15$ nM

6b, R = HO—⟨ ⟩—SCH$_2$CONHSO$_2$—

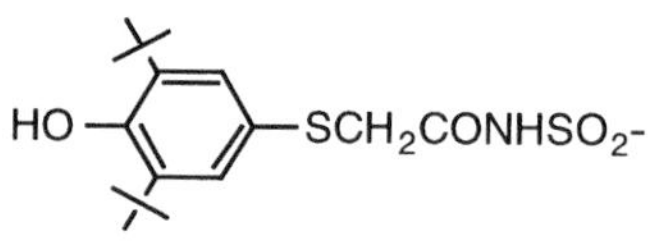

($ED_{50} = 2$ mg/kg). Inhibitors **3a** and **3b** are from the Marion Merrell Dow laboratories [63]. Although **3a** is a racemic mixture at P1, the pentafluoroethyl ketone moiety imparts good binding activity ($K_i = 20$ nM) and oral availability. It is speculated that the pentafluoroethyl ketone has a lower capacity for hydration, which gives it an advantage over the trifluoromethyl ketones with respect to oral activity. The α-keto ester enol acetate **3b** was designed as a prodrug to simplify the parent drug by eliminating the diastereomeric center. Cleavage of these prodrugs with esterase efficiently converts them to the parent pentafluoroethyl ketones. A group at

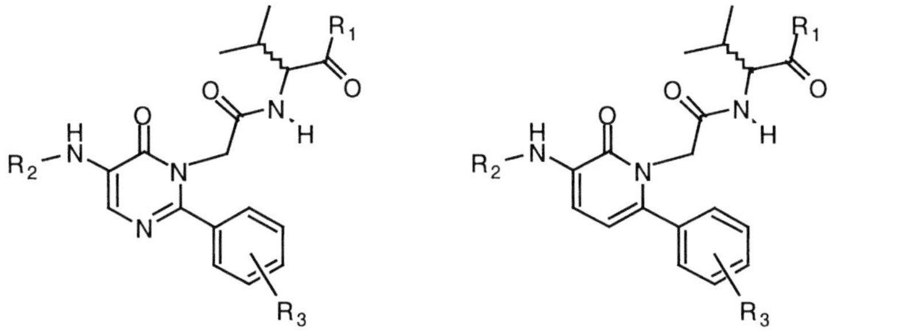

7a R = CF$_3$, R$_2$ = H, R$_3$ = 4-F   **8a** R = CF$_3$, R$_2$ = Cbz, R$_3$ = H
7b R = B(OH)$_2$ **8b** R = B(OH)$_2$

Boehringer Ingelheim has published a series of inhibitors in which the P2–P3 residues have incorporated a restricted lactam as a dipeptide replacement [64]. Lactam sulfoxide 4 is reported to be a 6.8 nM inhibitor of HNE. Fujisawa inhibitor 5 (K$_i$ = 4.2 nM) [65] is a water-soluble inhibitor of HNE with a slow-binding inhibition. It can therefore be administered either intratracheally or intravenously. Inhibitor 6a (IC$_{50}$ = 15 nM) [66] is a trifluoromethyl ketone inhibitor that substitutes the central proline residue of the valine-proline-valine tripeptide portion with an azabicyclo[2.2.2]octane. Modification of the lipophilic N-terminal side chain, previously designed into Zeneca's compound 1 and Boehinger's compound 4, with a di-tertiarybutylphenol ring, imparts antioxidant properties to the molecule. This inhibitor was found to inhibit lipid peroxidation while maintaining HNE inhibition. It was suggested that this added feature could be relevant in order to gain *in vivo* potency in a chronic model of lung injury.

Workers at Zeneca have described a series of inhibitors (7 and 8) wherein the P2-proline and P3-valine residues of the typical tripeptide sequence are replaced by a heterocycle. The heterocycle contains a hydrogen bond donor and acceptor that interacts with valine 216 of elastase. Pyrimidinone 7a is reported to have good oral activity with an ED$_{50}$ of 7.5 mg/kg [28b].

Replacement of the trifluoromethyl group with boronic acid enhanced the *in vitro* potency [28b, 31a]. In this case the boron atom covalently bonds to serine 195 with the tetrahedral geometry forming about the boron atom. Both pyrimidinone 7b and pyridinone 8b are reported to have a very high affinity for elastase with some analogs having K$_i$ values of less than 1.0 nM. However, they lack the oral activity of their trifluoromethyl ketone counterparts. It has also been observed that these boronic acid inhibitors actually advance the progression of elastase-induced emphysema in animal models. It is proposed that this may occur via the migration of boronate-complexed HNE to an environment free of an effective concentration of

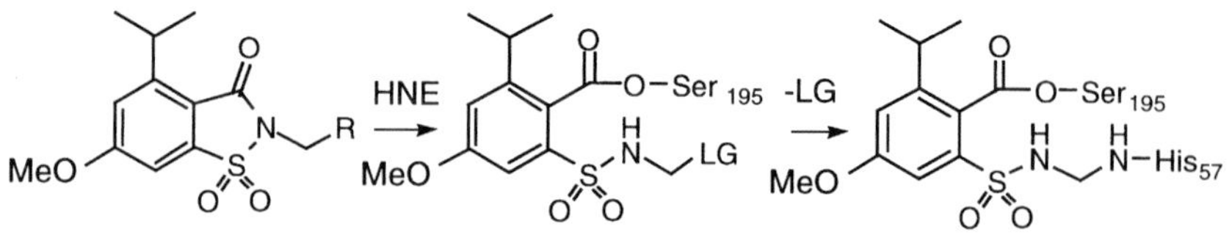

Scheme 3
Hydrolysis of acyl-enzyme complex

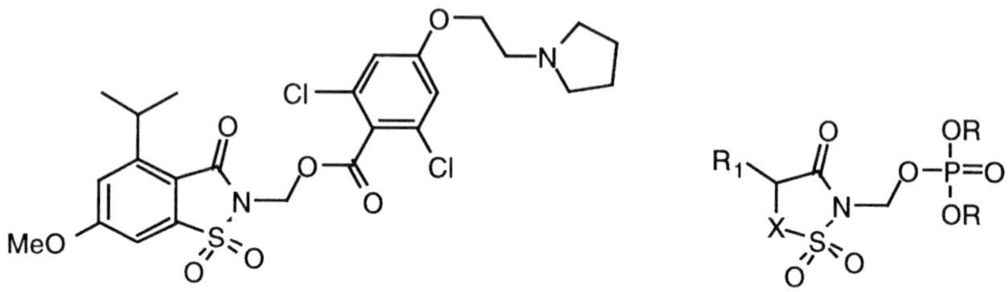

9   **10**

inhibitor. Once there, the inhibitor-enzyme complex may dissociate to release active elastase. Therefore, it is unlikely that these inhibitors will advance to clinical trials.

Among the many types of HNE inhibitors described in the literature, the tripeptide perfluoro ketones remain one of the most promising series of small molecule, orally active elastase inhibitors.

Irreversible inhibitors

The majority of acylating and alkylating agents interact irreversibly with HNE. They form a covalent bond with either the serine 195 or histidine 57 of the enzyme or both, and the adducts are converted to an inactive form of the inhibitor and enzyme. Irreversible inhibitors are generally more difficult to develop into a viable therapeutic agent because of selectivity issues.

Benzoisothiazolones 9 [67] and 10 [68] activate HNE by the mechanism shown in Scheme 3. The catalytic site serine hydroxyl group opens the isothiazolone ring by attack at the carbonyl center to form the acyl-enzyme intermediate. The leaving group tethered to the sulfonamide functionality is then displaced by the histidine 57 residue that inactivates the enzyme. The enzyme-inhibitor complex undergoes decomposition slowly to regenerate the active enzyme. Inhibitor **9** was reported by researchers at Sterling Winthrop and has an ED_{50} value of 1 to 3 mg/kg. A series of phosphonate derivatives of thiadiazolidinones (X = NR_2) and isothiazolidinone (X = CH_2) **10**, were designed [68] based on the observation [67b] that both potency and selectivity could be optimized by incorporating a phosphonate leaving group.

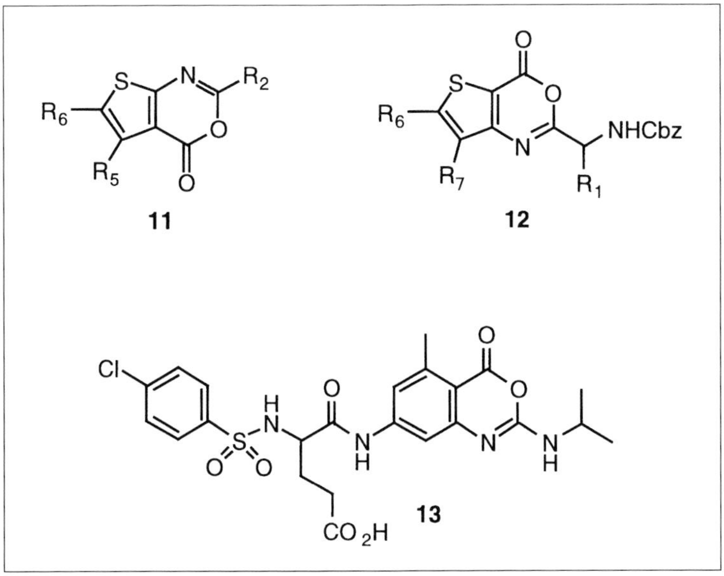

Thienooxazinones **11** and **12** have also been described as inhibitors which acylate elastase [69, 70]. Compound **12**, a proteinase inhibitor designed by SmithKline Beecham for inhibition of herpes proteinases, was found to be effective against HNE. These heterocyclic inhibitors usually interact with the serine 195 of the enzyme in such a manner that the heterocyclic ring is opened in the course of binding covalently to the enzyme. 3,1-Benzoxazin-4-one **13** and thienooxazinones **11** and **12** are irreversible inhibitors. Although benzoxazinones are known to have serine proteinase activity, modification at the 7-position was observed to increase the hydrolytic stability of the molecule and improve inhibitory activity. Inhibitor **13**, reported by a group at the Teijin Institute [71], incorporated an amino acid side chain at the 7-position which improved the HNE binding activity (K_i = 7 nM).

The mechanism by which cephalosporins and other β-lactams inhibit HNE is still uncertain. It is known that for cephalosporin-derived elastase inhibitors **14**, there are several key features that seem to be essential for activity. The oxidation state of the sulfur at the C-5 position, an electron withdrawing substituent at the C-7 position (R) and a good leaving group at the 3' position (R_3) are all important structural features. In most cases it was found that sulfones were more active inhibitors than sulfides or sulfoxides [72]. This may be due to the electronegative sulfone that is believed to enhance the electrophilicity of the lactam carbonyl group much the same way as an electron withdrawing group does at C-7. The increased electron withdrawl by the sulfone activates the lactam carbonyl toward nucleophilic addition by serine 195. Usually a carboxylic acid exists at the C-2 position (R_2) which is derivatized to optimize elastase inhibition.

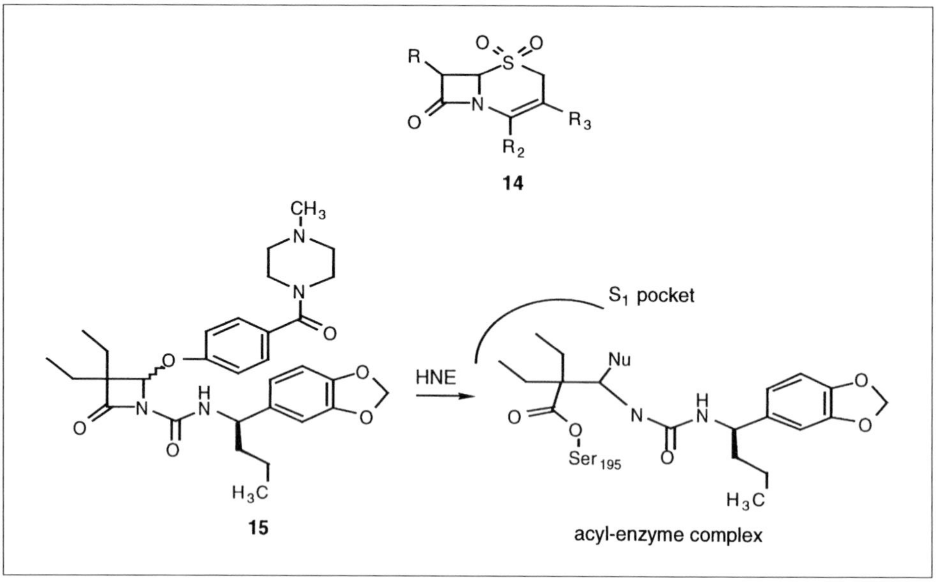

A series of monocyclic β-lactams were developed by researchers at Merck [73], based on earlier work with cephalosporins. The Merck group found that azetidinones were weak inhibitors of HNE and that the activity could be enhanced by varying the leaving group at the C-4 position of the lactam ring. Inhibitor 15 is currently being developed. Both inhibitors 14 and 15 are acylating agents and are irreversible inhibitors of elastase.

There is at least one case where cephalosporin-based elastase inhibitors showed optimum inhibitory activity with sulfur at the sulfide oxidation state. A series of 7-alkylidene-cephalosporin esters 16 were described [74] that were found to be potent, irreversible inhibitors of HNE. They are presumed to dock at the active site of HNE with the alkylidene substituent in the S1 pocket. Subsequent formation of the acyl-enzyme complex is followed by isomerization of the alkylidene double bond as shown in Scheme 4.

Some isocoumarin elastase inhibitors are also believed to form either an acyl-enzyme complex with the serine 195 of the enzyme or undergo double covalent bond formation with serine 195 and histidine 57 of the enzyme as shown in Scheme 5. In this dual attachment mechanism the electrophilic carbonyl group undergoes

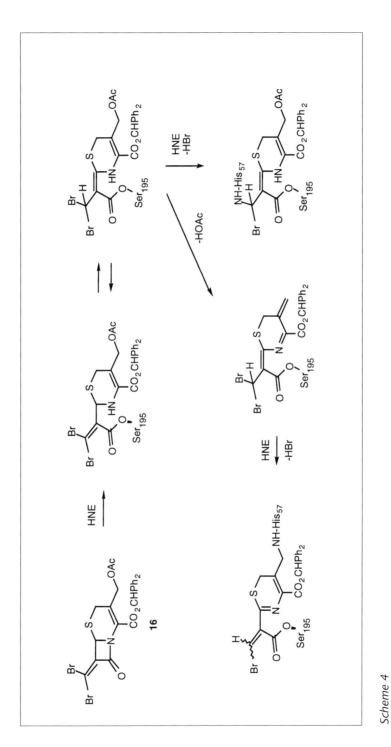

Scheme 4
*The proposed mechanism of inhibition for **16**.*

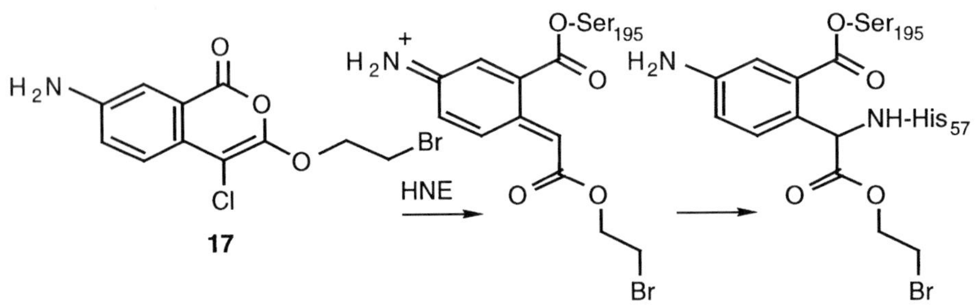

Scheme 5
Double-linked isocoumarin inhibitor.

nucleophilic addition by the the active site serine hydroxyl group to form the acyl enzyme that then undergoes a second reaction to generate a reactive intermediate that reacts further with the histidine of the active site [75]. The x-ray crystal structure was solved with **17** complexed with PPE which comfirmed this binding mode [76].

As mentioned, most β-lactams are irreversible enzyme inhibitors. There is at least one example of reversible acylation of elastase by γ-lactam inhibitors [77]. Researchers at Oxford and Zeneca found that unlike β-lactam inhibitors, which irreversibly interact to form a stable acyl-enzyme complex, monocyclic γ-lactams bind via reversible formation of a hydrolytically labile acyl-enzyme complex. This interaction is believed to occur by the mechanism illustrated in Scheme 6.

Researchers at Glaxo Wellcome recently reported a series of pyrrolidine *trans-γ*-lactams and *trans-γ*-lactones [78]. The lactams are observed to be more stable than the lactones to aqueous acid and bases, and human plasma half-lives of the lactams are much longer than those of the lactones. This suggests that the lactams are metabolically more stable than the lactones, but there is no mention of a reversible, labile acyl-enzyme mechanism. Inhibition appears to be effectively irreversible since reactivation of the enzyme occurs over a period of days.

Use of combinatorial methods to synthesize small molecule inhibitors

The rapid identification of prospective novel synthetic targets for biological evaluation is of paramount importance in the increasingly competitive arena of pharmaceutical research. Combinatorial chemistry, a term coined to describe a means of

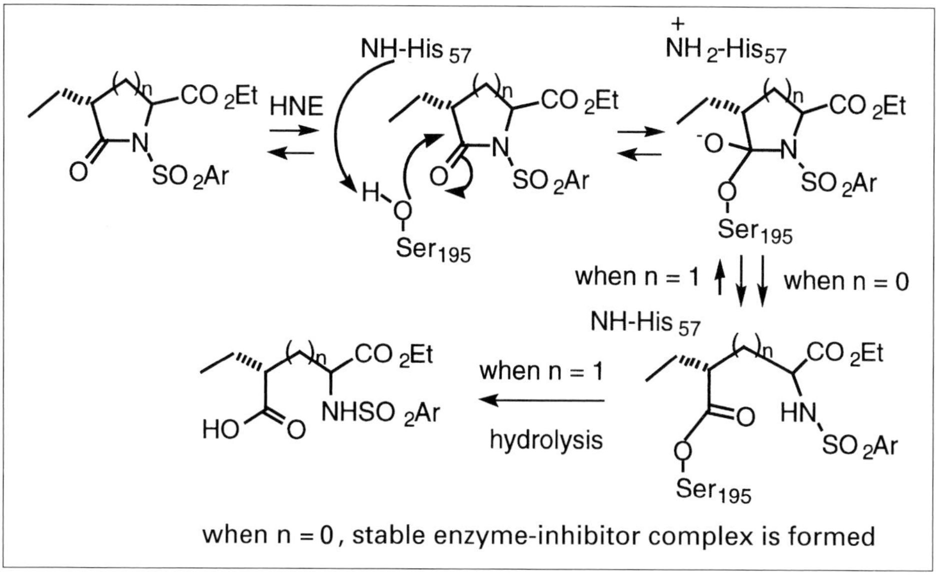

Scheme 6

rapidly creating a varied array of novel new compounds, whether it be by solid phase organic synthesis (SPOS), solution phase synthesis in parallel or liquid phase combinatorial synthesis (LPCS), has come of age as a powerful tool to fulfill this need. Combinatorial strategies have become increasingly important in generating collections of diverse chemical libraries of small organic molecules which serve as a valuble source of future new drugs [79].

In this section we review a few representatve examples from published research whereby a combinatorial method has been developed to create a rational, directed or pharmacophore-based library of potential elastase inhibitors. When applicable, solid phase syntheses of drug-like substances offers a significant advantage over conventional syntheses. It is a highly efficient method to produce a large number of compounds, either as mixtures or in parallel, which can be manipulated by split pool methods and released from resin in high purity to provide small amounts of compound.

Benzoxazoles have been shown to be small molecule inhibitors of elastase [80] and are therefore attractive targets for optimization using combinatorial methods. A recent report describes the synthesis of this structure type on solid phase support in a limited library format [81]. Wang resin was modified with an acid-labile carbamate linker [82] and treated with different diamines to provide amino-functionalized resin. Subsequent treatment with dicarboxylic anhydrides afforded carboxy-funtionalized resin **18** (Scheme 7). 4-Substituted-2-aminophenols were then coupled

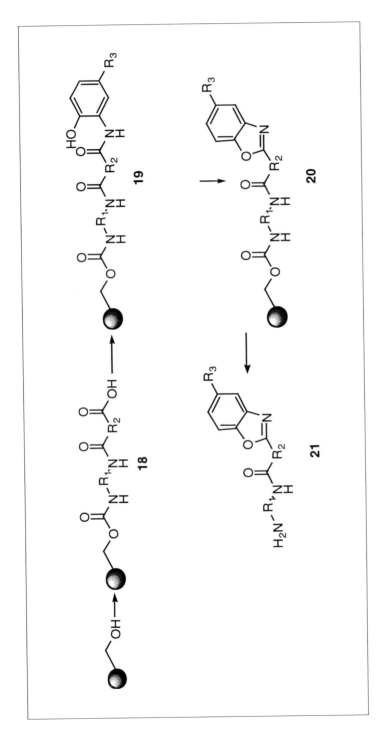

Scheme 7

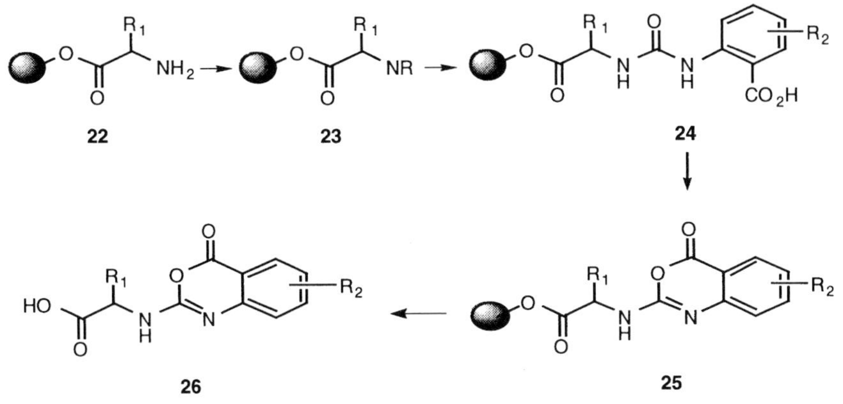

Scheme 8

to the resin-bound linker, using standard coupling methods, to provide the desired amide **19** with none of the ester observed. Intermolecular cyclization was then performed using Mitsunobu conditions to give the bound benzoxazole **20**. Upon release with TFA, high yields of pure benzoxazole **21** were obtained.

An efficient solid phase synthesis of 3,1-benzoxazine-4-ones was also performed on Wang support, functionalized with an amino acid-linked urea [83]. The benoxazine-4-one scaffold is a proven pharmacophore for the synthesis of elastase inhibitors with *in vivo* activity [84]. These HNE acylating agents were prepared from an immobilized isocyanate or activated carbamate **23** that was generated from the resin-based amino acid **22** on Wang resin. Intermediate **23** was then treated with substituted anthranilic acids to afford functionalized ortho-carboxyphenyl urea derivative **24**, which was easily cyclized under mild conditions to the benzoxazine-4-one **25** with diisopropylcarbodiimide (DIC). This intramolecular acylation proceeds regioselectively at the urea oxygen and none of the intramolecular N-acylation product is observed. Cleavage with TFA afforded the desired benzoxazine-4-one **26** (Scheme 8).

The development of solution phase synthetic methodologies for preparing an array of small molecules in a library format [85] is another tool in the chemist's arsenal of useful synthetic methods. A small chemical library biased as proteinase inhibitors was created based on the benzoxazinone scaffold using solution phase parallel synthesis [86]. This 5-step solution-phase synthesis was unique in that it used resin-based scavengers for trapping excess reagents and by-products to simplify purification of all intermediates and final products. An earlier report described a complementary molecular reactivity and molecular recognition (CMR/R) sequester-

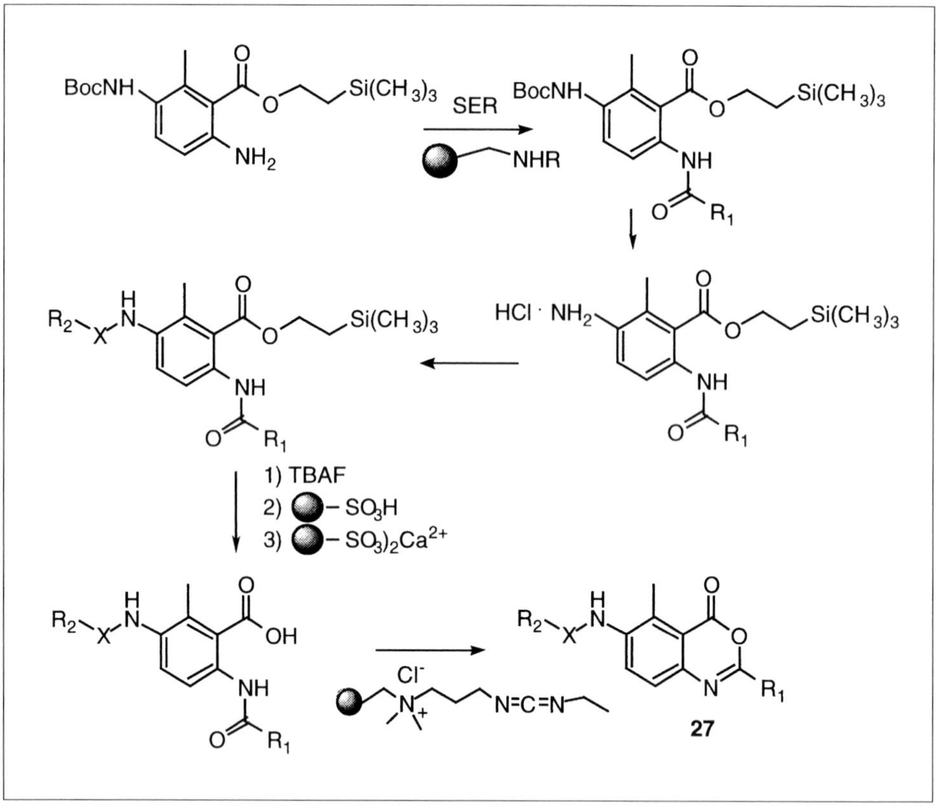

Scheme 9

ing resin and a sequestering-enabling-reagent (SER), which allowed simple filtration for purification [87]. The library synthesized by these methods was adapted for high-throughput production using automation. The reactions were performed in a reaction block with a 6X8 array in 48 reaction chambers, each having a 9-mL capacity. The 5-step reaction sequence is shown in Scheme 9.

The last step in the synthesis is the formation of the benzoxazinone ring. Since the benzoxazinone is susceptible to nucleophilic attack, an amine CMR/R resin was used to scavenge the acid-containing impurities. Good to excellent yields and purity were obtained for each step (82–99%) and an overall 60% yield of **27** was obtained.

Another illustration of the use of solution phase combinatorial synthesis is the synthesis [88] of a moncyclic β-lactam library using the Ugi reaction [89]. The authors describe a combinatorial approach to generate a library using a multi-component condensation reaction to efficiently generate a diverse array of monocyclic

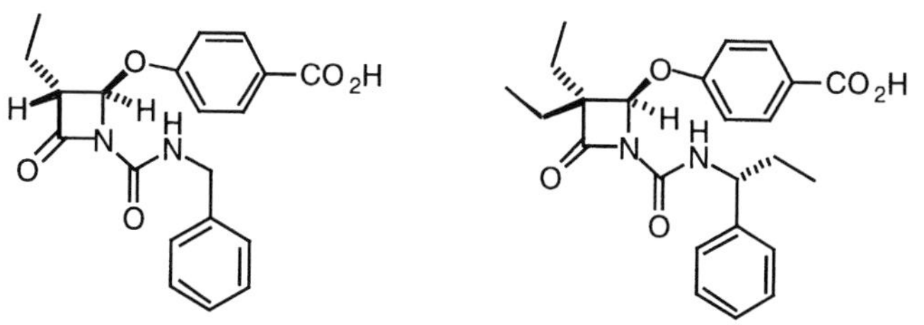

28   **29**

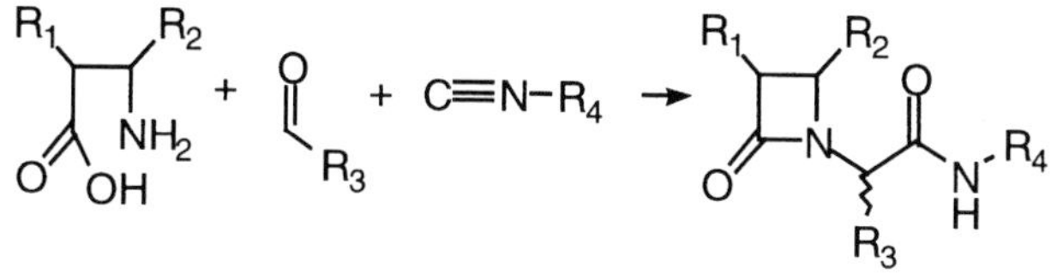

30

Scheme 10

β-lactams related to structures **28** and **29**. These inhibitors were reported by Merck researchers [90] and found to be potent inhibitors of HNE.

The urea backbone of the Merck inhibitor was replaced with a peptide-like backbone which possessed similar hydrogen bonding characteristics but facilitated the combinatorial approach. Using the Ugi reaction for combining β-amino acids, aldehydes, and isocyanides, the oligopeptide-like backbone and β-lactam scaffold were created in one step as illustrated in Scheme 10.

Twenty diverse compounds of type **30** were prepared in varying purity and yields to be evaluated for HNE activity.

Lastly, a recent article describes a homologation protocol to prepare an aromatic 16-mer as a scaffold for the synthesis of oligomers found to be potent inhibitors of HNE [91]. A functionalized diphenylmethane building block (Fig. 3) [92] was prepared for extending the aromatic scaffold, which allowed for selective derivatization. By this means, various functional groups could be incorporated in a variety of spatial configurations.

Selective activation of the corresponding *ortho*-positions of the aromatic rings was accomplished by unmasking individual phenol groups, making them vulnerable

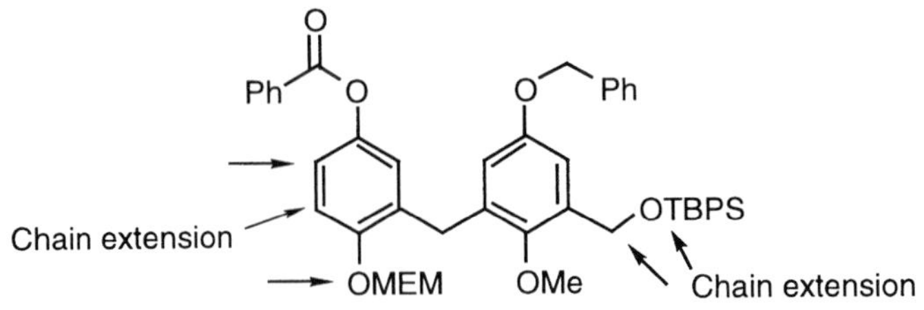

Figure 3

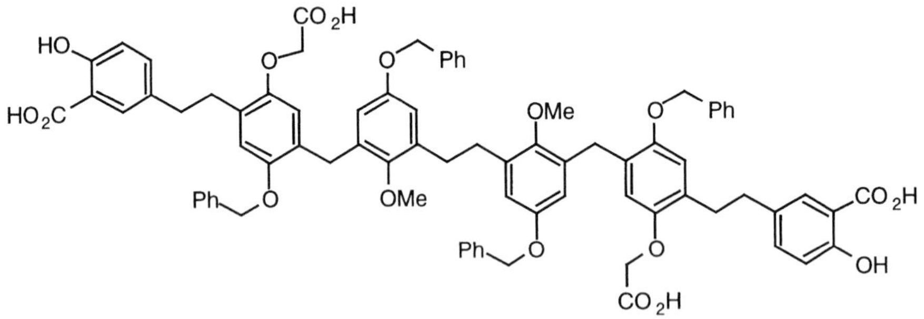

Figure 4

to electrophilic attack by a halogen. The benzylic silyl ether allows for a solid support if desired or chain extension for higher order oligomers. Functional group manipulation using direct alkylation, Mitsunobu etherfication and transition metal-mediated carbon-carbon bond formation strategies provide access to a variety of multifunctional molecules of the structure type shown in Figure 4.

Using this approach, libraries were designed for screening to provide compounds that were used for molecular recognition. The amount of chemical information built into this type of structure could provide information on the interaction of the many functional groups present in a varied spacial array with the enzyme. Thus, increased molecular size is used to raise the information content of the molecule. The hexamer in Figure 4 was found to be a potent inhibitor of HNE with a K_i value of 18 nM. Little is known about the mechanism of action or any other biological interactions.

Future outlook

Matrix metalloproteinases (MMPs) are a family of structurally related enzymes that differ from serine proteinases in that they utilize zinc at the catalytic site for activity. They are involved in the normal turnover and maintenance of extracellular matrix (ECM) proteins in connective tissue and basement membranes such as elastin [93]. ECM degradation is necessary for normal tissue remodeling and repair associated with development. During inflammation and injury the amount of MMP production increases, presumably to repair damaged extracellular matrix [94]. If there is abnormal up-regulation, excessive MMP production is associated with a variety of diseases characterized by tissue destruction. There are currently fourteen MMPs which have been identified and found to be uniquely genetically encoded. All of the MMPs, except for MMP-11 (stromolysin-3), are stored as inactive proenzymes (proMMPs) that are activated extracellularly through an initial cleavage by the action of proteinases such as neutrophil elastase. Therefore, their activation and catalytic activity is an important step in the exploration of up-regulation of MMP activity [95].

While the role of MMPs in the normal pathological turnover of tissues and membranes is not completely understood, their proteolytic activity is known to be regulated by endogenous tissue inhibitors of metalloproteinases (TIMPS) [96]. Disruption in this regulation leads to overproduction of MMPs and degradation of the matrix and connective tissue damage. As a consequence, MMPs have been implicated in several diseases [97], and therefore inhibition of MMPs is a significant strategy in the development of novel therapeutic agents.

Recently, Shapiro and coworkers [98–104] reported a matrix metalloproteinase, identified as matrix metalloelastase (MME or MMP-12) [EC-3.4.24.65], which exists in macrophages. It is believed that this elastase can exert just as much destructive degradation of tissue as neutrophil elastase, but extracellurally. MMP-12 has been implicated in tissue destruction related to emphysema [105].

Although there have been no reports to date of synthetic inhibitors of matrix metalloelastase (MMP-12), a vast amount of work has been reported for the other matrix metalloproteinases (MMPs) and their inhibitors. Since MMPs are often co-expressed in many pathological conditions, inhibitors of MMPs could be useful for the treatment of a range of inflammatory disorders [106, 107]. We expect that a future research direction may focus on broad spectrum inhibitors of MMPs or possibly on a selective inhibitor of MMP-12 which may provide the next generation of elastase inhibitors.

In summary, the use of HNE inhibitors for the treatment of pulmonary diseases is still being investigated. Proteinaceous inhibitors are presently being used as replacement therapy in patients with emphysema and cystic fibrosis. The efficacy of this treatment is still uncertain. A number of orally active, small molecule HNE inhibitors are in clinical trails. While none of these inhibitors has progressed beyond the clinic, their therapeutic potential could be enormous for the treatment of pulmonary diseases.

References

1   Dewald B, Rindler-Ludwig R, Bretz U, Baggiolini M (1975) Subcellular localization and heterogeneity of neutral proteases in neutrophilic polymorphonuclear leukocytes. *J Exp Med* 141: 709–723
2   Taylor JC, Mittman C (eds) (1987) *Pulmonary emphysema and proteolysis.* Academic Press, New York
3   Janoff A, Blondin J (1973) The effect of human granulocyte elastase on bacterial suspensions. *Lab Invest* 29: 454–457
4   a) Bieth JG (1986) Possible biological functions of protein proteinase inhibitors. In: V Turk (ed): *Cysteine proteinases and their inhibitors*, Proc. Int. Symp., 1st deGruyter, Berlin, 693–703
     b) Travis J, Salvesen GS (1983) Human plasma proteinase inhibitors. *Annu Rev Biochem* 52: 655–709
5   Janoff A, Scherer J (1968) Mediators of inflammation in leukocyte lysosomes. IX. Elastinolytic activity in granuales of human polymorphonuclear leukocytes. *J Exp Med* 128: 1137–1155
6   Sandberg LB, Gray WR, Franzblau C (eds) (1977) *Elastin and elastic tissue.* Plenum Press, New York
7   Hoidal JR, Niewoehner DE (1983) Pathogenesis of emphysema. *Chest* 83: 679–685
8   Henson PM, Henson JE, Kimani G, Bratton DL, Riches DWH (1988) Phagocytic cells: Degranulation and secretion. In: JL Gallin, IM Goldstein R Snyderman (eds): *Inflammation: Basic principles and clinical correlates.* Raven Press, New York, 363–380
9   a) Janoff A (1985) Elastases and emphysema. Current assessment of the protease-antiprotease hypothesis. *Am Rev Respir Dis* 132: 417–433
     b) Snider GL (1992) Emphysema: The first two centuries and beyond. A historical overview, with suggestions for future research: Part 2. *Am Rev Respir Dis* 146: 1615–1622
     c) Gadek JE (1992) Adverse effects of neutrophils on the lung. *Am J Med* 92: 27S–31S
10   a) Malech HL, Gallin JI (1987) Current concepts: Immunology. Neutrophils in human diseases. *N Eng J Med* 317: 687–694
     b) Henson PM, Johnson RB Jr (1987) Tissue injury in inflammation. Oxidants, proteinases, and cationic proteins. *J Clin Invest* 79: 669–674

11   a) Janusz MJ, Doherty NS (1991) Degradation of cartilage matrix proteoglycan by human neutrophils involves both elastase and cathepsin G. *J Immunol* 146: 3922–3928

b) Moore AR, Iwamura H, Larbre JP, Scott DL, Willoughby DA (1993) Cartilage degradation by polymorphonuclear leucocytes: *In vitro* assessment of the pathogenic mechanisms. *Ann Rheum Dis* 52: 27–31

c) Janusz MJ, Durham SL (1997) Inhibition of cartilage degradation in rat collagen-induced arthritis but not adjuvant arthritis by the neutrophil elastase inhibitor MDL 101,146. *Inflamm Res* 46: 503–508

d) Breedveld FC, Lafeber GJM, Siegert CEH, Vleeming LJ, Cats A (1987) Elastase and collagenase activities in synovial fluid of patients with arthritis. *J Rheumatol* 14: 1008–1012

12   a) McDonald JA, Kelly DG (1980) Degradation of fibronectin by human leukocyte elastase. Release of biologically active fragments. *J Biol Chem* 255: 8848–8858

b) McDonald JA, Baum BJ, Rosenberg DM, Kelman JA, Brin SC, Crystal RG (1979) Destruction of a major extracellular adhesive glycoprotein (fibronectin) of human fibroblasts by neutral proteases from polymorphonuclear leukocyte granules. *Lab Invest* 40: 350–357

13   Dal Nogare AR, Toews GB, Pierce AK (1987) Increased salivary elastase precedes gram-negative bacillary colonization in postoperative patients. *Am Rev Respir Dis* 135: 671–675

14   Kittelberger R, Neale TJ, Francky KT, Greenhill NS, Gibson GJ (1992) Cleavage of type VIII collagen by human neutrophil elastase. *Biochim Biophys Acta* 1139: 295–299

15   a) Janoff A, Blondin J (1970) Depletion of cartilage matrix by a neutral protease fraction of human leukocyte lysosomes. *Proc Soc Exp Biol Med* 135: 302–306

b) Gadek JE, Fells GA, Wright DG, Crystal RG (1980) Human neutrophil elastase function as a type III collagen "collagenase". *Biochem Biophys Res Commun* 98: 1815–1822

c) Starkey PM (1977) The effect of human neutrophil elastase and cathepsin G on the collagen of cartilage, tendon, and cornea. *Acta Biol Med* 36: 1549–1554

d) Mainardi CL, Dixit SN, Kang AH (1980) Degradation of type IV (basement membrane) collagen by a proteinase isolated from human polymorphonuclear leukocyte granules. *J Biol Chem* 225: 5435–5441

e) Janoff A (1985) Elastase in tissue injury. *Annu Rev Med* 36: 207–216

16   Gross P, Pfitzer E, Tolker E, Babyak M, Kaschak M (1965) Experimental emphysema: Its production with papain in normal and silicotic rats. *Arch Environ Health* 11: 50–58

17   Laurell CB, Ericksson S (1963) The electrophoretic alpha-globulin pattern of serum in alpha-antitrypsin deficiency. *Scand J Clin Invest* 15: 132–140

18   a) Eriksson S (1991) The potential role of elastase inhibitors in emphysema treatment. *Eur Respir J* 4: 1041–1043

b) Crystal RG, Brantly ML, Hubbard RC, Curiel DT, States DJ, Holmes MD (1989) The alpha 1-antitrypsin gene and its mutations. Clinical consequences and strategies for therapy. *Chest* 95: 196–208

c) Kuhn C, Senior RM (1975) The role of elastase in the development of emphysema. *Lung* 155: 185

d) Janoff A (1983) Biochemical links between cigarette smoking and pulmonary emphysema. *J Appl Physiol* 55: 285–293

19 Wewers MD, Casolaro MA, Crystal RG (1987) Comparison of alpha 1-antitrypsin levels and antineutrophil elastase capacity of blood and lung in a patient with the alpha 1-antitrypsin phenotype null-null before and during alpha 1-antitrypsin augmentation therapy. *Am Rev Respir Dis* 135: 539–543

20 a) Meyer KC, Lewandoski JR, Zimmerman JJ, Nunley D, Calhoun WJ, Dopico GA (1991) Human neutrophil elastase and elastase/alpha 1-antiprotease complex in cystic fibrosis. Comparison with interstitial lung disease and evaluation of the effects of intravenously administered antibiotic therapy. *Am Rev Respir Dis* 144: 580–585

b) Meyer KC, Zimmerman JJ (1993) Neutrophil mediators, Pseudomonas, and pulmonary dysfunction in cystic fibrosis. *J Lab Clin Med* 121: 654–661

c) Jackson AH, Hill SL, Afford SC, Stockley RA (1984) Sputum sol-phase proteins and elastase activity in patients with cystic fibrosis. *Eur J Respir Dis* 65: 114–124

21 a) Lee CT, Fein AM, Lippmann M, Holtzman H, Kimbel P, Weinbaum G (1981) Elastolytic activity in pulmonary lavage fluid from patients with adult respiratory-distress syndrome. *N Engl J Med* 304: 192–196

b) Merritt TA, Cochrane CG, Holcomb K, Bohl B, Hallman M, Strayer D, Edwards D, Gluck L (1983) Elastase and alpha 1-proteinase inhibitor activity in tracheal aspirates during respiratory distress syndrome. Role of inflammation in the pathogenesis of bronchopulmonary dysplasia. *J Clin Invest* 72: 656–666

c) Hyers TM, Fowler AA (1986) Adult respiratory distress syndrome: Causes, morbidity, and mortality. *Fed Proc Fed Am Soc Exp Biol* 45: 25–29

22 Stockley RA, Hill SL, Morrison H-M, Starkie CM (1984) Elastolytic activity of sputum and its relation to purulence and to lung function in patients with bronchiectasis. *Thorax* 39: 408–413

23 Boat TF, Welsh MJ, Beaudet AL (1989) Cystic fibrosis. In: CR Scriver, AL Beaudet, WS Sly, D Valle (eds): *The metabolic basis of inherited disease*. 6th ed McGraw-Hill, New York, 2649–2682

24 The P1, P2, P3 and S1 nomenclature has been described in: Schechter I, Berger A (1967) On the size of the active site of proteases. I. Papain. *Biochem Biophys Res Commun* 27: 157–162

25 a) Cregge RJ, Durham SL, Farr RA, Gallion SL, Hare CM, Hoffman RV, Janusz MJ, Kim HO, Koehl JR, Mehdi S et al (1998) Inhibition of human neutrophil elastase. 4. Design, synthesis, X-ray crystallographic analysis and structure-activity relationships for a series of P_2 modified, orally active peptidyl pentafluoroethyl ketones. *J Med Chem* 41: 2461–2480

b) Cregge RJ, Curran TT, Metz WA (1998) A convenient synthesis of peptidyl perfluoroalkyl ketones. *J Fluor Chem* 88: 71–77

26 a) Edwards PD, Anisik DW, Bryant CA, Ewing B, Gomes B, Lewis JJ, Rakiewicz D,

Steelman G, Strimpler A, Trainor DA et al (1997) Discovery and biological activity of orally active peptidyl trifluoromethyl ketone inhibitors of human neutrophil elastase. *J Med Chem* 40: 1876–1885

b) Edwards PD, Wolanin DJ, Anisik DW, Davis MW (1995) Peptidyl α-ketoheterocyclic inhibitors of human neutrophil elastase. 2. Effect of varying the heterocyclic ring on *in vitro* potency. *J Med Chem* 38: 76–85

c) Edwards PD, Meyer EF, Vijayalakshmi J, Tuthill PA, Andisik DA, Gomes B, Strimpler A (1992) Design, synthesis and kinetic evaluation of a unique class of elastase inhibitors, the peptidyl α-ketobenzoxazoles, and the X-ray crystal structure of the covalent complex between porcine pancreatic elastase and the Ac-Ala-Pro-Val-2-benzoxazole. *J Am Chem Soc* 114: 1854–1863

27 Williams JC, Falcone RC, Knee C, Stein RL, Strimpler AM, Reaves B, Giles RE, Krell RD (1991) Biologic characterization of ICI 200,880 and ICI 200,355, novel inhibitors of human neutrophil elastase. *Am Rev Respir Dis* 144: 875–883

28 a) Bernstein PR, Gomes BC, Kosmider BJ, Vavek EP, Williams JC (1995) Nonpeptidic inhibitors of human leukocyte elastase. 6. Design of a potent, intratracheally active, pyridone-based trifluoromethyl ketone (1995) *J Med Chem* 38: 212–215

b) Veale CA, Bernstein PR, Byrant C, Ceccarelli C, Damewood JR, Earley R, Feeney SW, Gomes B, Kosmider BJ, Steelman GB et al (1995) Non-peptidic inhibitors of human leukocyte elastase. 5. Design, synthesis and X-ray crystallography of a series of orally active 5-aminopyrimidin-6-one-containing trifluoromethyl ketones. *J Med Chem* 38: 98–108

c) Veale CA, Damewood JR, Steelman GB, Byrant C, Gomes B, Williams J (1995) Non-peptidic inhibitors of human leukocyte Elastase. 4. Design, synthesis and *in vitro* and *in vivo* activity of a series of b-carboline- containing trifluoromethyl ketones. *J Med Chem* 38: 86–97

d) Bernstein PR, Andisik D, Bradley PK, Bryant CB, Ceccarelli C, Damewood JR, Earley R, Edwards PD, Fenney S, Gomes, B et al (1994) Nonpeptidic inhibitors of human leukocyte elastase. 3. Design, synthesis, X-ray crystallographic analysis, and structure-activity relationships for a series of orally active 3-amino-6-phenylpyridin-2-one trifluoromethyl ketones. *J Med Chem* 37: 3313–3326

29 Groutas WC, Kuang R, Venkataraman R (1994) Substituted 3-oxo-1,2,5-thiadiazolidine 1,1-dioxides: A new class of potential mechanism-based inhibitors of human leukocyte elastase and cathepsin G. *Biochem and Biophys Res Comm* 198: 341–349

30 Player MR, Sowell JW, Patil GS, Kam CM, Powers JC (1994) 1,3-Oxazino-4,5-bindole-2,4-(1H, 9H)-diones and 5,6-dimethylpyrrolo2,3-d-1,3-oxazin-2,4-(1H, 7H)-diones as serine protease inhibitors. *Bioorg Med Chem Lett* 4: 949–954

31 For review of both peptide-based and non-peptidic inhibitors see:

a) Edwards PD, Bernstein PR (1994) Synthetic inhibitors of elastase. *Med Res Rev* 14: 127–194

b) Hlasta DJ, Pagani ED (1994) Human leukocyte elastase inhibitors. *Ann Rep Med Chem* 29: 195–204

32 a) Schrebli HP (1991) Recombinant elastase inhibitors for therapy. *Ann NY Acad Sci* 624: 212–218

b) Shinguh Y, Yamazaki A, Inamura N, Fujie K, Okamoto M, Nakahara K, Notsu Y, Okuhara M, Ono T (1998) Biochemical and pharmacological characteristics of FR134043, a novel elastase inhibitor. *Eur J Pharm* 345: 299–308

c) Yavin EJ, Fridkin M (1998) Peptides from human c-reactive protein inhibit the enzymatic activities of human leukocyte elastase and cathepsin G: Use of overlapping peptide sequences to identify a unique inhibitor. *Int J Pept Protein Res* 51: 282–289

d) Bingle L, Richards RJ, Fox B, Masek L, Guz A, Tetly TD (1997) Susceptibility of lung epithelium to neutrophil elastase-protection by native inhibitors. *Med Inflamm* 6: 345–354

e) Minagawa S, Ishida M, Shimakura K, Nagashima Y, Shiomi K (1997) Isolation and amino acid sequences of two Kunitz-type protease inhibitors from the sea anemone *Anthopleura aff. xanthogrammica*. *Comp Biochem Phys B Biochem Molec Bio* 118: 381–386

33 a) Crystal RG (1992) α_1-Antitrypsin augmentation therapy for chronic obstructive lung disorders. *Drugs of the Future* 17: 387–393

b) Travis J, Salvesen GS (1983) Human plasma proteinase inhibitors. *Ann Rev Biochem* 52: 655–709

34 a) Seemüller U, Meier M, Ohlsson, K, Müller H-P, Fritz H (1977) Isolation and characterization of low molecular weight inhibitor (of chymotrypsin and human granulocyte elastase and cathepsin G) from leeches. *Hoppe-Seyer's Z Physiol Chem* 358: 1105–1107

b) Baici A, Seemüller U (1984) Kinetics of the inhibition of human leukocyte elastase by eglin from the leech *Hirudo medicinalis*. *Biochem J* 218: 829–833

35 a) Gauthier F, Fryksmark U, Ohlsson K, Bieth JG (1982) Kinetics of the inhibition of leukocyte elastase by the bronchial inhibitor. *Biochim Biophys Acta* 700: 178–183

b) Rice WG, Weiss SJ (1990) Regulation of proteolysis at the neutrophil-substrate interface by secretory leukoprotease inhibitor. *Science* 249: 178–181

36 Wiedow O, Schröder J-H, Gregory H, Young JA, Christophers E (1990) Elafin: An elastase-specific inhibitor of human skin. *J Biol Chem* 265: 14791–14795

37 Rosenberg S, Barr PJ, Najarian RC, Hallewell RA (1984) Synthesis in yeast of a functional oxidation-resistant mutant of human alpha-antitrypsin. *Nature* 312: 77–80

38 a) Laurell CB, Eriksson S (1963) The electrophoretic a1-globulin pattern of serum in a1-antitrypsin deficiency. *Scand J Clin Lab Invest* 15: 132–140

b) Garver RI, Mornex JF, Nukiwa T, Brantly M, Courtney M, Lecocq JP, Crystal RG (1986) Alpha1-antitrypsin deficiency and emphysema caused by homozygous inheritance of non-expressing alpha1-antitrypsin genes. *New Engl J Med* 314: 762–766

39 Janus ED, Phillips NT, Carrell RW (1985) Smoking, lung function and α_1-antitrypsin deficiency. *Lancet* 152–154

40 Ohlsson K (1975) In: E Reich, E Shaw, E (eds): *Proteases and biological control*. Cold Spring Harbor Laboratory, New York, 591–612

41 Boudier C, Bieth JG (1989) Mucus proteinase inhibitor: A fast acting inhibitor of leukocyte elastase. *Biochim Biophys Acta* 995: 36–41

42 a) Rosenberg S, Barr PJ, Najarian R C, Hallewell, RA (1984) Synthesis in yeast of a functional oxidation-resistant mutant of human alpha-antitrypsin. *Nature* 312: 77–80
b) Courtney M, Buchwalder A, Tessier LH, Jaye M, Benavente A, Balland A, Kohli V, Lathe R, Tolstoshev P, Lecocq JP (1984) High level production of biologically active human alpha 1-antitrypsin in *Escherichia coli*. *Proc Natl Acad Sci USA* 81: 669–673

43 Travis J, Owen M, George P, Carrell R, Rosenberg S, Hallewell RA, Barr PJ (1985) Isolation and properties of recombinant DNA produced variants of human alpha 1-proteinase inhibitor. *J Biol Chem* 260: 4384–4389

44 a) Wewers MD, Casolaro MA, Sellers SE, Swayze SC, McPhaul KM, Wittes JT, Crystal RG (1987) Replacement therapy for alpha 1-antitrypsin deficiency associated with emphysema. *N Engl J Med* 316: 1055–1062
b) Hubbard RC, Sellers S, Czerski D, Stephens L, Crystal RG (1988) Biochemical efficiency of monthly augmentation therapy for alpha-1-antitrypsin deficiency. *JAMA* 260: 1259–1264

45 a) Sallenave JM, Har MS, Cox G, Chignard M, Gauldie J (1997) Secretory leukocyte proteinase inhibitor is a major leukocyte elastase inhibitor in human neutrophils. *J Leukocyte Biol* 61: 695–702
b) Boudier C, Bieth JG (1989) Mucus proteinase inhibitors: A fast acting inhibitor of leukocyte elastase. *Biochim Biophys Acta* 995: 36–41
c) Thompson RC, Ohlsson K (1986) Isolation, properties and complete amino acid sequence of human leukocyte proteases inhibitor, a potent inhibitor of leukocyte elastase. *Proc Natl Acad Sci USA* 83: 6692–6696

46 Grütter MG, Fendrich G, Huber R, Bode W (1988) The 2.5 Å X-ray crystal structure of the acid-stable proteinase inhibitor from human mucous secretions analyzed in its complex with bovine α-chymotrypsin. *EMBO J* 7: 345–351

47 Lucey EC, Stone PL, Ciccolella DE, Breuer R, Christensen TG, Thompson RC, Snider GL (1990) Recombinant human secretory leukocyte-protease inhibitor: *In vitro* properties, and amelioration of human neutrophil elastase-induced emphysema and secretory cell metaplasia in the hamster. *J Lab Clin Med* 115: 224–232

48 McElvaney NG, Donjaji B, Moan MJ, Burham MR, Wu MC, Crystal RG (1993) Pharmacokinetics of recombinant secretory leukoprotease inhibitor aerosolized to normals and individuals with cystic fibrosis. *Am Rev Respir Dis* 148: 1056–1060

49 a) Wiedow O, Schroeder JM, Gregory H, Young JA, Christophers E (1990) Elafin: An elastase-specific inhibitor of human skin. *J Biol Chem* 265: 14791–14795
b) Ying QL, Simon SR (1993) Kinetics of the inhibition of human leukocyte elastase by elafin, a 6-kilodalton elastase-specific inhibitor from human skin. *Biochemistry* 32: 1866–1874

50 Sallenave JM, Silva A, Marsden ME, Ryle AP (1993) Secretion of mucus protein inhibitor and elafin by Clara cell and type II pneumocyte cell lines. *Am J Respir Cell Mol Biol* 8: 126–133

51 a) Tsunemi M, Kato H, Nishiuchi Y, Kumagaye S, Sakakibara S (1993) Synthesis and structure-activity relationship of elafin, an elastase-specific inhibitor. *Biochem Biophys Res Commun* 185: 967–973

b) Ying QL, Simon SR (1993) Kinetics of the inhibition of human leukocyte elastase by elafin, a 6-kilodalton elastase-specific inhibitor from human skin. *Biochemistry* 32: 1866–1874

c) Francart C, Dauchez M, Alix AJP, Lippens G (1997) Solution structure of R-elafin, a specific inhibitor of elastase. *J Mol Biol* 268: 666–677

52 Alkemade HA, Molhuizen HO, van Vlijmen-Willems IM, van Haelst UJ, Schwalkwijk J (1993) Differential expression of SKALP/elafin in human epidermal tumors. *Am J Pathol* 146: 1679–1687

53 Knecht R, Seemüller U, Liersch M, Fritz H, Braun DG, Chang TJ (1983) Sequence determination of eglin c using combined microtechniques of amino acid analysis, peptide isolation and automated Edman degradation. *Anal Biochem* 130: 65–71

54 Hipler K, Priestle JP, Rahuel J, Grütter MG (1992) X-ray crystal structure of the serine proteinase inhibitor eglin c at 1.95 Å resolution. *FEBS Lett* 309: 139–145

55 Snider GL, Stone PJ, Lucey EC, Breuer R, Calore JD, Seshadri T, Catanese A, Maschler R, Schnebli HP (1985) Eglin c, a polypeptide derived from the medicinal leech, prevents human neutrophil elastase-induced emphysema and bronchial secretory cell metaplasia in the hamster. *Am Rev Respir Dis* 132: 1155–1161

56 Janoff A, Blondin J (1971) Further studies on an esterase inhibitor in human leukocyte cytosol. *Lab Invest* 25: 565–571

57 Remold-O'Donnell E, Chin J, Alberts M (1992) Sequence and molecular characterization of human monocyte/neutrophil elastase inhibitor. *Proc Natl Acad Sci USA* 89: 5635–5639

58 a) Farley D, Faller B, Nick H (1997) Therapeutic protein inhibitors of elastase. *Drugs Pharma Sci* 84: (Pharmaceutical Enzymes), 305–334

b) Bernstein PR, Edwards PD, Williams JC (1994) Inhibitors of human leukocyte elastase. *Prog Med Chem* 31: 59–120

59 a) Thompson RC, Blout ER (1973) Dependence of the kinetic parameters for elastase-catalyzed amide hydrolysis on the length of peptide substrates. *Biochemistry* 12: 57–65

b) Thompson RC, Blout ER (1973) Elastase-catalyzed amide hydrolysis of tri- and tetrapeptide amides. *Biochemistry* 12: 66–71

c) Nakajima K, Powers JC, Ashe BM, Zimmerman M (1979) Mapping the extended substrate binding site of cathepsin G and human leukocyte elastase. Studies with peptide substrates related to the alpha 1-protease inhibitor reactive site. *J Biol Chem* 254: 4027–4032

60 Navia M A, McKeever BM, Springer JP, Lin TY, William HR, Fluder EM, Dorn CP, Hoogsteen K (1989) Structure of human neutrophil elastase in complex with a peptide chloromethyl ketone inhibitor at 1.84-Å resolution. *Proc Nat Acad Sci USA* 86: 7–11

61 Wei AZ, Mayr I, Bode W (1988) The refined 2.3 Å crystal structure of human leukocyte elastase in a complex with a valine chloromethyl ketone inhibitor. *FEBS Lett* 234: 367–373

62   a) Edwards PD, Andisik DW, Bryant CA, Ewing B, Gomes B, Lewis JJ, Rakiewicz D, Steelman G, Strimpler A, Trainor DA et al (1997) Discovery and biological activity of orally active peptidyl trifluoromethyl ketone inhibitors of human neutrophil elastase. *J Med Chem* 40: 1876–1885

b) Veale CA, Bernstein PR, Bohnert CM, Brown FJ, Bryant C, Damewood JR, Earley R, Feeney SW, Edwards PD, Gomes B et al (1997) Orally active trifluoromethyl ketone inhibitors of human leukocyte elastase. *J Med Chem* 40: 3173–3181

63   a) Burkhart JP, Koehl JR, Mehdi S, Durham SL, Janusz MJ, Huber EW, Angelastro MR, Sunder S, Metz WA, Shum PW et al (1995) Inhibition of human neutrophil elastase. 3. An orally active enol acetate prodrug. *J Med Chem* 38: 223–233

b) Angelastro MR, Baugh LE, Bey P, Burkhart JP, Chen TM, Durham SL, Hare CM, Huber EW, Janusz MJ, Koehl JR et al (1994) Inhibition of human neutrophil elastase with peptidyl electrophilic ketones. 2. Orally active PG-val-pro-val pentafluoroethyl ketones. *J Med Chem* 37: 4538–4554

c) Durham SL, Hare CM, Angelastro MR, Burkhart JP, Koehl JR, Marquart AL, Mehdi S, Peet NP, Janusz MJ (1994) Pharmacology of N-4-(4-morpholinylcarbonyl)benzoyl-L-valyl-N-3,3,4,4-pentafluoro-1-(1-methylethyl)-2-oxobutyl-L-prolinamide (MDL 101,146); A potent orally active inhibitor of human neutrophil elastase. *J Pharmacol Exp Ther* 270: 185–191

d) Burkhart JP, Mehdi S, Koehl JR, Angelastro MR, Bey P, Peet, NP (1998) Preparation of alpha-keto ester enol acetates as potential prodrugs of human neutrophil elastase inhibitors. *Bioorg Med Chem Lett* 8: 63–64

64   Skiles JW, Sorcek R, Jacober S, Miao C, Mui PW, McNeil D, Rosenthal AS (1993) Elastase inhibitors containing lactams as P3-P2 dipeptide replacements. *Bioorg Med Chem Lett* 3: 773–778

65   Shinguh Y, Imai K, Yamazaki A, Inamura N, Shima I, Wakabayashi A, Higashi Y, Ono T (1997) Biochemical and pharmacological characterization of FK706, a novel elastase inhibitor. *Eur J Pharm* 337: 63–71

66   Portevin B, Lonchampt M, Canet E, Denanteuil G (1997) Dual inhibition of human leukocyte elastase and lipid peroxidation: *In vitro* and *in vivo* activities of azabicyclo2.2.2octane and perhydroindole derivatives. *J Med Chem* 40: 1906–1918

67   a) Hlasta DJ, Subramanyam C, Bell MR, Carabateas, PM, Court JJ, Desai, RC, Drozd, ML, Eickhoff WM, Freguson EW et al (1995) Orally bioavailable benzisothiazolone inhibitors of human leukocyte elastase. *J Med Chem* 38: 739–744

b) Desai RC, Court JC, Freguson E, Gordon RJ, Hlasta DJ, Dunlap RP, Franke CA (1995) Phosphonates and phosphinates: Novel leaving groups for benzisothiazolone inhibitors of human leukocyte elastase. *J Med Chem* 38: 1571–1574

68   Kuang RZ, Venkataraman R, Ruan SM, Groutas WC (1998) Use of the 1,2,5-thiadiazolin-3-one 1,1 dioxide and isothiazolidin-3-one 1,1 dioxide scaffolds in the design of potent inhibitors of serine proteinases. *Bioorg Med Chem Lett* 8: 539–544

69   Gütschow M, Neumann U (1998) Novel thieno[2,3-*d*]-1,3-oxazin-4-ones as inhibitors of human leukocyte elastase. *J Med Chem* 41: 1729–1740

70   Jarvest RL, Connor SC, Gorniak JG, Jennings LJ, Serafinowska HT, West A (1998) Potent selective thienoxazinone inhibitors of herpes proteases. *Bioorg Med Chem Lett* 7: 1733–1738

71   Uejima Y, Kokubo M, Oshida J, Kawabata H, Kato Y, Fujii, K (1993) 5-Methyl-4H-3-1-benzoxazin-4-one derivatives: Specific inhibitors of human leukocyte elastase. *J Pharmacol Exp Ther* 265: 516–523

72   Doherty JB, Ashe BM, Argenbright LA, Lawrence W, Barker PL, Bonney RJ, Chandler GO, Dahlgren ME, Dorn CP Jr, Finke PE et al (1986) Cephalosporin antibiotics can be modified to inhibit human leukocyte elastase. *Nature* 322: 192–194

73   a) Doherty JB, Shah SK, Finke PE et al (1993) Chemical biomedical pharmacokinetic an biological properties of L-680,833: A potent orally-active monocyclic β-lactam inhibitor of human polymorphonuclear leukocyte elastase. *Proc Natl Acad Sci USA* 90: 8727–8731

b) Vincent SH, Painter SK, Lufferatlas D, Karanam BV, McGowan E, Cioffe C, Doss G,Chiu SH (1997) Orally active inhibitors of human leukocyte elastase. 2. Disposition of L694,458 in rats and rhesus monkeys. *Drug Met Disp* 25: 932–939

74   Buynak JD, Rao AS, Ford GP, Carver C, Adam G, Geng B, Bachmann B, Shobassy S, Lackey S (1997) 7-Alkylidenecephalosporin esters as inhibitors of human leukocyte elastase. *J Med Chem* 40: 3423–3433

75   Hernandez MA, Powers JC, Glinski J, Oleksyszyn J, Vijayalakshmi J, Meyer EF Jr (1992) Effect of the 7-amino substituent on the inhibitory potency of mechanism-based isocoumarin inhibitors for porcine pancreatic and human neutrophil elastases: A 1.85-Å X-ray structure of the complex between porcine pancreatic elastase and 7-9N-tosylphenylalanyl)amino-4-chloro-3-methoxyisocoumarin. *J Med Chem* 35: 1121–1129

76   Vijayalakshmi J, Meyer EF Jr, Kam CM, Powers JC (1991) Structural study of porcine pancreatic elastase complexed with 7-amino-3-(2-bromoethoxy)-4-chloroisocoumarin as a nonreactivatable doubly covalent enzyme-inhibitor complex. *Biochemistry* 30: 2175–2183

77   Westwood NJ, Claridge TDW, Edwards PN, Schofield CJ (1997) Reversible acylation of elastase by gamma-lactam analogues of beta-lactam inhibitors. *Bioorg Med Chem Lett* 7: 2973–2978

78   Macdonald SJF, Belton DJ, Buckley DM, Spooner JE, Anson MS, Harrison LA, Mills K, Upton RJ, Dowle MD, Smith RA, Molloy CR, Risley C (1998) Syntheses of trans-5-oxo-hexahydro-pyrrolo3,2-bpyrroles and trans-5-oxo-hexahydro-furo3,2-bpyrroles (pyrrolidine trans-lactams and trans-lactones): New pharmacophore for elastase inhibition. *J Med Chem* 41: 3919–3922

79   For a review on polymer supported reactions see:
a) Brown RC (1998) Recent developments in solid-phase organic synthesis. J *Chem Soc Perkin Trans* I: 3293–3320

b) Thompson LA, Ellman JA (1996) Synthesis and applications of small molecule libraries. *Chem Rev* 96: 555–600

c) Hermkens PH, Ottenheijm HC, Rees DC (1997) Solid-phase organic reactions. II: A review of the literature Nov 95-Nov 96. *Tetrahedron* 53: 5643–5678

d) Chaiken IM, Janda KD (1996) Molecular diversity and combinatorial chemistry, libraries and drug design. ACS Washington DC Conference Proceedings Series III

e) Wilson SR, Czarnik AM (eds) (1997) Combinatorial chemistry. Synthesis and application. John Wiley and Sons, New York

80 a) Edwards PD, Meyer EF Jr, Vijayalakshmi J, Tuthill PA, Andisik DW, Gomes B, Strimpler A (1992) Design, synthesis and kinetic evaluation of a unique class of elastase inhibitors, the peptidyl α-ketobenzoxazoles, and the X-ray crystal structure of the covalent complex between porcine pancreatic elastase and Ac-Ala-Pro-Val-2-benzoxazole. *J Am Chem Soc* 114: 1854–1863

b) Edwards PD, Wolanin DJ, Andisik DW, Davis MW (1995) Peptidyl α-ketoheterocyclic inhibitors of human neutrophil elastase. 2. Effect of varying the heterocyclic ring on *in vitro* potency. *J Med Chem* 38: 76–85

c) Edwards PD, Zottola MA, Davis M, Williams J, Tuthill PA (1995) Peptidyl α-ketoheterocyclic inhibitors of human neutrophil elastase. 3. *In vitro* and *in vivo* potency of a series of peptidyl α-ketobenzoxazoles. *J Med Chem* 38: 3972–3982

81 Wang F, Hauske JR (1997) Solid-phase synthesis of benzoxazoles via Mitsunobu reaction. *Tet Lett* 38: 6529–6532

82 Hauske JR, Dorff P (1995) A solid phase CBZ chloride equivalent. A new matrix specific linker. *Tet Lett* 36: 1589–1592

83 Gordeev MF (1998) Combinatorial approaches to pharmacophoric heterocycles: A solid-phase synthesis of 3,1-benzoxazine-4-ones. *Biotech Bioeng* 61: 13–16

84 a) Uejima Y, Oshida, JI, Kawabata H, Kokubo M, Kato Y, Fujii K (1994) Inhibition of human sputum elastase by 7-substituted 5-methyl-2-isopropylamino-4H-3,1-benzoxazin-4-ones. *Biochem Pharmacol* 48: 426–428

b) Uejima Y, Kokubo M, Oshida JI, Kawabata H, Kato Y, Fujii K (1993) 5-Methyl-4H-3,1-benzoxazin-4-one derivatives: Specific inhibitors of human leukocyte elastase. *J Pharmacol Exp Ther* 265: 516–523

c) Krantz A, Spencer RW, Tam TF, Liak TJ, Copp LJ, Thomas EM, Raffety SP (1990) Design and synthesis of 4H-3,1-benzoxazin-4-ones as potent alternate substrate inhibitors of human leukocyte elastase. *J Med Chem* 33: 464–479

d) Abood NA, Schretzman LA, Flyn DL, Houseman KA, Wittwer AJ, Dilworth VM, Hippenmeyer PJ, Holwerda BC (1997) Inhibition of human cytomegalovirus protease by benzoxazinones and evidence of antiviral activity in cell culture. *Bioorg Med Chem Lett* 7: 2105–2108

85 a) Gayo LM, Suto MJ (1997) Ion-exchange resins for solution phase parallel synthesis of chemical libraries. *Tet Lett* 38: 513–516

b) Parlow JJ, Mischke DA, Woodard SS (1997) Utility of complementary molecular reactivity and molecular recognition (CMR/R) technology and polymer-supported reagents in the solution-phase synthesis of heterocyclic carboxamides. *J Org Chem* 62: 5908–5919

c) Studer A, Hadida S, Ferritto R, Kim SY, Jeger P, Wipf P, Curran DP (1997) Fluorous synthesis: A fluorous-phase strategy for improving separation efficiency in organic synthesis. *Science* 275: 823–826

d) Cheng S, Comer DD, Williams JP, Myers PL, Boger DL (1996) Novel solution phase strategy for the synthesis of chemical libraries containing small organic molecules. *J Am Chem Soc* 118: 2567–2573

86   Parow JJ, Flynn DL (1998) Solution-phase parallel synthesis of a benzoxazinone library using complementary molecular reactivity and molecular recognition (CMR/R) purification technology. *Tetrahedron* 54: 4013–4031

87   Parlow JJ, Naing W, South MS, Flynn DL (1997) *In situ* chemical tagging: tetrafluorophthalic anhydride as a "Sequestration Enabling Reagent" (SER) in the purification of solution-phase combinatorial libraries. *Tet Lett* 38: 7959–7962

88   Pitlik J, Townsend CA (1997) Solution-phase synthesis of a combinatorial monocyclic β-lactam library: Potential protease inhibitors. *Bioorg Med Chem Lett* 7: 3129–3134

89   Ugi I, Lohberger S, Karl R (1991) In: BM Trost, CH Heathcock (eds) *Comprehensive organic synthesis for synthetic efficiency*. Pergamon Press, Oxford, , vol 2, 1083–1109

90   a) Hagmann WK, Kissinger AL, Shah SK, Finke PE, Dorn CP, Brause KA, Ashe BM, Weston H, Maycock AL, Knight WB et al (1993) Orally active β-lactam inhibitors of human leukocyte elastase. 2. Effect of C-4 substitution. *J Med Chem* 36: 771–777

b) Hagmann WK, Thompson KR, Shah SK, Finke PE, Ashe BM, Weston H, Maycock AL, Doherty JB (1992) The effect of N-acyl substituents on the stability on moncyclic β-lactam inhibitors of human leukocyte elastase. *Bioorg Med Chem Lett* 2: 681–684

91   a) Bruno JG, Chang MN, Choi-Sledeski YM, Green DM, McGarry DG, Regan JR, Volz FA (1997) Synthesis of functionalized aromatic oligomers from a versatile diphenylmethane template. *J Org Chem* 62: 5174–5190

b) Regan J, McGarry D, Bruno J, Green D, Newman J, Hsu CY, Kline J, Barton J, Travis J, Choi Y M Volz F, Pauls H, Harrison R, Zilberstein A, Bensasson SA, Chang M (1997) Anionic- and lipophilic-mediated surface binding inhibitiors of human leukocyte elastase. *J Med Chem* 40: 3408–3422

92   Pavia MR, Cohen MP, Dilley GJ, Dubuc GR, Durgin TL, Forman FW, Hedigier ME, Milot G, Powers TS, Sucholeiki I et al (1996) The design and synthesis of substituted biphenyl libraries. *Bioorg Med Chem Lett* 4: 659–666

93   For reviews, see:

a) Birkedal-Hansen H, Moore WGI, Bodden MK, Windsor LJ, Birkedal-Hansen B, DeCarlo A, Engler JA (1993) Matrix metalloproteinases: A review. *Crit Rev in Oral Biol and Med* 4: 197–250

b) Hagmann WK, Lark MW, Becker JW (1996) Inhibition of matrix metalloproteinases. *Ann Rep in Med Chem* 31: 231–240

c) Zask A, Levin JI, Killar LM, Skotnicki JS (1996) Inhibition of matrix metalloproteinases: Structure based design. *Curr Pharma Design* 2: 624–661

d) Greenwald RA, Golub LM (eds) (1994) *Inhibition of matrix metalloproteinases*. The New York Academy of Sciences, New York, vol 732

94 a) Makowski GS, Ramsby ML (1998) Binding of latent matrix metalloproteinase 9 to fibrin: Activation via a plasmin-dependent pathway. *Inflammation* 22: 287–305
    b) Woessner JF Jr (1991) Matrix metalloproteinases and their inhibitors in connective tissue remodeling. *FASEB J* 5: 2145–2154

95 Ohuchi E, Imai K, Fujii Y, Sato H, Seiki M, Okada Y (1997) Membrane type 1 matrix metalloproteinase digests interstitial collagens and other extracellular matrix macromolecules. *J Biol Chem* 272: 2446–2451

96 Docherty AJ, Lyons A, Smith BJ, Wright EM, Stephens PE, Harris TJ, Murphy G, Reynolds JJ (1985) Sequences of human tissue inhibitors of metalloproteinases and its identity to erythroid-potentiating activity. *Nature* 318: 66–69

97 White AD, Bocan TM, Boxer PA, Peterson JT, Schrier, D (1997) Emerging therapeutic advances for the development of second generation matrix metalloproteinase inhibitors. *Curr Pharm Design* 3: 45–58

98 Hautamaki RD, Kobayashi DK, Senior RM, Shapiro SD (1997) Requirement for macrophage elastase for cigarette smoke-induced emphysema in mice. *Science* 277: 2002–2004

99 Shapiro SD, Griffin GL, Gilbert DJ, Jenkins NA, Copeland NG, Welgus HG, Senior RM, Ley TJ (1992) Molecular cloning, chromosomal localization, and bacterial expression of a murine macrophage metalloelastase. *J Biol Chem* 267: 4664–4671

100 Shapiro SD, Kobayashi DK, Ley TJ (1993) Cloning and characterization of a unique elastolytic metalloproteinase produced by human alveolar macrophages. *J Biol Chem* 268: 23824–23829

101 Shipley JM, Wesselschmidt RL, Kobayashi DK, Ley TJ, Shapiro SD (1996) Metalloproteinase is required for the macrophage-mediated proteolysis and matrix invasion in mice. *PNAS* 93: 3942–3946

102 Gronski TJ Jr., Martin RL, Kobayashi, DK, Walsh, BC, Holman MC, Huber M, Van Wart HE, Shapiro SD (1997) Hydrolysis of a broad spectrum of extracellular matrix proteins by human macrophage elastase. *J Biol Chem* 272: 12189–12194

103 Mecham RP, Broekelmann TJ, Fliszar CJ, Shapiro SD, Welgus HG, Senior RM (1997) Elastin degradation by matrix metalloproteinases. *J Biol Chem* 272: 18071–18076

104 Pagenstecher A, Stalder AK, Kincaid CL, Shapiro SD, Campbell IL (1998) Differential expression of matrix metalloproteinase and tissue inhibitor of matrix metalloproteinase genes in the mouse central nervous system in normal and inflammatory states. *Am J Path* 152: 729–741

105 Shapiro S (1995) The pathogenesis of emphysema: The elastase:antielastase hypothesis 30 years later. *Proc Assoc Amer Physicians* 107: 346–352

106 Baxter AD, Bird J, Bhogal R, Massil T, Minton KJ, Montana J, Owen DA (1997) A novel series of matrix metalloproteinase inhibitors for the treatment of inflammatory disorders. *Bioorg Med Chem Lett* 7: 897–902

107 Hirayama R, Yamamoto M, Tsukida T, Matsuo K, Obata Y, Sakamoto F, Ikeda S (1997) Synthesis and biological evaluation of orally active matrix metalloproteinase inhibitors. *Bioorg Med Chem* 5: 765–778

A high throughput assay for the TNF converting enzyme

M. Anthony Leesnitzer, D. Mark Bickett, Marcia L. Moss and J. David Becherer

Department of Molecular Biochemistry, Glaxo Wellcome Research and Development Inc., 5 Moore Drive, P.O. Box 13998, Research Triangle Park, NC 27709, USA

Introduction

Tumor necrosis factor-α (TNFα) has been implicated in cancer and inflammatory diseases since it was first characterized and eventually identified by researchers in several laboratories in the mid-1980s [1–5]. However, only recently has the pathological role of TNF in arthritis and Crohn's disease been demonstrated in the clinic with the FDA's approval of Enbrel and Remicade [6–8]. The recent success of these biological agents that neutralize TNF has led to intense efforts to find small molecule TNF antagonists that will mimic the consequences, if not the mechanism, of these agents. Because TNF interacts at multiple contact points with either of its two receptors, researchers have struggled to find small molecular weight inhibitors that antagonize this interaction. Therefore, most efforts have focused on targets upstream of TNF synthesis or secretion and downstream of TNF receptor engagement since these targets appear more amenable to modulation by small molecular weight inhibitors [9].

In this chapter, we focus on high throughput assays for the TNFα converting enzyme, or TACE, a recently identified protease that modulates TNFα. TACE activity is essential for secretion of TNF from the cell [10]. Several labs initially demonstrated inhibition of TNF secretion with metalloproteinase inhibitors [11–13]. These inhibitors not only blocked *in vitro* production of TNF from assorted cell types in response to various stimuli, but they also blocked TNF secretion *in vivo* in response to LPS. However, TIMP-1 and TIMP-2, potent endogenous inhibitors of metalloproteinases, were ineffective in blocking TNF release. Additionally, not all synthetic metalloproteinase inhibitors were effective at blocking the cellular release of TNF. Together, this suggested the involvement of another metalloprotease distinct from the known matrix metalloproteases (MMPs). Eventually, the TNFα converting enzyme (ADAM-17) was cloned [14, 15]. This enzyme is related to MMPs in that it contains the characteristic Zn^{2+} binding motif HEXXH. However, significant sequence differences exist elsewhere in the catalytic domain of the molecule. Adjacent to the catalytic domain is a disintegrin domain followed by a short cysteine rich

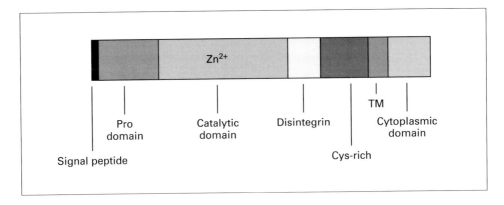

Figure 1
A schematic representation of the domain structure of TACE.

domain, a transmembrane domain and a cytosolic tail (Fig. 1). This domain structure clearly places TACE in the reprolysin or adamalysin family of metalloproteases [16]. Many of the mammalian members of this metalloproteinase family are currently being characterized, and their physiological substrates are yet to be identified [17–19].

The fact that some MMP inhibitors block TNF secretion, coupled with the well-established role of TNF in arthritis and Crohn's disease, makes the development of small molecular weight inhibitors of TACE very attractive. The first step in establishing a clear knowledge of the structure-activity relationship between TACE and its inhibitors is to develop an enzyme assay suitable for screening a significant number of inhibitors.

TACE assay development history

Initially, TACE activity was qualitatively characterized by SDS-PAGE analysis of digested recombinant proTNF. However, to facilitate the assessment of activity in fractions during purification of TACE from cell sources, a more facile and quantitative HPLC assay supplemented this cumbersome method. The substrate for this HPLC assay, Dnp-SPLAQAVRSSSR, when digested with TACE, produced the N-terminal product Dnp-SPLAQA. The product peptide easily separated from the substrate peptide on a C18 column with a heptafluorobutyric acid/acetonitrile gradient. Measuring the absorbance of the Dnp group at 350 nm made screening crude enzyme fractions practical. Furthermore, the HPLC assay was necessary for characterization of TACE during purification since it provided confirmation that cleavage occurred at the correct site, between Ala[76]–Val[77]. While this assay was valuable during TACE purification, the level of throughput was unacceptable for screening for inhibitors of TACE.

Scintillation proximity technology

Traditionally, isotopic labeling of a ligand or substrate has allowed researchers to quantitate receptor binding or substrate turnover. Isotope counting is typically accomplished by addition of soluble isotope to scintillation cocktail. The necessity to separate bound ligand from unbound, or product from substrate, in assays involving traditional isotope counting has limited their use as high throughput inhibitor screens. Scintillation proximity assays (SPA) have overcome these limitations in that no separation of product and substrate is required, thus yielding a homogenous assay format. In the SPA, the scintillant is embedded in the polyvinyl toluene bead and emits light only when a beta emitter is in close proximity to achieve efficient energy transfer. Isotopes free in solution are not within the required proximity to effect the scintillant, thereby, in essence, effecting a phase separation between bound and unbound radiolabel.

Introduction of radioisotopes into the ligand or substrate peptide has been accomplished through a variety of methods. These include synthetic incorporation of ^{3}H proline as demonstrated here, modification of cysteine with ^{3}H–N-ethylmaleimide [20], iodination of substrate peptide [21], and ^{33}P phosphorylation of peptides to be used as proteolytic substrate [22]. Capture mechanisms which sequester the isotope near the SPA bead include coating beads with wheat germ agglutinin for (glycosylated) membrane bound receptors, polylysine for ionic interactions, protein A for antibodies and, as in the TACE assay design below, streptavidin for capture of a biotinylated substrate or protein. The streptavidin/biotin interaction is of particularly high affinity and ensures rapid, efficient substrate capture and excellent signal stability. Together, these attributes make SPA a suitable format for automation. Indeed, the SPA has been well established for high throughput screening and has been used in a multitude of assay types, including assays for proteases [23] kinases [22], protein/protein interactions [24, 25], membrane receptor binding assays [26], and nuclear receptor assays [27]. For a thorough review, see Cook [28].

TACE scintillation proximity assay characterization

Thus, to fill the need for a high throughput assay of TACE suitable for automation, a scintillation proximity assay (SPA) was developed. Incorporation of a ^{3}H label into the SPA substrate required C-terminal elongation of the HPLC peptide substrate to include a tritiated proline. Also, biotin with a linker replaced the Dnp-group result-

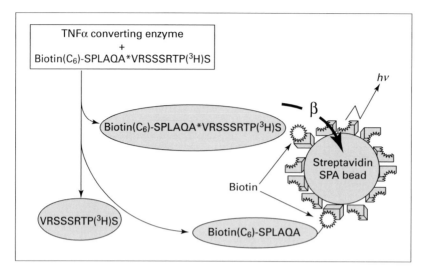

Figure 2
A schematic representation of the TACE scintillation proximity assay. TACE is incubated with the tritiated substrate and the reaction is stopped by the addition of SPA beads in buffer containing EDTA.

ing in a substrate sequence of biotin–$(CH_2)_6$–SPLAQA*VRSSSRTP(^{3}H)S. The biotin facilitates capture by the streptavidin coated SPA bead. The binding of the intact peptide results in a signal from the scintillant impregnated bead as depicted in Figure 2. Following cleavage of the substrate peptide, a decrease in signal is observed since the ^{3}H-labeled C-terminal peptide fragment remains in the media.

This assay format was evaluated using a microsomal fraction of TACE (mTACE) activity isolated from Mono Mac 6 cells [29]. Mass spectrometry verified the cleavage site of a non-tritiated peptide and confirmed that the above modifications did not alter the cleavage specificity of mTACE for this substrate (Fig. 3). Microsomal and rTACE were used to establish assay parameters suitable for screening inhibitors. Linearity of rate with dilution of mTACE was established over a four-fold range of enzyme concentration. The dilute concentration and microsomal nature of the preparation limited the range. However, rTACE showed linearity over a wider dilution range as shown in Figure 4. Both the mTACE and rTACE preparations were stable over the assay incubation period (data not shown). Excellent reproducibility and favorable signal relative to noise was observed at an enzyme concentration that yielded 50% substrate turnover in one hour. Under first order conditions, substrate turnover in the range of 50% was not linear with respect to time and required correction to assess percent inhibition accurately. Corrected turnover was defined in

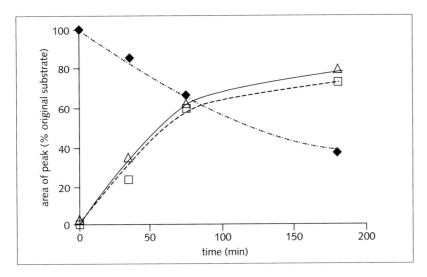

Figure 3
TACE specific cleavage of biotin-SPLAQA*VRSSSRTPS. Mass spectral analysis of products generated by TACE digestion of the SPA substrate verified the expected TACE specific cleavage (substrate (◆), N-terminal product. (Δ), C-terminal product (□)).

Equation 1,
Corrected turnover = $-\ln(S_t/S_o)$ (Eq. 1)

where S_t was substrate concentration remaining at time t, and S_o was initial substrate concentration. The one hour incubation also reduced the probability that slow binding inhibitors could be overlooked. Furthermore, longer incubations permitted more interleaving of assay steps in automated procedures, and resulted in increased efficiency when scheduling software was used. As a guide for assessing assay performance, Equation 2 was used to calculate a "response ratio", where 100% and 0% responses referred to counts detected in the presence and absence of enzyme respectively.

Response ratio = $\dfrac{(100\% \text{ response} - 0\% \text{ response})}{3\times \text{ Standard deviation}_{100\%} + 3\times \text{ Standard deviation}_{0\%}}$ (Eq. 2)

From empirical observations in our labs, a response ratio of 2.5 or greater indicated an acceptable assay. For the TACE SPA with either rTACE or mTACE, the ratio ranged from 4 to 6.

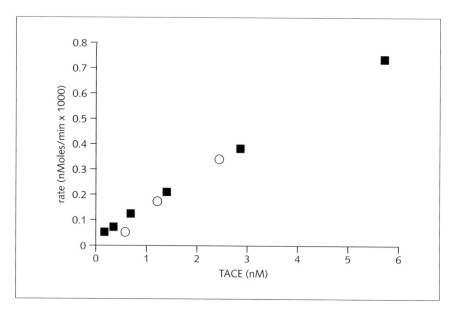

Figure 4

Linearity of TACE activity with dilution. Recombinant TACE (■) was serially diluted in 2-fold increments before assaying. Each point represents the average slope of duplicate progress curves generated at that enzyme concentration. Recombinant enzyme concentration was titrated with an inhibitor to determine concentration. Microsomal TACE (O) concentration was extrapolated from the rTACE concentration on the basis of turnover rates. TACE activity was linear with dilution.

Robustness of the assay was assessed using a panel of metalloproteinase inhibitors with different metal chelating groups – hydroxamates, thiols, and carboxylates. All were compatible with the SPA format. An IC_{50} was generated for each TACE inhibitor by testing the compound with 3-fold serial dilutions, 11 concentrations per curve. Microsomal TACE typically was assayed at 37 °C to conserve enzyme (activity approximately doubled with a ten degree increase in temperature). Recombinant TACE, for convenience or to facilitate automation, was typically assayed at room temperature. The pIC_{50}s of compounds tested against mTACE and rTACE were strongly correlated as were the pIC_{50}s of compounds tested against rTACE at room temperature and at 37 °C (Fig. 5). Figure 6 compares pIC_{50}'s determined on the same day and pIC_{50}s determined on different days and demonstrates minimal intra-and interassay variability. Finally, the IC_{50}s determined by HPLC were comparable to those generated by SPA. Figure 7 shows a representative compound, GW 9471 [11], assayed in both formats.

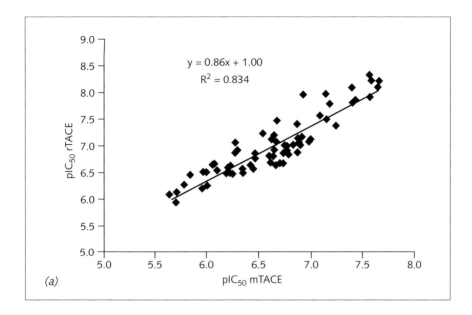

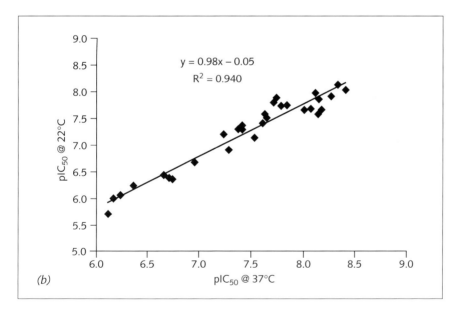

Figure 5
Inhibitor pIC$_{50}$ comparison. (a) Comparison of pIC$_{50}$s between mTACE (37°C) and rTACE (22°C). (b) Comparison of inhibitor pIC$_{50}$s against rTACE at 22°C and 37°C. In both examples, a panel of inhibitors was serially diluted and tested in the TACE SPA at either room temperature or 37°C against either mTACE or rTACE.

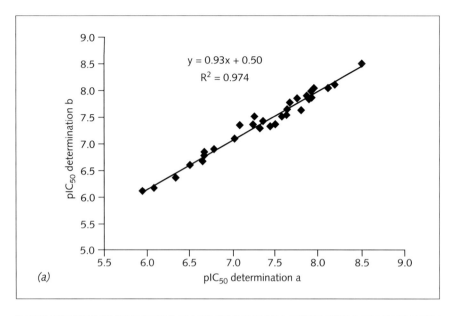

(a)

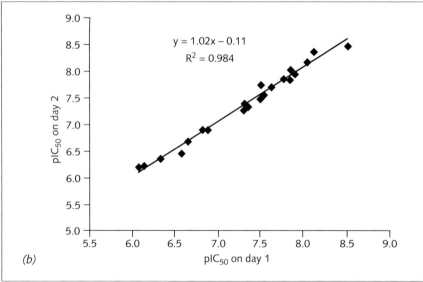

(b)

Figure 6
Inter and intra-assay variability. $pIC_{50}s$ were compared from the same day and from a different day to assess reproducibility of the assay. In panel (a), determinations a and b represent independent values from single IC_{50} curves generated on the same day. Panel (b) compares single values generated on different days. Variability in this assay is acceptable for generating structure activity relationships with inhibitors.

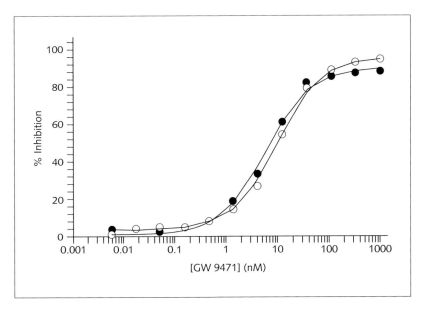

Figure 7

IC_{50} curves generated by SPA (●) and HPLC (O) assays. The IC_{50} value for the inhibition of mTACE determined by the SPA assay (10.2 nM) was in good agreement with the IC_{50} generated using the HPLC assay (6.1 nM). TACE inhibitor GW 9471 is shown here as an example.

Alternatives to SPA for proteinase screening

Alternative assay formats to SPA include the use of substrates incorporating fluorophores or chromophores to monitor hydrolysis. Recently, two fluorescent peptide substrates for TACE became commercially available (BACHEM Biosciences Inc.). Both rely on internal quenching by resonance energy transfer to provide low background signals, good sensitivity and a homogeneous format. M-2155 (DABCYL-Leu-Ala-Gln-Ala-Val-Arg-Ser-Ser-Ser-Arg-EDANS) incorporated a donor/acceptor pair of DABCYL (4-(4-dimethylaminophenylazo)benzoyl) and EDANS (5-[(2-aminoethyl)amino]napthalene-1-sulfonic acid). M2255 (Mca-Pro-Leu-Ala-Gln-Ala-Val-Dpa-Arg-Ser-Ser-Ser-Arg-NH$_2$) incorporated Mca ((7-methoxycoumarin-4-yl) acetyl) and Dpa (N-3-(2,4-dinitrophenyl)-L-2,3-diaminopropionyl) as described previously [30]. The resonance energy transfer for M2155 was less efficient than for M2255. The background signal of M2155 contributed 30% of the fluorescence signal produced at 20% substrate turnover. With comparable turnover, M2255 background was 15%. The response ratios, using Equation 2, were 6 and 12, respectively. No differences in pIC$_{50}$s were observed when these two substrates were compared to each other or when compared with IC$_{50}$s generated by SPA (Figs. 8a–c).

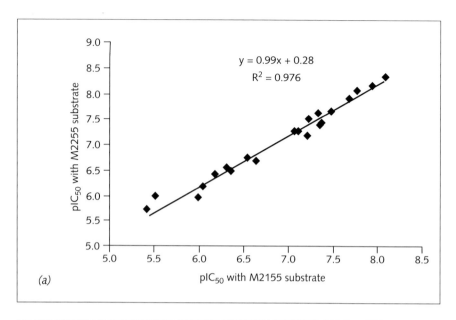

(a)

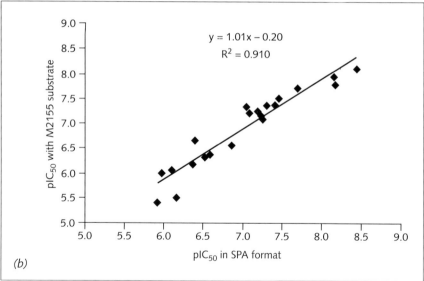

(b)

Figure 8

TACE activity assayed in a fluorescence format. Inhibitors of TACE were assayed using fluo-rescent substrates M-2155 and M-2255. Each pIC_{50} value is determined from an 11-point titration curve of the inhibitor. Single pIC_{50}s generated from each substrate were compared (panel a) and were in excellent agreement. pIC_{50} values from single determinations by SPA were compared to pIC_{50}s generated with substrates M-2155 (panel b) and M-2255 (panel c).

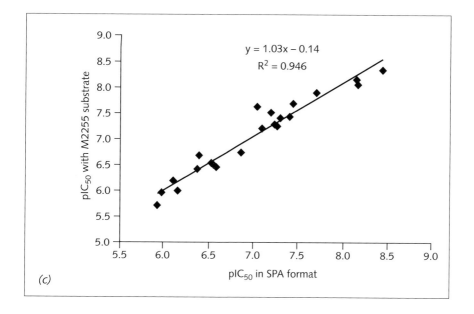

$$y = 1.03x - 0.14$$
$$R^2 = 0.946$$

(c)

The downside to using fluorescent substrates in high throughput assays is that some compounds tested may quench the fluorescence signal resulting in a false positive "hit". Also, depending on the substrate concentration, intrinsically fluorescent compounds may result in a "false negative" observation. Increasing the substrate concentration may significantly decrease the prevalence of "false negatives". The amount of interference by these inhibitors is a direct function of the emission/excitation spectra of the fluorescent groups of the particular substrate.

Summary

Our understanding of the molecular mechanisms contributing to various disease states and associated symptoms has increased dramatically over the past decade. Advances in molecular biology, genetics and combinatorial chemistry as well as our ability to screen a large number of compounds quickly and cost effectively have driven this mechanistic understanding. As new targets are identified, it is imperative that assay formats be applied quickly to screen these targets. We have demonstrated a straightforward method for identifying protease substrates, initially using HPLC techniques, and then translating that into a format for high throughput screening. Of the potential formats discussed for protease assays, the SPA described herein is used routinely in our lab. This assay performs within our criteria for high throughput assays despite the fact that we are measuring a decrease in signal. Furthermore, SPA technology is easily transferred to an automated environment. The

utility of the SPA as an enzyme activity and receptor binding assay is well documented. The TACE SPA described herein has also been applied as a bioassay to
assess compound plasma stability, plasma levels for *in vivo* testing and solubility in
simulated body fluids. The assay is much faster than traditional HPLC assays that
are slowed by methods development time and low throughput. As stated previously, many metalloproteinases related to TACE have no clearly defined physiological
substrate. In due time, these substrates will be identified and similar assays can be
developed to identify potent and specific inhibitors of these enzymes as well.

References

1   Beutler B, Mahoney J, Nguyen LT, Pekala P, Cerami A (1985) Purification of cachectin,
     a lipoprotein lipase-suppressing hormone secreted by endotoxin-induced RAW 264.7
     cells. *J Exp Med* 161: 984–995
2   Haranaka K, Carswell EA, Williamson BD, Prendergast JS, Satomi N, Old LJ (1986)
     Purification, characterization, and antitumor activity of non-recombinant mouse tumor
     necrosis factor. *Proc Natl Acad Sci USA* 83: 3949–3953
3   Aggarwal BB, Kohr WJ, Hass PE, Moffat B, Spencer SA, Henzel WJ, Bringman TS, Ned-
     win GE, Goeddel DV, Harkins RN (1985) Human tumor necrosis factor. Production,
     purification, and characterization. *J Biol Chem* 260: 2345–2354
4   Pennica D, Hayflick JS, Bringman TS, Palladino MA, Goeddel DV (1985) Cloning and
     expression in *Escherichia coli* of the cDNA for murine tumor necrosis factor. *Proc Natl
     Acad Sci USA* 82: 6060-6064
5   Wang, AM, Creasey AA, Ladner MB, Lin LS, Strickler J, Van Arsdell JN, Yamamoto R,
     Mark DF (1985) Molecular cloning of the complementary DNA for human tumor
     necrosis factor. *Science* 228: 149–154
6   Moreland LW, Baumgartner SW, Schiff MH, Tindall EA, Fleischmann RM, Weaver AL,
     Ettlinger RE, Cohen S, Koopman WJ, Mohler K et al (1997) Treatment of rheumatoid
     arthritis with a recombinant human tumor necrosis factor receptor (p75)-Fc fusion pro-
     tein. *N Engl J Med* 337: 141–147
7   Weinblatt ME, Kremer JM, Bankhurst AD, Bulpitt KJ, Fleischmann RM, Fox RI, Jack-
     son CG, Lange M, Burge DJ (1999) A trial of etanercept, a recombinant tumor necro-
     sis factor receptor: Fc fusion protein, in patients with rheumatoid arthritis receiving
     methotrexate. *N Engl J Med* 340: 253–259
8   Targan SR, Hanauer S., Van Deventer SJH, Mayer L, Present DH, Braakman T,
     Dewoody KL, Schaible TF, Rutgeerts PJ (1997) A short-term study of chimeric mono-
     clonal antibody cA2 to tumor necrosis factor a for Crohn's disease. *N Engl J Med* 337:
     1029–1035
9   Shire MG, Muller GW (1998) TNF-α inhibitors and rheumatoid arthritis. *Expert Opin
     Ther Pat* 8: 531–544
10   Peschon JJ, Slack JL, Reddy P, Stocking KL, Sunnarborg SW, Lee DC, Russell WE, Cast-

ner BJ, Johnson RS, Fitzner JN et al (1998) An essential role for ectodomain shedding in mammalian development. *Science* 282: 1281–1284

11 McGeehan GM, Becherer JD, Bast RC, Boyer CM, Champion B, Connolly K, Conway J, Furdon P, Karp S, Kidao S et al (1994) Regulation of tumor necrosis factor-a processing by a metalloproteinase inhibitor. *Nature* 370: 558–561

12 Mohler KM, Sleath PR, Fitzner JN, Cerretti DP, Alderson M, Kerwar SS, Torrance DS, Otten-Evans C, Greenstreet T, Black RA (1994) Protection against a lethal dose of endotoxin by an inhibitor of tumor necrosis factor processing. *Nature* 370: 218–221

13 Gearing AJH, Beckett P, Christodoulou M, Churchill M, Clements J, Davidson AH, Drummond AH, Galloway WA, Gilbert R (1994) Processing of tumor necrosis factor-a precursor by metalloproteases. *Nature* 370: 555–558

14 Moss ML, Jin SC, Milla ME, Burkhart W, Carter HL, Chen W., Clay WC, Didsbury JR, Hassler D, Hoffman CR et al (1997) Cloning of a disintegrin metalloproteinase that processes precursor tumor necrosis factor-α. *Nature* 385: 733–736

15 Black RA, Rauch CT, Kozlosky CJ, Peschon JJ, Slack JL, Wolfson MF, Castner BJ, Stocking KL, Reddy P, Srinivasan S et al (1997) A metalloproteinase disintegrin that releases tumor necrosis factor-a from cells. *Nature* 385: 729–733

16 Hooper NM (1994) Families of zinc metalloproteases. *FEBS Lett* 354: 1–6

17 Blobel CP (1997) Metalloprotease-disintegrins: links to cell adhesion and cleavage of TNF-α and Notch. *Cell* 90: 589–592

18 Hooper NM, Karran EH, Turner AJ (1997) Membrane protein secretases. *Biochem J* 321: 265–279

19 Black RA, White JM (1998) ADAMs: focus on the protease domain. *Curr Opin Cell Biol* 10: 654–659

20 Brown AM, George SM, Blume AJ, Dushin RG, Jacobsen JS, Sonnenberg-Reines J (1994) Biotinylated and cysteine-modified peptides as useful reagents for studying the inhibition of cathepsin G. *Anal Biochem* 217: 139–147

21 Basak A, Boudreault A, Jean F, Chretien M, Lazure C (1993) Radiolabeled biotinyl peptides as useful reagents for the study of proteolytic enzymes. *Anal Biochem* 209 (2): 306–314

22 Baum EZ, Hohnston SH, Bebernitz GA, Gluzman Y (1996) Development of a scintillation proximity assay for human cytomegalovirus protease using [33]Phosphorus. *Anal Biochem* 237: 129–134

23 Cook ND, Jessop RA, Robinson PS, Richards AD, Kay J (1991) Structure and function of the aspartic proteinases. In: BM Dunn (ed): *Scintillation proximity enzyme assay: a rapid and novel assay technique applied to HIV proteinase.* Plenum Press, London, 525–528

24 Jones AE, Saksela K, Game SM, O'Beirne G, Cook ND (1998) Screening assay for the detection of the protein-protein interaction between HIV-1 Nef protein and SH3 domain of Hck. *J Biomolec Screening* 3 (1): 37–41

25 Pernelle C, Clerc FF, Dureuil C, Bracco L, Tocque B (1993) An efficient screening assay

for the rapid and precise determination of affinities between leucine zipper domains. *Biochemistry* 32 (43): 11682–11687

26 Nelson N (1987) A novel method for the detection of receptors and membrane proteins by scintillation proximity radioassay. *Anal Biochem* 165: 287–293

27 Nichols JS, Parks DJ, Consler TG, Blanchard SG (1998) Development of a scintillation proximity assay for peroxisome proliferator-activated receptor gamma ligand binding domain. *Anal Biochem* 257: 112–119

28 Cook ND (1996) Scintillation proximity assay: A versatile high-throughput screening technology. *Drug Discovery Today* 1 (7): 287–294

29 Ziegler-Heitbrook HWL, Thiel E, Fuetter A, Herzog V, Wirtz A, Reithmueller G (1988) Establishment of a human cell line (Mono Mac 6) with characteristics of mature monocytes. *Int J Cancer* 41: 456–461

30 Van Dyk DE, Marchand P, Bruckner RC, Fox JW., Jaffee BD, Gunyuzlu PL, Davis GL, Nurnberg S, Covington M, Decicco CP et al (1997) Comparison of snake venom reprolysin and matrix metalloproteinases as models of TNF-α converting enzyme. *Bioorg Med Chem Lett* 7: 1219-1224

Tryptase inhibitors

Kenneth D. Rice[1] and William R. Moore[2]

Department of [1]Medicinal Chemistry and [2]Biology, Axys Pharmaceuticals Inc., 180 Kimball Way, South San Francisco, CA 94080, USA

Introduction

Human tryptase is a structurally unique trypsin-like serine protease expressed exclusively by mast cells. Recent biological and clinical research suggest that this enzyme may function as a mediator of several mast cell related allergic and inflammatory conditions, including most notably, asthma, conjunctivitis and rhinitis [1–5]. Tryptase activity has also recently been implicated in some adverse drug reactions [6, 7]. The scope of this role in allergic and inflammatory disease is determined in part by the heterogeneous and widely distributed nature of the mast cell population throughout the human body [8, 9]. Two primary mast cell phenotypes have been identified and distinguished based on either their levels of both tryptase and chymase or by ultrastructural analysis [10, 11]. The MC_{TC} subset expresses both enzymes while the MC_T type expresses only tryptase. A single report of a third human mast cell phenotype containing only chymase remains to be confirmed [12]. Tryptase is the major protease expressed in either phenotype and along with chymase may represent up to 25% of the total protein content of the mast cell [13].

Mast cell activation by either IgE-dependent or IgE-independent stimuli affords the secretion of tryptase, along with other mediators, as a non-covalent, tetrameric assembly of four conserved monomers. Each monomer is of individual molecular mass in the range of 31–38 kDa, with roughly 70–110 kDa of the total enzyme mass attributable to glycosylation and heparin association [14–19]. In the absence of heparin and at neutral pH, the tetramer rapidly dissociates through a multi-step sequence affording enzymatically inactive monomers [20, 21]. The general resistance of tryptase activity to inhibition by endogenous circulating protease inhibitors suggests that this dissociative mechanism may play a significant role in insuring the regulation of tryptase activity *in vivo*.

The recently solved crystal structure of β-tryptase provides insight into the enzyme's unique substrate specificity and resistance to endogenous inhibitors [22]. A central cavity on the tetramer surface, which contains the active site domain, has limited accessibility due to the proximity and arrangement of adjacent monomers.

High Throughput Screening for Novel Anti-Inflammatories, edited by M. Kahn
© 2000 Birkhäuser Verlag Basel/Switzerland

This structural feature limits the substrate family to small, conformationally flexible peptides and to proteins that can project cleavable surface loops into the active site cavity. The active site domain of the tetramer features a unique assembly of four functional S1 sites, contributed by each of the four monomers. The individual S_1 sites are defined by monomer Asp^{189} residues positioned at the base of two peptide planes comprised of residues 215-216 and 190-192. The thermodynamically favorable salt-bridge interaction of an organic nitrogen base conjugate acid with the side chain carboxylate oxygens of Asp^{189}, and the size of the S_1 pocket, allows for the weak inhibition of tryptase by a range of simple amines, amidines and guanidines, and accounts for the tendency of tryptase to cleave substrates at the C-terminus of Arg and Lys residues. Early structure determination efforts focused on the construction of active site monomer models based on trypsin homology, however, the successful application of such models to inhibitor design has not been realized since they are not predictive of the active tetramer structure [23]. Despite this fact, such models correctly predict the close analogy of the S_1 specificity pockets of tryptase and trypsin. Indeed, both proteases demonstrate a similar preference for simple organic nitrogen bases at S_1. For example, phenylguanidine, benzamidine, and benzylamine are all weakly active and competitive inhibitors of both tryptase and trypsin.

Although very limited knowledge of the active tryptase structure has been available during recent years, the discovery and optimization of lower molecular weight peptidic and non-peptidic inhibitors of tryptase has been achieved at Axys Pharmaceuticals, Inc. through the systematic development of a structure-activity relationship (SAR) database and the application of a proprietary zinc-mediated inhibitor design technology. The availability of these novel, highly potent and selective inhibitors, described herein, should significantly impact the continued understanding of the pathophysiology of this unique serine protease as well as provide opportunities for the future development of new and effective drugs for the treatment of tryptase-mediated diseases.

Pathological functions of tryptase

In broad terms, the scope of biological functions and the corresponding physiological consequences of tryptase proteolytic activity *in vivo* is defined by its substrate specificity, regulation, and by the complex distribution of mast cells throughout the body. Researchers have identified a number of endogenous substrates, which may be classified into the following general types; neuropeptides, other proteases and zymogen proteins, and cell surface receptors. Independently, the development of a sensitive and specific radio-immunoassay for tryptase has allowed for detection of the enzyme in a variety of complex biological media, including serum, urine, nasal and bronchoalveolar lavage, cerebrospinal fluid and tears [24–30]. While a direct correlation of these and more recent clinical observations to specific proteolytic activities of tryptase remains to be achieved, a knowledge of the endogenous substrates of this enzyme provides insight into the potential scope of tryptase pathological function in allergic and inflammatory disease.

Neuropeptides

The potent bronchodilating neuropeptides, vasoactive intestinal peptide (VIP) and peptide histidine methionine (PHM), are readily cleaved by tryptase *in vitro*, however, the bronchoconstricting peptide, substance P, is not [31–34]. Calcitonin gene related peptide (CGRP), a potent vasodilator *in vivo* as well as a bronchoconstrictor *in vitro*, is similarly cleaved by tryptase [35, 36]. While the degradation of VIP, PHM and CGRP have been proposed as potential mechanisms by which tryptase might enhance bronchoconstriction, the physiological relevance of these mechanisms in the context of asthma pathology remains in question. However, the close association of mast cells with nerve tissue and blood vessels suggests that tryptase-mediated neuropeptide cleavage may indeed have physiological relevance. For instance, CGRP has been shown to have a protective effect against gastric ulceration [37–39]. As a result, the cleavage of CGRP by tryptase could be relevant to the development and progression of some gastrointestinal inflammatory diseases. Recently, a correlation between intestine mucosal mast cell concentration and gastritis in humans has been reported [40], although a connection to CGRP cleavage activity was not made.

Proteases and zymogen proteins

One of the first proteolytic activities demonstrated for tryptase is the cleavage of fibrinogen, leading to the loss of thrombin-induced blood clotting [41–43]. Tryptase has been shown to cleave fibrinogen at specific positions along both the α and β chains of fibronogen with similar efficacy. β-Chain cleavage takes place primarily at Lys^{21}, resulting in the removal of a key thrombin cleavage site at Arg^{14} and the fragmentation of a DKKREE sequence, a critical fibrin polymerization site [44]. α-Chain cleavage takes place initially at Arg^{572}, resulting in the removal of an endothelial cell-recognizing RGD sequence defined by residues 572-574. Thus, tryptase may block integrin αvβ3 mediated endothelial cell binding to fibrin, and as a result, promote capillary tube formation. Such a role for tryptase is supported by recent studies conducted by Gruber et al. who reported that significant angiogenic activity in a human mast cell line (HMC-1) and human dermal microvascular endothelial cell (HDMEC) co-culture could be attenuated, by up to 80%, by pretreatment with tryptase inhibitors [45]. While blood vessel formation is an essential feature of normal tissue growth and wound healing [46, 47], Gruber has suggested that tryptase mediated angiogenic activity may also function in the progression of some pathological conditions associated with vascular proliferation, including tumor growth, rheumatoid arthritis, and diabetic retinopathy.

Single-chain urinary type plasminogen activator (uPA or urokinase) is a serine protease indirectly implicated in the degradation and remodeling of extracellular matrix and is activated by tryptase *in vitro* [48]. Once activated, the cleavage of plasminogen by uPA affords the matrix degrading enzyme plasmin. Though the physiological importance of the tryptase-mediated pathway relative to alternative proteolytic routes remains unclear, the above observation provides a link between mast cell tryptase activity and the pathology of aberrant matrix degradation, cell migration and invasion.

Another pathway by which tryptase may promote extracellular matrix degradation is through the activation of matrix metalloproteases. In this case, the cleavage of prostromolysin (pro-matrix metalloprotease-3 or proMMP-3) by tryptase would result in the degradation proteoglycans, fibronectin and laminin as well as type IV and type IX collagen. Gruber et al. demonstrated that synovial procollagenase is activated by tryptase *in vitro*, and furthermore, that this process is entirely dependent upon the activation of MMP-3 [49, 50]. More recent studies by Sepper et al. demonstrated a potential connection between tryptase activation of pro-matrix metalloprotease-8 and bronchiectasis, a chronic lung disorder characterized by degradation of airway and lung tissue extracellular matrix [51]. In this study, a comparison of the bronchoalveolar lavage (BAL) fluid from subjects with bronchiectasis and healthy controls showed a strong correlation of tryptase activity with endogenous collagenase activation. Independently, tryptase has been shown to cleave 72 kDa gelatinase, fibronectin and intact type IV collagen microfibrils [52, 53], suggesting that tryptase may also function directly in the turnover of extracellular matrix.

The ability of tryptase to act as a kininogenase has been more controversial. Initially it was reported that tryptase did not generate bradykinin from either high molecular weight kininogen (HMWK) or low molecular weight kininogen (LMWK) and in related studies tryptase was also unable to convert either plasma prekallikrein or urinary prekallikrein to active kallikrein [54–56]. However, more recent independent studies by both Proud and Walls contradict these observations [57–59]. Clearly, the ability to generate bradykinin, through either a direct or indirect pathway, could be an important component of tryptase-mediated inflammatory activity, particularly in the lung [60].

Cell surface receptors

An additional substrate target for tryptase is the protease-activated receptor 2 (PAR-2), a G-protein-coupled receptor which is the second member identified in a growing family of cell surface receptors. Like the thrombin receptor (PAR-1), PAR-2 is activated by either proteolytic release of a tethered ligand from the N-terminus of the receptor, or by direct interaction of the receptor with peptides that mimic the newly generated N-terminus [61, 62]. PAR-2 is a tissue- and cell-specific receptor associated with several human cell lines, including vascular endothelial cells, keratinocytes, intestinal epithelial cells, and colonic myocytes [63–66]. Currently, tryptase and trypsin are the only two proteases known to activate PAR-2 [67], however, given the limited biodistribution of trypsin, only activation by tryptase may be of physiological relevance. The activation of this receptor is associated primarily with the induction of a mitogenic response [63, 68–70].

Tryptase, as well as the PAR-2 activating peptide SLIGRL, have measurable effects on human fibroblasts, including the stimulation of cell proliferation and collagen m-RNA synthesis, as well as the induction of fibroblast chemotaxis [71–73]. Though the importance of these observations *in vivo* is unclear at present, the data at hand suggests that tryptase may play a role in the early stages and progression of fibrotic disease. Fibrotic disease, or fibrosis, is a characteristic feature of chronic inflammation and is defined by the progressive accumulation of extracellular matrix collagen [74]. Diseases of this type include fibrotic lung disease, scleroderma, atherosclerosis and related cardiomyopathic disorders, some of which have a direct association with mast cell activity and hyperplasia at specific tissue sites [75–77].

The ability of tryptase to stimulate eosinophil and neutrophil chemotaxis and degranulation *in vitro* and in animal models is well documented [78–82], and provides a compelling link to the proteolytic activity of this enzyme and human asthma, a recently reviewed subject [83–85]. Additional asthma related findings include the potent mitogenic activity of tryptase on airway smooth muscle cells and epithelial cells *in vitro*, as well as the activation of epithelial cell interleukin-8 (IL-8) release and the associated up-regulation of ICAM-1 [86–88]. These findings are consistent with the tissue hyperplasia observed in the airways of asthmatic patients and suggest the possible involvement of a tryptase-mediated PAR-2 activation pathway. Most notably, the ability of tryptase to directly stimulate mast cell degranulation *in vitro* and in animal models suggests further that a tryptase-mediated amplification mechanism of the allergic inflammatory response may also operate *in vivo* [89, 90].

Inhibitors of tryptase

Although the rational design of potent tryptase inhibitors based solely on a detailed knowledge of the active enzyme structure has not been realized in recent years, several unique inhibitors of the enzyme have been reported. In general terms, the known tryptase inhibitors can be classified into four general types; peptides or modified peptides, zinc-mediated inhibitors, synthetic dibasic inhibitors, and heparin antagonists. The latter two classes of inhibitors take advantage of unique structural features of the active tetrameric enzyme and as a result are typically exquisitely selective for tryptase over related proteases.

Peptidic inhibitors

APC-366 is an N-terminal acylated dipeptide derivative, $RC(O)$-Arg-Pro-NH_2, where R is 1-hydroxynaphthylene-2-yl. This optimized peptidic inhibitor is proposed to bind tryptase and related trypsin-like proteases through interaction of the arginyl side chain with the S1 pocket Asp189, with the flanking residues occupying the prime and non-prime sides of the substrate cleft, although the preferred orientation is unknown. SAR studies around APC-366 indicate that a free hydroxyl group on the N-terminal aroyl ring is required for potency. However, a range of aromatic permutations are tolerated with variable activity loss [91, 92]. At the C-terminus an unsubstituted (L)-prolinamide moiety is preferred. Characteristic of APC-366 inhibition *in vitro*, is a pronounced time-dependent onset of potency. The free hydroxyl group on the naphthyl ring appears to be a structural necessity for the time-dependence. At very short incubation times the K_i' of APC-366 is 450 μM, but after 3 h of preincubation with tryptase, a K_i' value of 330 nM is obtained. The time-dependence is due to a kinetically slow and irreversible multi-step inhibition mechanism, in which (presumably an active site) nucleophile adds to the inhibitor hydroxynaphthoyl ring, leading to the formation of a covalent derivative of the enzyme [93]. Unrelated mechanism-based inhibitors for trypsin-like proteases are known [94], however the extension of such approaches to tryptase inhibition has not been reported.

In a previously published study, APC-366 effectively prevented the late airway responses in allergic sheep when delivered by aerosol [95]. However, the most direct evidence for the involvement of tryptase proteolytic activity in human asthma pathology has been obtained by Axys Pharmaceuticals, Inc. using the tryptase inhibitor APC-366 in clinical studies. A recent phase IIa study was conducted with 16 mild asthmatics who were dosed with either placebo or a nebulized formulation of the tryptase inhibitor [96]. When treated with APC-366, patients had a statistically significant improvement in the mean area under the curve for the late airway response of 33% ($\rho = 0.012$) and a mean maximum fall in FEV1 (forced expiratory volume in 1 s) of 21% ($\rho = 0.007$) for LAR (late airway hyperresponsiveness), as compared to the results from the same patients treated with placebo.

Dibasic inhibitors

The presence of an acidic surface loop in the active site region of tryptase, comprised of residues Asp[143] and Asp[147], and the unique pseudo 222 symmetry of the active tryptase tetramer, which places the individual active sites within a close proximity (20–40 Å) of one another, suggests that relatively simple dibasic structures with C_2 symmetry may have potent tryptase inhibitory activity. Thus, one end of the inhibitor would anchor in the S_1 pocket of one active site, and the second base would interact with either an acidic surface loop or a second monomer active site S_1 pocket. Indeed, a number of small dibasic inhibitors have been independently reported by Sommerhoff and Tidwell including pentamidine, (1), 2,5-bis-(3-amidinobenzylidene)-cyclopentanone (BABCP), (2), and [1,1',3',1'']terphenyl-3,3''-dicarbamidinium (TPDCA), (3) (see Tab. 1). Compounds of this class are generally only modestly active tryptase inhibitors with K_i values in the low micromolar range [97, 98]. This family of inhibitors, is proposed to interact with tryptase at both the active site S_1 pocket and at an acidic surface loop defined by residues Asp[143]-Asp[147] [23]. Inhibitors of this type, including leech-derived tryptase inhibitor (LDTI) [99], which is proposed to interact with the same tryptase acidic loop through its Lys[1]-Lys[2] N-terminus, are generally not selective for tryptase, presumably due to the presence of similar loops near the active site of related proteases such as trypsin.

A novel series of far more potent and selective dibasic inhibitors of human tryptase have been synthesized at Axys Pharmaceuticals, Inc. using longer nitrogen base linking scaffolds that are in the range of 20 Å in length as an extended conformer. This class of inhibitors is tight-binding and inhibits tryptase with a four to one stoichiometry (i.e. one inhibitor per enzyme active site), suggesting that an active site bridging mode of binding may not be operative. Compound (4) is a representative tryptase inhibitor in this series, which is selective versus trypsin and related proteases by nearly a factor of 10^5. The inhibitor utilizes a flexible peptide-like scaffold of C_2 symmetry to link two benzylamine nitrogen bases. Compound (4) has a K_i value of 3.0 nM, while the corresponding asymmetric analog, which lacks only a second aminomethyl group, is over 10^3-fold less potent [91]. This observation suggests that the free energy of inhibitor binding in this series is primarily due to specific interactions of the two basic termini with tryptase.

A closely related series of dibasic tryptase inhibitors, which retains the optimal extended conformer length is exemplified by benzylamine (5). This glycine derived inhibitor, which differs only in the replacement of the internal amide bond with a carbamate linkage, has a sub-nanomolar K_i value and is extremely selective over trypsin. Overall, the SAR in both benzylamine inhibitor classes illustrates a general trend of increasing intolerance for substitution along the scaffold on proceeding from the central arene to the terminal nitrogen base [91]. In an analogous phenylguanidine series, substitution of the central arene with unsubstituted alicyclic functionality, as in the case of cyclooctylene analog (6), is well tolerated and affords a slight improvement in potency over similar inhibitors of this type.

As an additional modification to the scaffold, we focused on replacement of the external amide linkage in lead cyclooctylene analog (6). The piperazine ring was

Table 1 - Dibasic inhibitor SAR

Compound		Inhibitory activity K_i (μM)	
		Tryptase	Trypsin
1[a]	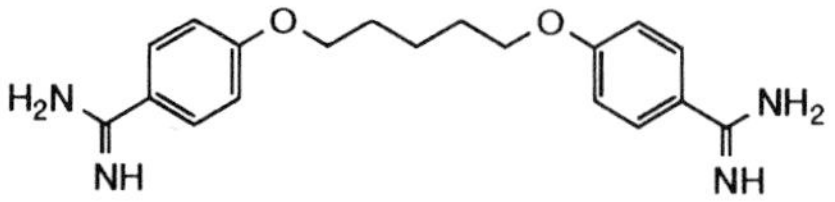	1.2	2.3
2[b]	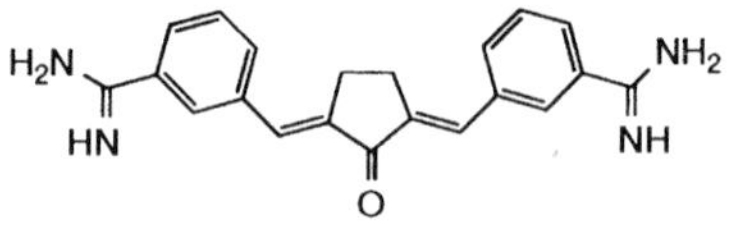	0.92	0.63
3[c]	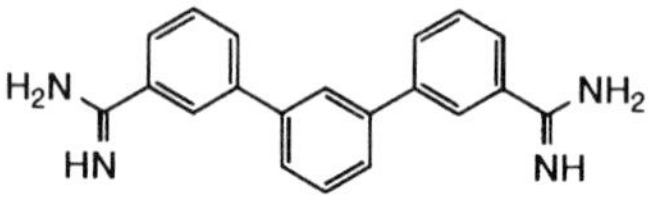	0.85	n.d.
4[d]	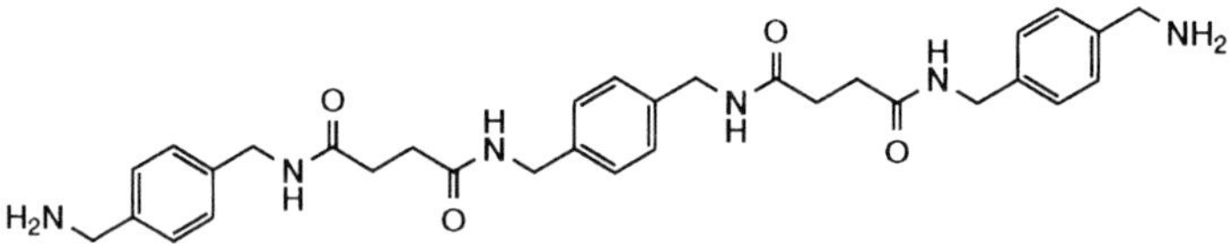	0.003	237
5[d]	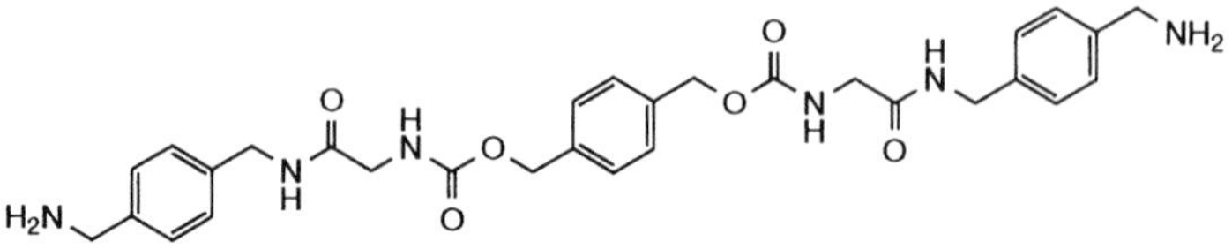	0.0006	84
6[d]	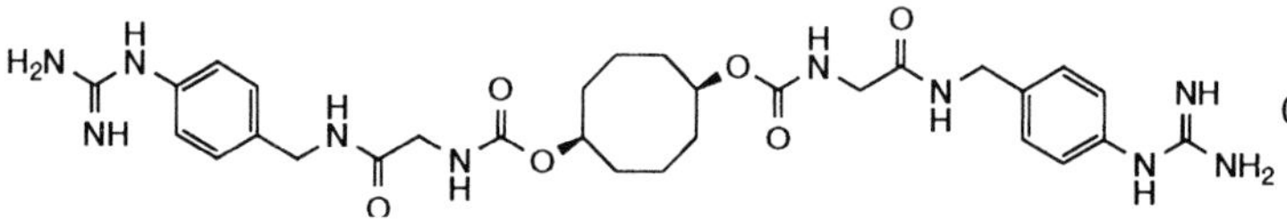	0.002	78

[a]Caughy et al. [98]; [b]Stürzebecher et al. [97]; [c]Stubbs et al. [99]; [d]Rice et al. [91]

chosen as a conformationally rigid glycyl mimetic which would serve to introduce a urea linkage in place of the external amide. Table 2 summarizes the *in vitro* activity and selectivity for this optimized series. For lead arylguanidine (7) a K_i' value of 0.07 nM was measured, with selectivity over trypsin approaching 10^6-fold. Replace-

Table 2 - Dibasic inhibitor SAR

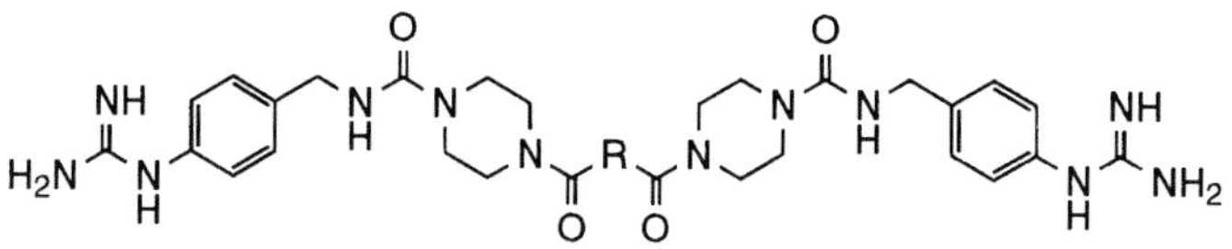

Compound	R	Inhibitory activity K_i (μM)	
		Tryptase	Trypsin
7	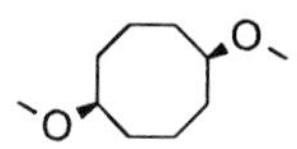 (structure)	0.00007[a]	38.9
8	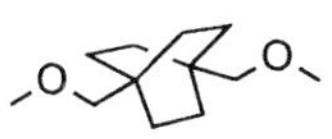 (structure)	0.0004	19.8
9	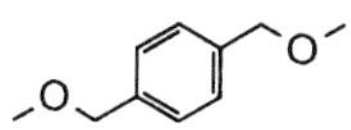 (structure)	0.0004	16.9
10	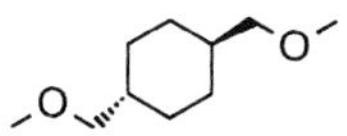 (structure)	0.0034	28.1
11	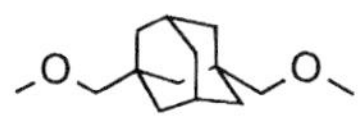 (structure)	0.0122	16.6
12	$-(CH_2)_4-$	0.044	54.1
13	$-(CH_2)_5-$	0.004	51.5
14	$-(CH_2)_6-$	0.0001	34.3
15	$-(CH_2)_7-$	0.0005	29.4
16	$-(CH_2)_8-$	0.0007	20.3

[a]K_i value for this tight binding inhibitor was calculated from the apparent dissociation constant obtained from a replot of IC_{50} values (ordinate) versus tryptase concentration (abscissa) measured at variable inhibitor and tryptase concentrations.

ment of the central cyclooctylene with alternative alicyclic, aliphatic and aromatic functionality is well tolerated in this series. The most potent examples are the relatively rigid and extended [2.2.2]bicyclooctylene and aromatic analogs (8) and (9), which should disfavor hydrophobic collapse of the inhibitor scaffold in a polar environment. Significant tolerance for steric bulk is also apparent in the central alkylene region, as illustrated by adamantane derivative (11). Of particular interest is the diacid derived series exemplified by inhibitors (12–16). On proceeding from the four methylene linker (12) to the six methylene homologue (14), a greater than 100-fold improvement in activity is obtained. Increasing the chain length further is tolerated without a significant loss in activity. Surprisingly, these relatively flexible inhibitors are similar in potency to the alicyclic and aromatic analogs.

Zinc-mediated inhibitors

The discovery of a novel approach to the design of serine protease inhibitors has recently been reported by Katz et al. in which the inhibitor interacts with the catalytic Ser[195] and His[57] residues through an intermediary divalent zinc ion (Tab. 3) [100]. BABIM [bis-(5-amidino-2-benzimidazolyl)methane] is an example of such an inhibitor. In analogy to simple benzamidine, BABIM (17) interacts with Asp[189] in the S_1 pocket of both tryptase and trypsin. However, the heterocyclic core of the inhibitor forms a distorted tetrahedral zinc ion complex just outside the S_1 pocket with Ser[195] and His[57]. This zinc-mediated inhibition mechanism is entirely suppressed in the presence of an excess of the metal-chelating agent ethylenediaminetetraacetic acid (EDTA). This zinc-dependence helps explain the SAR data of Caughey and Tidwell [98], because even trace concentrations of ambient zinc ion will enhance the *in vitro* potency of these inhibitors substantially.

The K_i of BABIM for tryptase is 0.005 μM in the presence of zinc ion but only 2.5 μM in the presence of EDTA. The EDTA value corresponds closely to the K_i values obtained for the related dibasic inhibitors of Stürzebecher and Sommerhoff [97], which are incapable of metal chelation. In the presence of zinc ion, BABIM is nearly 102 fold selective for tryptase over trypsin. However, the selectivity is diminished to nearly ten-fold in the absence of zinc ion. The asymmetric ketone analog (18), which lacks the second amidine moiety of BABIM, has a similar dependence on zinc ion for potent inhibition, but loses its tryptase selectivity over trypsin. In this case, removal of the second amidine to give the parent bis-(1*H*-benzimidazol-2-yl)methanone (19), results in a complete loss of activity for the trypsin-like proteases with or without zinc ion present.

This zinc-mediated technology is applicable to a range of serine protease targets, including tryptase, and represents a new approach to the design of serine protease inhibitors. Using this technology, we have recently designed a BABIM analog which is extremely potent and entirely selective for tryptase. In general, appropriate func-

Table 3 - Zinc-dependent inhibitor SAR

| Inhibitory activity[a,b] | Inhibitory activity K_i (μM) | | | |
| | Zn²⁺ | | EDTA | |
Compound	Tryptase	Trypsin	Tryptase	Trypsin
17	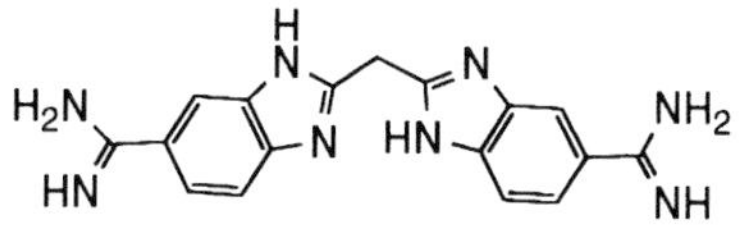 0.005	0.09	2.5	18.8
18	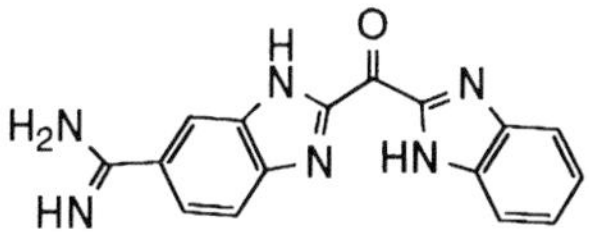 0.05	0.005	5.7	87.5
19	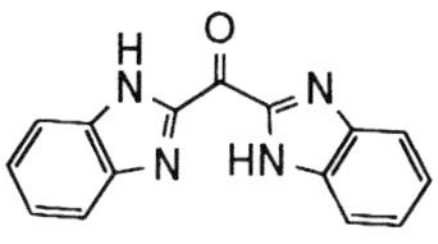 >1000	>1000	>1000	>1000

[a]*Zinc assay carried out with 150 μM Zn^{2+} present;* [b]*Non-zinc assay carried out with 10 mM EDTA present.*

tionalization of the chelating heterocyclic "master key" allows for optimization of both potency and selectivity for a targeted enzyme.

Heparin antagonists

Another strategy that we have employed for the design of human tryptase inhibitors takes advantage of the heparin-dependence of tryptase activity. In theory, the irreversible inhibition of tryptase can be realized *in vitro* by agents that compete with tryptase for heparin. We initially focused on the cationic protein neutrophil lactoferrin as such a heparin antagonist, because it binds heparin tightly, and following its release from activated neutrophils, may regulate tryptase activity *in vivo*. We demonstrated that lactoferrin disrupts the quarternary structure of tryptase *in vitro* by competing heparin away from the enzymatically active tetramer. Lactoferrin selectively inhibits tryptase with a K_i' of 24 nM and when delivered by aerosol, blocks both late phase bronchoconstriction and airway hyperresponsiveness in an allergic sheep model of asthma [101].

Dibasic inhibitor synthesis

As illustrated in Figure 1, the synthesis of benzylamine (**4**), representative of this dibasic inhibitor series, is straightforward. Initial reaction of a two-fold excess of methyl succinyl chloride with *p*-xylylenediamine (**20**) affords the intermediate diester (**22**). Subsequent mild thermolysis in the presence of an excess of *p*-xylylene-diamine at 40 °C then yields the desired oligomer directly with minimal contamination by higher polymers. Alternatively, the external amide formation step may be carried out using 4-aminobenzylamine to provide an aniline. In this case, preferential acylation of the benzylamine nitrogen selectively generates the desired anilines. Direct guanylation of the aniline hydrochloride with cyanamide [102], or reaction with 1-*H*-pyrazole-1-[N,N'-bis(*tert*-butoxycarbonyl)]carboxamidine [103], followed by deprotection in the latter case, affords the corresponding phenylguanidine analog. Synthesis of the carbamate linking inhibitors may be carried out conveniently through the initial reaction of chloroformate (**21**) [104], or the corresponding alicyclic equivalent, with a two-fold excess of glycine methyl ester followed by direct benzylamine condensation as before.

Synthesis of the piperazine linked dibasic tryptase inhibitors may also be carried out straightforwardly using an alternative approach. For example, initial conversion of *tert*-butyl 1-piperazine carboxylate to the corresponding carbamyl chloride (**25**), followed by reaction with 4-guanidinobenzylamine [105], gives intermediate phenylguanidine (**26**). BOC-deprotection, followed by reaction with cis-1,5-cyclooctanediol dichloroformate, provides the phenylguanidine (**7**) directly. Carbamate formations of this type may be carried out efficiently without guanidine protection so long as the reaction pH is maintained below 10. In the case of (**7**), the final coupling step may be carried out in buffered aqueous THF at pH 7–8. This general approach is also useful for the preparation of analogs (**8–16**) by substitution of the appropriate chloroformate or acid chloride in the coupling step with guanidine (**26**). For [2.2.2]bicyclooctylene and adamantane analogs (**8**) and (**11**) the starting diols were prepared by reduction of the corresponding diester or diacid [106, 107].

Summary

Recent biological and clinical data strongly implicate tryptase as a key regulatory enzyme in the development and progression of both chronic and acute allergic, inflammatory, and immunological diseases, and as a potentially important target for therapeutic intervention. Research efforts at Axys Pharmaceuticals, Inc. have focused on the discovery of new potent and selective tryptase inhibitors that will help further define the role of tryptase in various diseases and provide leads for the clinical development of new pharmaceuticals. Significant advances in the under-

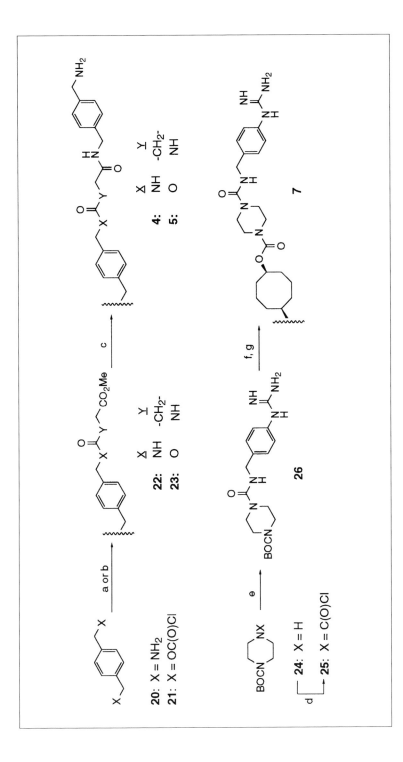

Figure 1

Synthetic approaches to dibasic inhibitors.

Reagents: (a) methyl succinyl chloride, diisopropylethylamine, CH$_2$Cl$_2$, 0°C; (b) glycine methyl ester, diisopropylethylamine, CH$_2$Cl$_2$, −78°C; (c) p-xylylenediamine, 40°C; (d) triphosgene, pyridine, CH$_2$Cl$_2$, 0°C; (e) 4-guanidinobenzylamine HCl, diisopropylethylamine, CH$_2$Cl$_2$, MeOH; (f) TFA; (g) cis-1,5cyclooctanediol bis-chloroformate, aq. THF, pH 7–8.

standing of critical tryptase-inhibitor interactions, as well as the independently solved crystal structure of tetrameric tryptase, should further aid in the continued design of novel inhibitors of this enzyme. These advancements offer promise for the future availability of safe and effective drugs for the treatment of both chronic and acute mast cell-mediated disorders.

Acknowledgements

The authors wish to thank Chuck Johnson and Kerry Spear for the synthesis of APC-366 and analogs, Elaine Kuo, Robert Lum, Tony Gangloff, Jeff Dener and Vivian Wang for the synthesis of dibasic tryptase inhibitors, Daun Putnam and Robert Warne for assay data, Heinz Gschwend and Mike Venuti for project direction, and Bayer AG for their support of tryptase research at Axys Pharmaceuticals, Inc.

References

1   Jacobi HH, Skov PS, Kampen GT, Poulsen LK, Reimert CM, Bindslev-Jensen C, Praetorius C, Malling HJ, Mygind N (1998) Histamine and tryptase in nasal lavage fluid following challenge with methacholine and allergen. *Clin Exp Allergy* 28: 83–91

2   Turner G, Stevenson EC, Taylor R, Shields MD, Ennis M (1997) Histamine and tryptase in bronchoalveolar lavage fluid samples from asthmatic children. *Inflamm Res* 46 (1): S69–S70

3   Wilson SJ, Lau L, Howarth PH (1998) Inflammatory mediators in naturally occuring rhinitis. *Clin Exp Allergy* 28: 220–227

4   Di Lorenzo G, Mansueto P, Melluso M, Candore G, Colombo A, Pellitteri ME, Drago A, Potestio M, Caruso C (1997) Allergic rhinitis to glass pollen: Measurement of inflammatory mediators of mast cell and eosinophils in native nasal fluid lavage and in serum out of and during pollen season. *J Allergy Clin Immunol* 100: 832–836

5   Bonini S, Schiavone M, Bonini S, Magrini L, Lischetti P, Lambiase A, Bucci MG (1997) Efficacy of lodoxamide eye drops on mast cells and eosinophils after allergen challenge in allergic conjunctivitis. *Opthalmology* 104: 849–853

6   Fisher MM, Baldo BA (1998) Mast cell tryptase in anaesthetic anaphylactoid reactions. *Brit J Anaesthesia* 80: 26–29

7   Ordoqui E, Zubeldia JM, Aranzabal A, Rubio M, Herrero T, Tornero P, Rodriguez, VM, Prieto A, Baeza ML (1997) Serum tryptase levels in adverse drug reactions. *Allergy* 52: 1102–1105

8   Welle M (1997) Development, significance, and heterogeneity of mast cells with particular regard to the mast cell-specific proteases chymase and tryptase. *J Leukoc Biol* 61: 233–245

9   Yong LCJ (1997) The mast cell: origin, morphology, distribution, and function. *J Exp Toxic Pathol* 49: 409–424

10 Irani AA, Schechter NM, Craig SS, Deblois G, Shwartz LB (1986) Two types of human mast cells that have distinct neutral protease compositions. *Proc Natl Acad Sci USA* 83: 4464–4468

11 Craig SS, Schechter NM, Shwartz LB (1988) Ultrastructural analysis of human T and TC mast cells identified by immunoelectron microscopy. *Lab Invest* 58: 581–585

12 Weidner N, Austen KF (1993) Heterogeneity of mast cells at multiple body sites. Fluorescent determination of avidin binding and immunofluorescent determination of chymase, tryptase, and carboxypeptidase content. *Pathol Res Pract* 189: 156–162

13 Shwartz LB, Irani AA, Roller K, Castells MC, Schechter NM (1987) Quantitation of histamine, tryptase, and chymase in dispersed human T and TC mast cells. *J Immunol* 138: 2611–2615

14 Shwartz LB, Lewis RA, Austen KF (1981) Tryptase from human pulmonary mast cells. Purification and characterization. *J Biol Chem* 256: 11939–11943

15 Smith TJ, Hougland MW Johnson DA (1984) Human lung tryptase. *J Biol Chem* 259: 11046–11051

16 Shwartz LB, Bradford TR (1986) Regulation of tryptase from human lung mast cells by heparin: stabilization of the active tetramer. *J Biol Chem* 261: 7372–7379

17 Harvima IT, Schechter NM, Harvima RJ, Fräki JE (1988) Human skin tryptase: purification, partial characterization and comparison with human lung tryptase. *Biochim Biophys Acta* 957: 71–80

18 Cromlish JA, Siedah NG, Marcinkiewicz M, Hamelinm J, Johnson DA, Chretein M (1987) Human pituitary tryptase: molecular forms, NH_2-terminal sequence, immunocytochemical localization, and specificity with prohormone and fluorogenic substrates. *J Biol Chem* 262: 1363–1373

19 Butterfield JH, Weiler DA, Hunt LW, Wynn SR, Roche PC (1990) Purification of tryptase from a human mast cell line. *J Leukoc Biol* 47: 409–419

20 Shwartz LB, Bradford TR, Lee DC, Chlebowski JF (1990) Immunologic and physiochemical edivence for conformational changes occurring on conversion of human mast cell tryptase from active tetramer to inactive monomer. Production of monoclonal antibodies recognizing active tryptase. *J Immunol* 144: 2304–2311

21 Schechter NM, Grace YE, Darrell RM (1993) Human skin tryptase: kinetic characterization of its spontaneous inactivation. *Biochemistry* 32: 2617–2625

22 Barbosa Pereira PJ, Bergner A, Macedo-Ribeiro S, Huber R, Matschiner G, Fritz H, Sommerhoff CS, Bode W (1998) Human β-tryptase is a ring-like tetramer with active sites facing a central pore. *Nature* 392: 306–311

23 Di Marco S, Priestle JP (1997) Structure of the complex of leech-derived tryptase inhibitor (LDTI) with trypsin and modeling of the LDTI-tryptase system. *Structure* 5: 1465–1474

24 Wenzel S, Irani AA, Sanders JM, Bradford TR, Schwartz LB (1986) Immunoassay of tryptase from human mast cells. *J Immunol Methods* 86: 139–142

25 Enander I, Matsson P, Nystrand J et al (1991) A new radioimmunoassay for human mast cell tryptase using monoclonal antibodies. *J Immunol Methods* 138: 39–46

26 Schwartz LB, Metcalfe DD, Miller JS, Earl H, Sullivan T (1987) Tryptase levels as an indicator of mast-cell activation in systemic anaphylaxis and mastocytosis. *New Engl J Med* 316: 1622–1626

27 Wenzel SE, Fowler AA III, Schwartz LB (1988) Activation of pulmonary mast cells by bronchoalveolar allergen challenge: *in vivo* release of histamine and tryptase in atopic subjects with and without asthma. *Am Rev Respir Dis* 137: 1002–1008

28 Butrus SI, Ochsner KI, Abelson MB, Schwartz LB (1990) The level of tryptase in human tears: an indicator of activation of conjunctival mast cells. *Ophthalmology* 97: 1678–1683

29 Rozniecki JJ, Hauser SL, Stein M, Lincoln R, Theoharides TC (1995) Elevated mast cell tryptase in cerebrospinal fluid of multiple sclerosis patients. *Ann Neurol* 37: 63–66

30 Haak-Frendscho M, Okragly A, Niles A, Schmidt D, Moon TD, Jarrard DF, Uehling DT, Saban R (1998) Elevated NT-3, NGF, GDNF and tryptase levels in the urine of bladder cancer and interstitial cystitis patients. *FASEB J* 12: A596

31 Tam EK, Caughey GH (1990) Degradation of airway neuropeptides by human lung tryptase. *Am J Respir Cell Mol Biol* 3: 27–32

32 Lilly CM, Martins MA, Drazen JM (1993) Peptidase modulation of vasoactive intestinal peptide pulmonary relaxation in tracheal superfused guinea pig lungs. *J Clin Invest* 91: 235–243

33 Franconi GM, Graf PD, Lazarus SC, Nadel JA, Caughey GH (1989) Mast cell tryptase and chymase reverse airway smooth muscle relaxation induced by vasoactive intestinal peptide in the ferret. *J Pharmacol Exp Ther* 248: 947–951

34 Church MK, Lowman MA, Rees PH, Benyon RC (1989) Plenary lecture: mast cells, neuropeptides and inflammation. *Agents Actions* 27: 8–16

35 Walls AF, Brain SD, Desai A, Jose PJ, Hawkings E, Church MK, Williams TJ (1992) Human mast cell tryptase attenutes the vasodilatory activity of calcitonin gene-related peptide. *Biochem Pharmacol* 43: 1243–1248

36 Rosenfeld MG, Mermod JJ, Amara SG, Swanson LW, Sawchenko PE, Rivier J, Vala WW, Evans RM (1983) Production of a novel neuropeptide encoded by the calcitonin gene via tissue specific RNA processing. *Nature* 304: 129–135

37 Gray JL, Bunnett NW, Orloff SL, Mulvihill SJ, Debas HT (1994) A role for calcitonin gene-related peptide in protection against gastric ulceration. *Ann Surgery* 219: 58–64

38 Tache Y, Pappas T, Lauffenburger M, Goto Y, Walsh JH, Debas H (1984) Calcitonin gene-related peptide: Potent peripheral inhibitor of gastric acid secretion in rats and dogs. *Gastroenterology* 87: 344–349

39 Bauerfeind P, Hoff R, Hoff A et al (1989) Effects of hCGRP I and II on gastric blood flow and acid secretion in anesthetized rabbits. *Amer J Physiol* 256: G145–149

40 Beil WJ, Schultz M, McEuen AR, Buckley MG, Walls AF (1997) Number, fixation properties, dye-binding and protease expression of duodenal mast cells: Comparisons

between healthy subjects and patients with gastritis or Crohn's disease. *Histochemical J* 29: 759–773

41   Schwartz LB, Bradford TR, Littman BH, Wintroub BU (1985) The fibrinogenolytic activity of purified tryptase from human lung mast cells. *J Immunol* 135: 2762–2767

42   Ren S, Lawson AE, Carr M, Baumgarten CM, Schwartz LB (1997) Human tryptase fibronogenolysis is optimal at acidic pH and generates anticoagulant fragments in the presence of the anti-tryptase monoclonal antibody B12. *J Immunol* 159: 3540–3548

43   Thomas VA, Wheeless CJ, Stack MS, Johnson DA Human mast cell tryptase fibrinogenolysis: kinetics, anticoagulation mechanism, and cell adhesion disruption. *Biochemistry* 37: 2291–2298

44   Hsieh KH (1997) Localization of an effective fibrin β-chain polymerization site: implications for the polymerization mechanism. *Biochemistry* 36: 9381–9387

45   Blair RJ, Meng H, Marchese MJ, Ren S, Schwartz LB, Tonnesen MG, Gruber BL (1997) Human mast cells stimulate vascular tube formation. Tryptase is a novel, potent angiogenic factor. *J Clin Invest* 99: 2691–2700

46   Brooks P, Clark RAF, Cheresh, DA (1994) Requirement of vascular integrin $\alpha v \beta 3$ for angiogenesis. *Science* 264: 569–571

47   Findaly JK (1986) Angiogenesis in reproductive tissues. *J Endocrinol* 111: 357–366

48   Stack MS, Johnson DA (1994) Human mast cell tryptase activates single-chain urinary-type plasminogen activator (pro-urokinase). *J Biol Chem* 269: 9416–9419

49   Gruber BL, Marchese MJ, Suzuki K, Schwartz LB, Okada Y, Nagase H, Ramamurthy NS (1989) Synovial procollagenase activation by human mast cell tryptase dependence upon matrix metalloproteinase 3 activation. *J Clin Invest* 84: 1657–1662

50   Gruber BL, Schwartz LB, Ramamurthy NS, Irani A, Marchese MJ (1988) Activation of latent rheumatoid synovial collagenase by human mast cell tryptase. *J Immunol* 140: 3936–3942

51   Sepper R, Konttinen YT, Buo L, Eklund KK, Lauhio A, Sorsa T, Tschesche H, Aasen AO, Sillastu H (1997) Potentiative effects of neutral proteinases in an inflamed lung: relationship of neutrophil procollagenase (proMMP-8) to plasmin, cathepsin G and tryptase in bronchiectasis *in vivo. Eur Respir J* 10: 2788–2793

52   Lohi J, Harvima I, Keski-Oja J (1992) Pericellular substrates of human mast cell tryptase: 72,000 dalton gelatinase and fibronectin. *J Cell Biochem* 50: 337–349

53   Kielty CM, Lees M, Shuttleworth A, Woolley D (1993) Catabolism of intact type VI collagen microfibrils: Susceptibility to degradation by serine proteinases. *Biochem Biophys Res Commun* 191: 1230–1236

54   Maier M, Spragg J, Schwartz LB (1983) Inactivation of human high molecular weight kininogen by mast cell tryptase. *J Immunol* 130: 2352–2356

55   Schwartz LB, Bradford TR, Griffin JH (1985) The effect of tryptase from human mast cells on human prekallikrein. *Biochem Biophys Res Commun* 129: 76–81

56   Alter SC, Yates P, Margolius HS, Schwartz LB (1987) Tryptase and kinin generation: tryptase from human mast cells does not activate human urinary prekallikrein. *Int Archs Allergy Appl Immunol* 83: 321–324

57 Proud D, Siekierski ES, Bailey GS (1988) Identification of human lung mast cell kininogenase as tryptase and relevance of tryptase kininogenase activity. *Biochem Pharmacol* 37: 1473–1480

58 Walls AF, Bennett AR, Sueiras-Dias J, Olsson H (1992) The kininogenase activity of human mast cell tryptase. *Biochem Soc Trans* 22: 260S

59 Imamura T, Dubin A, Moore W, Tanaka R, Travis J (1996) Induction of vascular permeability enhancement by human tryptase: dependence on activation of prekallikrein and direct release of bradykinin from kininogens. *Lab Invest* 74: 861–870

60 Abraham WM, Burch RM, Farmer SG et al (1991) A bradykinin antagonist modifies allergen-induced mediator release and late bronchial responses in sheep. *Am Rev Respir Dis* 143: 787–796

61 Nystedt S, Emilsson K, Wahlestedt C, Sundelin J (1994) Molecular cloning of a potential proteinase activated receptor. *Proc Natl Acad Sci USA* 91: 9208–9212

62 Bohm SK, Kong WY, Bromme D, Smeekens SP, Anderson DC, Connolly A, Kahn M, Nelken NA, Coughlin RS, Payan DG, Bunnett NW (1996) Molecular cloning, expression and potential functions of the human proteinase-activated receptor-2. *Biochem J* 314: 1009–1016

63 Mirza H, Yatsula V, Bahou WF (1996) The proteinase activated receptor (PAR-2) mediates mitogenic responses in human vascular endothelial cells. Molecular characterization and evidence for functional coupling to the thrombin receptor. *J Clin Invest* 97: 1705–1714

64 Santulli RJ, Derian CK, Darrow AL, Tomko KA, Eckardt AJ, Seilbarg M, Scarborough RM, Andrade-Gordon P (1995) Evidence for the presence of a protease-activated receptor distinct from the thrombin receptor in human keratinocytes. *Proc Natl Acad Sci USA* 92: 9151–9155

65 Schechter NM, Barnathan ES, Brass LF, Lavker RM, Jensen PJ (1997) Mast cell protease activation of protease activated receptor 2 (PAR-2) on human keratinocytes. *J Invest Dermatol* 108: 618

66 Corvera CU, Dery O, McConalogue K, Khitin L, Böhm SK, Kong W, Raymond W, Caughy GH, Bunnett NW (1997) Mast cell tryptase regulates colonic myocytes through proteinase-activated receptor-2 (PAR-2). *Gastroenterology* 112: A1140

67 Fox MT, Harriott P, Walker B, Stone SR (1997) Identification of potential activators of proteinase-activated receptor-2. *FEBS Letters* 417: 267–269

68 Mirza H, Schmidt VA, Derian CK, Jesty J, Bahou WF (1997) Mitogenic responses mediated through the proteinase-activated receptor-2 are induced by expressed forms of mast cell α- or β-tryptases. *Blood* 90: 3914–2922

69 Molino M, Barnathan ES, Numerof R, Clark J, Dreyer M, Cumashi A, Hoxie JA, Schechter N, Woolkalis M, Brass LF (1997) Interactions of mast cell tryptase with thrombin receptors and PAR-2. *J Biol Chem* 272: 4043–4049

70 Mirza H, Schmidt V, Jesty J, Bahou WF (1997) Proteinase-activated receptor-2 (PAR-2)-mediated mitogenic responses are induced by human mast cell tryptases. *J Am Coll Cardiology* 29: 484A

71 Gruber BA, Kew RR, Jelaska A, Marchese MJ, Garlick J, Ren S, Schwartz LB, Korn JH (1997) Human mast cells active fibroblasts: Tryptase is a fibrogenic factor stimulating collagen messenger ribonucleic acid synthesis and fibroblast chemotaxis. *J Immunol* 158: 2310–2317

72 Cairns JA, Walls AF (1997) Mast cell tryptase stimulates the synthesis of type I collagen in human lung fibroblasts. *J Clin Invest* 99: 1313–1321

73 Akers IA, Laurent GJ, Sanjar S, McAnulty RJ (1998) Human lung fibroblasts express protease activated receptor-2 (PAR-2) which mediate the mitogenic effects of mast cell tryptase. *FASEB J* 12: A434

74 Kovacs EJ (1991) Fibrogenic cytokines: The role of immune mediators in the development of scar tissue. *Immmunol Today* 12: 17–23

75 Walls AF, Bennet AR, Godfrey RC, Holgate ST, Church MK (1991) Mast cell tryptase and histamine concentrations in bronchoalveolar lavage fluid from patients with interstitial lung disease. *Clin Sci* (Lond) 81: 183–188

76 Patella V, Marino I, Arbustini E, Lamparter-Schummert B, Verga L, Adt M, Marone G (1998) Stem cell factor in mast cells and increased mast cell density in idiopathic and ischemic cardiomyopathy. *Circulation* 97: 971–978

77 Jeziorska M, McCollum C, Woolley DE (1997) Mast cell distribution, activation, and phenotype in atherosclerotic lesions of human carotid arteries. *J Pathol* 182:115–122

78 He S, Peng Q, Walls AF (1997) Potent induction of a neutrophil and eosinophil-rich infiltrate *in vivo* by human mast cell tryptase: Selective enhancement of eosinophil recruitment by histamine. *J Immunol* 159: 6216–6225

79 Jung K-S, Shute JK, Cairns JA et al (1995) Human mast cell tryptase: a mediator of eosinophil chemotaxis. *Am J Respir Crit Care Med* 151: A530

80 Louis R, Shute J, Biagi S, Stanciu L, Marrelli F, Tenor H, Hidi R, Djukanovic R (1997) Cell infiltration, ICAM-1 expression, and eosinophil chemotactic activity in asthmatic sputum. *Am J Respir Crit Care Med* 155: 466–472

81 Numerof R, Moore W, Tanaka R (1996) Activation of human eosinophils, but not neutrophils, in response to mast cell tryptase. *Am J Respir Crit Care Med* 153: A202

82 Buckley MG, Teran LM, Walls AF (1997) Human mast cell tryptase stimulates neutrophil chemotaxis and degranulation. *J Allergy Clin Immunol* 99: S235

83 Numerof RP, Simpson PJ, Tanaka R (1997) Tryptase inhibitors: a novel class of anti-inflammatory drugs. *Exp Opin Invest Drugs* 6: 811–817

84 Rossi GL, Olivieri D (1997) Does the mast cell still have a key role in asthma? *Chest* 112: 523–529

85 Zhang M-Q, Timmerman H (1997) Mast cell tryptase and asthma. *Mediators of Inflammation* 6: 311–317

86 Kennedy JA, Wright CD (1998) Effect of mast cell tryptase on bronchial smooth muscle cell proliferation. *FASEB J* 12: A175

87 Cairns JA, Walls AF (1996) Mast cell tryptase is a mitogen for epithelial cells: Stimulation of IL-8 production and ICAM-1 expression. *J Immunol* 156: 275–283

88 Brown JK, Jones CA, Rooney LA, Caughey GH (1997) Early intracellular signals

induced by mast cell tryptase during mitogenesis in airway smooth muscle cells. *J Invest Med* 45: 285A

89 He S, Walls AF (1997) Human mast cell tryptase: a stimulus of microvascular leakage and mast cell activation. *Eur J Pharmacol* 328: 89–97

90 He S, Gaca MDA, Walls AF (1998) A role for tryptase in the activation of human mast cells: Modulation of histamine release by tryptase and inhibitors of tryptase. *J Pharmacol Exp Ther* 286: 289–297

91 Rice KD, Tanaka RD, Katz BA, Numerof RP, Moore WR (1998) Inhibitors of tryptase for the treatment of mast cell-mediated diseases. *Current Pharm Design* 4: 381–396

92 Radika K, Elrod KC, Kuo EY et al (1996) Inhibition of human tryptase by APC-366 and its analogs: structure-activity relationships. *FASEB J* 10: A1404

93 Moore WR, Elrod, KC, Johnson CR, Tanaka RD (1995) The chemical mechanism of human tryptase inhibition by the dipeptide APC-366. *FASEB J* 9: A1344

94 Kam C-M, Fujikawa K, Powers JC (1988) Mechanism-based isocoumarin inhibitors for trypsin and blood coagulation serine proteases: new anticoagulants. *Biochemistry* 27: 2547–2557

95 Clark JM, Abraham WM, Fishman CE, Forteza R, Ahmed A, Cortes A, Warne RL, Moore WR, Tanaka RD (1995) Tryptase inhibitors block ahhergen-induced airway and inflammatory responses in allergic sheep. *Am J Respir Crit Care Med* 152: 2076–2083

96 Krishna MT, Chauhan AJ, Little L, Sampson K, Mant TGK, Hawksworth R, Djukanovic R, Lee TH, Holgate ST (1998) Effect of inhaled APC-366 on allergen-induced bronchoconstriction and airway hyperresponsiveness to histamine in atopic asthmatics. *Am J Respir Crit Care Med* 157: A456

97 Stürzebecher J, Prasa D, Sommerhof CP (1992) Inhibition of human mast cell tryptase by benzamidine derivatives. *Biol Chem Hoppe-Seyler* 373: 1025–1030

98 Caughy GH, Raymond WW, Bacci E, Lombardy RJ, Tidwell RR (1993) Bis(5-amidino-2-benzimidazolyl)methane and related amidines are potent, reversible inhibitors of mast cell tryptases. *J Pharmacol Exp Ther* 264: 676–682

99 Stubbs MT, Morenweiser R, Stürzebecher J, Bauer M, Bode W, Huber R, Piechottka GP, Matschiner G, Sommerhof CP, Fritz H, Auerswald EA (1997) The three-dimensional structure of recombinant leech-derived tryptase inhibitor in complex with trypsin. *J Biol Chem* 272: 19931–19937

100 Katz BA, Clark JM, Finer-Moore JS, Jenkins TE, Johnson CR, Ross MJ, Luong C, Moore WR, Stroud RM (1998) Design of potent selective zinc-mediated serine protease inhibitors. *Nature* 391: 608–612

101 Elrod KC, Moore WR, Abraham WM, Tanaka RD (1997) Lactoferrin, a potent tryptase inhibitor, abolishes late-phase airway responses in allergic sheep. *Am J Respir Crit Care Med* 156: 375–381

102 Bannard RAB, Casselman AA, Cockburn WF, Brown GM (1958) Guanidine compounds II. Preparation of mono- and N,N-di-alkylguanidines. *Can J Chem* 36: 1541

103 Drake B, Patek M, Lebl M (1994) A convenient preparation of monosubstituted N,N'-di(BOC)-protected guanidines. *Synthesis* 579–582

104 Richter R, Tucker B (1983) Dimethylformamide-catalyzed decarboxylation of alkyl chloroformates. A synthesis of primary alkyl chlorides. *J Org Chem* 48: 2625–2627

105 Safier SR, Kushner S, Brancone LM, Subbarrow Y (1948) Experimental chemotherapy of trypanosomiasis II. The preparation of compounds related to p-phenylenediguanidine. *J Org Chem* 13: 924–930

106 Kumar K, Wang SS, Sukenik CN (1984) Synthesis, characterization, and chemistry of bridgehead-functionalized bicyclo[2.2.2]octanes: Reactions at neopentyl sites. *J Org Chem* 49: 665–670

107 Dohm J, Nieger M, Rissanen K, Vögtle F (1991) Adamantan als baustein neuer araliphane synthese, specktroskopie und kristallstrukturen. *Chem Ber* 124: 915–922

Selectin antagonists

Falguni Dasgupta

Bioorganic and Medicinal Chemistry, BioMarin Pharmaceuticals, Inc., 11 Pimentel Ct., Novato, CA 94949, USA

Selectins and inflammation

During the last fifteen years, research on various animal lectins and their specific roles in important biological functions have been under serious investigation [1–5]. This interest is not only to understand their physiological roles, but also due to the fact that the lectins, through their carbohydrate recognition domains (CRDs), recognize carbohydrate chains present on invading bacteria, viruses, and parasites. Manifestation and recognition of carbohydrate epitopes and their roles in various biological functions, mediated through enzymes and proteins, is well known [6–9]. CRDs in each group of lectins contain highly conserved amino acids at well-defined sites, a characteristic that has enabled their classification into now well recognized C-type lectins, P-type lectins or galectins (S-type). While the P-type and galectins recognize mannose-6-phosphate and β-D-galactosides respectively, the C-type lectins can recognize various monosaccharides as well as complex oligosaccharides. The C-types invariably require Ca^{2+} for binding, are typically found on the plasma membrane and share a common pattern of 14 invariant and 18 highly conserved amino acids uniquely spaced in the part of the polypeptide chain that forms the CRD. Unique among the C-type lectins are selectins [10], a class of cell adhesion molecules (CAMs), that have been implicated in the pathology of inflammatory diseases. Inflammation is the body's natural reaction to injury and infections. It is caused by the extravasation of white blood cells or the leukocytes, especially the neutrophil polymorphs, through the endothelium and their migration and accumulation at the appropriate sites under the influence of cytokine products/chemotactic factors [11–15]. The whole process is a dynamic and well coordinated, cyclic sequence of events (Fig. 1), that can cause pain due to unwanted proliferation of leukocytes in the tissues, under both acute as well as chronic disorders such as rheumatism, psoriasis, dermatitis and acute respiratory distress syndrome. The "adhesion" of leukocytes to the activated endothelium is the critical step that initiates the host defense as well as the progression of the inflammatory response. Adhesion or "locking on" is mediated through L-, E-, and P- selectin [16, 17].

High Throughput Screening for Novel Anti-Inflammatories, edited by M. Kahn
© 2000 Birkhäuser Verlag Basel/Switzerland

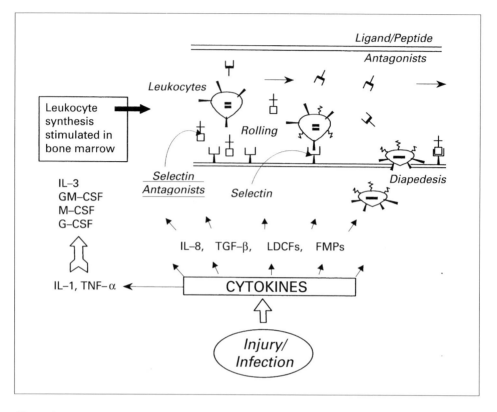

Figure 1
Generation and selectin-mediated infiltration of leukocytes under inflammatory conditions.

L-selectin (90–110 kDa), also known by LEXCAM-1, LAM-1, CD62L, gp90MEL, is constitutively expressed on the surface of the leukocytes and was the first to be identified by monoclonal antibodies raised against lymphoma cell lines. It is involved in the trafficking of the lymphocytes and granulocytes in the peripheral lymph nodes. This process exposes lymphocytes to foreign antigens within the lymphatic tissues and is important in the immune response. E-selectin or ELAM-1 (endothelial leukocyte adhesion molecule-1, 115 kDa) was also identified by monoclonal antibodies (developed against cytokine-activated endothelium), that specifically inhibit adhesion of myeloid cells to activated endothelium monolayers. Upon activation of the endothelium by endotoxins or cytokines, E-selectin is transiently expressed only on the surface of the capillary endothelial cells in a variety of acute and chronic inflammatory conditions. Thus, it is involved in the inflammatory response and mediates the recruitment of neutrophils and monocytes to sites of inflammation. The P-selectin (140 kDa), also known as GMP-140 (granule membrane protein-140), PADGEM (platelet activation dependent granule external membrane) protein, currently designated as CD62, was discovered as a component of the α-granules and is found on activated platelets as well as endothelium. P-selectin also occurs in the Weibel-Palade bodies of vascular endothelial cells and gets externalized rapidly upon activation by thrombin, histamine or phorbol esters. The CRDs of the three selectins show more than 60% homology at the amino acid level. The extracellularly exposed CRD at the extreme amino-terminus is connected through an epidermal growth factor (EGF)-like domain to a number of tandemly repeated complement regulatory protein-like units called CR-repeats. Typically, the number of these repeats are different for each selectin and these are connected to a hydrophobic transmembrane domain of approximately 25 amino acids that anchors the selectin molecules in the cell membrane through a type I orientation. There is a short cytoplasmic tail at the carboxy terminus (Fig. 2). Both transmembrane and the cytosolic domains show less than 20% homology. The genes coding for the three selectins are all located between the q22 and q25 bands on human chromosome 1.

Since all three selectins express overlapping amino acid sequence in their CRD, as expected, there exists considerable overlap in the carbohydrate structures that they recognize. However, E-selectin seems to be more specific in its choice of carbohydrate ligands (Tab. 1). As is evident, all three selectins recognize a family of sialylated, sulfated, and fucosylated oligosaccharides that constitute the glycolipids and glycoproteins of the leukocyte membrane [5]. The smallest carbohydrate epitopes recognized by the selectins are sialyl Lewis x (sLe^x), sulfo-Lewis x and sialyl Lewis a (sLe^a) [18–23]. More recently, a sulfatide [Gal(3-SO$_4$)β1-1Cer] was found to inhibit the binding of the natural ligand (sLe^x) to all three selectins and also exhibited anti-inflammatory activity *in vivo* [24–26]. Also, protein C, the human agglutinin factor was found to bind to E-selectin through a polylactosamine carbohydrate epitope [27]. Renkonen et al. reported a multi-sLe^x substituted oligolactosamine with nanomolar binding for L-selectin [28, 29]. Although these and a number of polyanions are known to inhibit the adhesion of selectins to its natural ligand [30, 31], the sialic acid and sulfate substituted smallest epitope [18–23] have remained the most attractive target for the discovery of small molecule antagonists.

The extravasation process of the leukocytes is initiated with their "rolling" caused by the interaction of their cell surface carbohydrates with the cytokine activated endothelium expressing E- and P-selectins. The initial attachment is followed by firm adherence of the leukocytes onto the endothelium with the help of other CAMs, e.g. intercellular adhesion molecules (ICAMs), which is followed by their migration through the endothelium into the neighboring tissues. It was firmly believed and subsequently shown that modulation of any of the steps during the "adhesion-firm adhesion-migration" could help control acute and/or chronic inflammatory problems [32, 33]. Selectin antagonism has been considered as one of

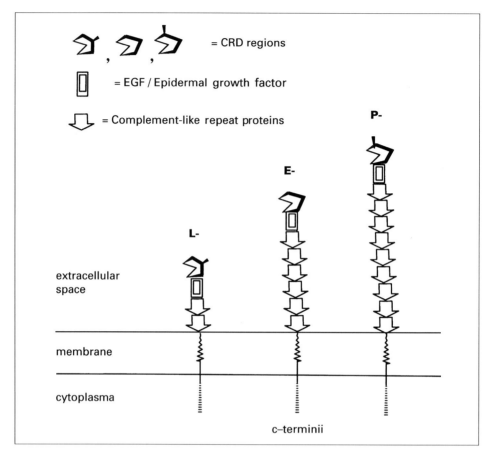

Figure 2
Selectins and their membrane organization.

the most efficient ways to develop novel therapeutics that could be used to control adhesion-related disorders at a very early stage of the process. It is evident that for the identification of a small molecule-selectin antagonist, its synthesis and subsequent development as a possible therapeutic agent, either the selectins (the receptor-a-peptidic approach) or their ligands (a carbohydrate approach) can be good starting points. In this article these areas of research and development will be mainly discussed.

It is worthwhile to note here that use of monoclonal antibodies (Mab) raised against one or the other selectin has also been well documented in the literature, with animal studies described, in which good protective effects have been observed

Table 1: Oligosaccharide sequences and other polysaccharides recognized by human selectins

Oligosaccharide	Structure	L-	E-	P-
Sialyl-Lewis[x]	NeuAcα-(2-3)-Galβ-(1-4)-GlcNAcα1-R [Fucα-(1-3)]	*	**	**
VIM-2 (CD65)	NeuAcα-(2-3)-Galβ-(1-4)-GlcNAcβ-(1-3)=Galβ-(1-4)-GlcNAcβ1-R [Fucα-(1-3)]	*	*/-	*
Sialyl dimeric Le[x]	NeuAcα-(2-3)-Galβ-(1-4)-GlcNAcβ-(1-3)-Galβ-(1-4)-GlcNAcβ1-R [Fucα-(1-3)] [Fucα-(1-3)]	*	**	**
Sialyl-Lewis[a]	NeuAcα-(2-3)-Galβ-(1-3)-GlcNAcβ-1-R [Fucα-(1-4)]	*	**	**
3'-sulfo-Lewis[x]	SO$_4$-3-Galβ-(1-4)-GlcNAcβ-1-R [Fucα-(1-3)]	**	*	**
Sulfatide	SO$_4$-3-Galβ-1'-Ceramide	**	–	*
HNK-1	SO$_4$-3-GlcAβ-(1-4)-Galβ-(1-4)-GlcNAcβ-1-R	*	–	
Heparin sulfate proteoglycan		****	–	****
Polyphosphomannan		**	–	**
Fucoidin		**	–	**
Dextran sulfate		**	–	**

*Recognition scale: best = ****; none = –*

[32–36]. Thus, anti E-selectin Mab was found to reduce the late-phase bron-choconstriction in primate and reduced permeability edema in acute lung inflam-mation in rats. Anti P-selectin antibody was shown to protect rat lung from injury induced by cobra venom. Neutralizing Mabs to murine E- and P-selectins, when administered together, effectively inhibited the migration of the polymorphonuclear granulocytes. In another detailed study in mice, it was demonstrated that blocking the L- and P-selectins with relevant antibodies almost completely stopped the neu-trophil migration in the peritonium. However, blocking of each selectin alone inhibited neutrophil migration to a similar partial degree ranging from 63 to 72% [17].

Peptides as antagonists

With the successful discovery of small peptides and their mimics as novel therapeu-tic agents, e.g. ACE inhibitors, AT-II receptor antagonists and perhaps of more rel-evance, adhesion-associated, gpIIb/IIIa antagonist (RGD mimics), it was reasoned that it would be possible to identify a family of small peptides with the ability to inhibit the binding of leukocytes to immobilized selectins. It was also argued that a peptide-based approach is necessary in order to overcome the inherently weak inter-action between carbohydrates and proteins. The natural ligands also contain pro-teins [37, 38] and other molecular epitopes that recognize selectins. Thus, a peptide that recognizes regions other than the CRD region may form the basis for a new lead. This is particularly true in the case of E-selectin for which it is clear that sLe^x is not the entire ligand. On the other hand, many cells which express sLe^x do not adhere to E-selectin and sLe^x containing glycoproteins do not necessarily bind to P- or E- selectins [20, 23, 39].

Since libraries of combinatorial peptides could be quickly generated through recombinant techniques [40–43] and rapidly screened by phage ELISA assay, this method was adopted by researchers at the Affymax Research Institute [44]. Several active peptides were isolated, one of which AF 10166 (H$_2$N-DITWDOLWDLMK-COOH) and its corresponding amide (AF 10185) bound to selectins, especially E-, with high selectivity and affinity. The structure activity relationship of this family was quite clear and the active peptides appeared to require tryptophan at the 4 and 8 positions, leucine at position 7 and methionine at position 11. Although the pep-tide bound to E-selectin in both static and flow-cell assays, it did not compete with sLe^x and did not require calcium for its binding activity, thus leading to the hypoth-esis that it might be involved in binding to regions other than the CRD of E-selectin. It is also noteworthy that although there is no homology of AF 10166 with the pri-mary structure of L-selectin, the first four residues of the mature PSGL-1 that binds to both E- and P-selectin [45], are identical to the four amino acid residues underlined above. With an IC_{50} of 4 nM (Phage display ELISA assay) and 10 μM in the static cell adhesion assay, AF 10166 was considered a lead compound worthy of further improvement.

In a more "structure-based" approach, amino acid sequences were selected from the consensus region of the CRD of E-, L- and P-selectin, synthesized and evaluated in cell binding assays [46–51]. On several occasions, it was demonstrated that synthetic peptides based on amino acid sequence from the CRD of selectins could block neutrophil adhesion to immobilized P-selectin. *In vivo* efficacy of one such heptapeptide, RIGIWYY, was demonstrated by Briggs et al. in thioglycollate and IL-1α induced neutrophil infiltration models in mice [52]. This peptide was derived from a consensus, highly conserved nonapeptide, consisting of amino acid sequence 47–55 from the CRD of E-, P- and L-selectins. Various positional substitutions, substitution with D-isomers, as well as truncation of the heptapeptide suggested this to be the optimum sequence for the best inhibitory activity. Isothermal titration calorimetry with the natural carbohydrate ligands indicated non-polar interactions between the two ligands encompassing the N-terminal segment of the peptide. It was also observed that the sialic acid did not contribute towards the stability of the peptide/saccharide complex. The tryptophan and the neighboring tyrosine residues were found to be absolutely essential for the activity of this peptide [53] which is currently being investigated for the treatment of inflammatory bowel disease [54].

Natural carbohydrate ligands and their analogues as antagonists

With a clear understanding that the carbohydrate ligands (Fig. 3) are indeed capable of inhibiting adhesion in appropriate *in vitro* assays, synthesis of the sulfated trisaccharide, the sialic acid containing tetrasaccharide and larger oligosaccharides were carried out using known synthetic methods [55–64]. Unique chemoenzymatic synthesis [65] utilizing enzymatic routes [66, 67] were also developed in order to access these natural ligands in larger quantities. However, it was soon clear that although synthetic methods could be refined and scaled up to obtain kilogram quantities of various oligosaccharides, the short half lives of these "natural" ligands disqualified them as candidates for further development into useful pharmaceuticals. By this time screening studies with some of the simpler, modified ligands (Fig. 3) had indicated that the carboxylic acid function of sialic acid and the three contiguous hydroxyl groups of L-fucose were essential for recognition of these complex carbohydrate ligands by selectins. This biochemical information and NOE studies of sLe^x in solution suggested that the essential pharmacophore of a selectin ligand consisted of these two ingredients placed at a distance of ~10–11 Å apart in space [33, 68–73].

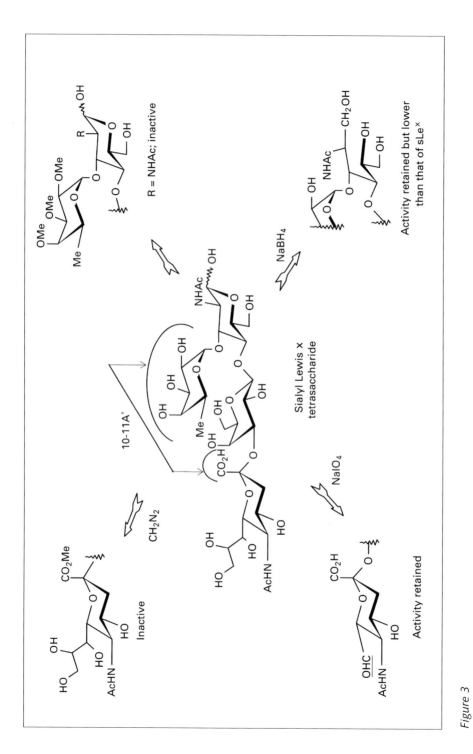

Figure 3
Sialyl Lewis x tetrasaccharide and its minimum pharmacophore region.

These observations formed the basis for synthesis and screening of next generation of compounds in which the sialic acid was substituted for acetic acid, lactic acid, mandelic acid and phenyl acetic acid, the disaccharide (lactosamine) scaffold was also replaced with lactose, 1-O-(2-hydroxyethyl)-β-D-galactopyranoside, 1-O-(2-hydroxycyclohexyl)-β-D-galactopyranoside, and L-fucose with a glyceryl residue [73–77]. A number of these first line of glycomimetics exhibited antagonism to selectins in cell based assays and inhibited cytokine induced leukocyte infiltration in isolated rabbit heart. However, the IC_{50} values of these compounds did not reach significantly lower than that of sLe^x-glc and the question confronting the investigators was whether multivalent interactions observed in nature, was necessary for improving the IC_{50} and efficacy of these selectin ligands. Multivalency has been known to improve the binding activity of carbohydrate ligands towards their natural substrates [80].

Synthesis of multivalent sLe^x with putative therapeutic activity could be carried out by several methods [78, 79]. A carbohydrate ligand having 1-O-$(CH_2)^8$.CO.NH.NH. CO.CH=CH$_2$ was copolymerised with 5 equivalent of acrylamide to afford a water soluble poly(acrylamide-co-3'-sulfo-Le^x-glc). The compound exhibited inhibitory activities against E- and L-selectins with IC_{50}s in the μM range, a value at which a simple copolymer of sialic acid also showed inhibition! Novel cell free binding assays and scintillation proximity assays have been developed using such copolymers [81, 82]. Sulfated neoglycopolymers as well as the acrylamide-sLe^x homopolymers have shown good inhibitory effects during cell adhesion [83–85]. The synthesis and evaluation of multivalent sLe^x and sialic acid has been reviewed [86]. Dendrimeric sulfo-Le^x was synthesized using a chemoenzymatic strategy to give di-, tetra- and octa-valent sLe^x, which are being investigated as selectin antagonists [87]. Nanomolar P-selectin inhibitors were synthesized using the concept that a polymerised bilamellar assembly containing multivalent sLe^x or its mimics can behave like neutrophils with respect to adhesion. Indeed such compounds were prepared using a trisaccharide mimic having acetic acid instead of the sialic acid as well as those having only the lactose core to produce "glycoliposomes" having a high degree of inhibitory activity (IC_{50} 2 nM) towards P-selectin IgG chimera binding to HL-60 cells [88].

Bristol-Meyers Squibb had selected to develop an antagonist using the natural sulfatide ligand 3-O-sulfo-β-D-Gal-1-O-ceramide [25] as a template for new drug development. The approach is also consistent with the observation that natural hyaluronates induced rolling of lymphocytes under physiologic flow conditions [31]. The lead compound BMS-190394 (Fig. 4) inhibited the binding of both E- and P-selectin with IC_{50}s of 9.5 μM and 11 μM respectively. The compound was tested by i.v. and i.p. routes in rats for vascular permeability/PMN infiltration and was found to be as potent as dexamethasone [89]. For molecules with a long chain hydrophobic aglycone, their liposomal assembly resulting in multivalent presentation of the epitopes can not be ruled out.

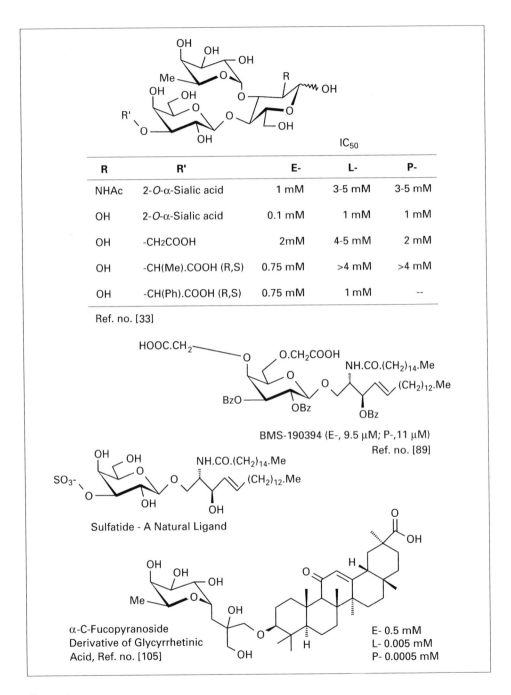

R	R'	E-	L-	P-
			IC$_{50}$	
NHAc	2-O-α-Sialic acid	1 mM	3-5 mM	3-5 mM
OH	2-O-α-Sialic acid	0.1 mM	1 mM	1 mM
OH	-CH2COOH	2mM	4-5 mM	2 mM
OH	-CH(Me).COOH (R,S)	0.75 mM	>4 mM	>4 mM
OH	-CH(Ph).COOH (R,S)	0.75 mM	1 mM	--

Ref. no. [33]

BMS-190394 (E-, 9.5 μM; P-,11 μM)
Ref. no. [89]

Sulfatide - A Natural Ligand

α-C-Fucopyranoside
Derivative of Glycyrrhetinic
Acid, Ref. no. [105]

E- 0.5 mM
L- 0.005 mM
P- 0.0005 mM

Figure 4
Some natural antagonists and their synthetic and semisynthetic analogues.

Novel glycomimetics as antagonists

Problems with the natural oligosaccharides as therapeutic agents are manyfold, particularly those related to cost, stability, and pharmacokinetic profile. Thus, optimizing the carbohydrate scaffold region (lactose/lactosamine) of sLe^x through tethering, synthesis of small molecular weight glycopeptides as well as introduction of various organic molecular bridges between the essential pharmacophores, L-fucose and a carboxylate function, has been extensively carried out during the last decade [90–104]. In many of these compounds either α-L-fucose in conjuction with β-D-galactopyranose, or only the L-fucose residue persisted since, as per the early SAR studies, at least L-fucose was essential for selectin recognition (Fig. 5). Even the simplest molecules, i.e. O-sulfonate or 2-O-α-sialic acid tethered to 1-O-α-L-fucopyranoside exhibited moderate/comparable (to the natural ligand) binding to P-selectins and inhibited P-selectin-IgG binding to HL-60 cell lines [90–92]. Allanson et al. tethered the 2-position of sialic acid with the 4-position of L-fucose (6-deoxy-L-galactopyranose) by coupling methy 2,3-di-O-benzoyl-4-(3'-dimethylphosphono-2'-oxo-propan-1-yl)-6-deoxy-β-L-O-galactopyranoside with appropriate sialosides to give disaccharide mimics of sLe^x [93, 94].

α-L-fucopyranoside containing glycopeptides were also synthesized with good success. N-(2-tetradecylhexadecanoyl)-O-(α-L-fucopyranosyl)-D-seryl-L-glutamic acid 1-methylamide, a fucosylated dipeptide with a type II β-turn showed 50–100 times more potent *in vitro* activity than sLe^x and sulfo-Le^x. Combination of various L- and D-forms of the two amino acids were tested for efficacy. Dipeptides having L-, D- and D-, L-combinations had μM to sub-μM activities against all three selectins [95]. However, the other two with L-, L- and D-, D-combinations exhibited poor activity against E-selectin, although they were as good antagonists as the L-, D-combinations against L- and P-selectins. This reconfirmed the fact that specific structural requirements need to be considered in designing E-selectin ligands. Several other glycopeptides have been synthesized in which both O- and C-linked fucoses were incorporated into the peptidic backbones. Several of these exhibited ten to twenty times greater affinities for E-selectin than sLe^x [96, 97]. The C-glycoside approach has been adopted for the synthesis of libraries of glycopeptides on solid support using a combinatorial strategy [98]. Thus using one of the components as an appropriate C-fucoside, four-component Ugi reactions were carried out on a Rink type solid support to provide a "directed library" from which isomeric mixtures of active compounds could be isolated (Fig. 6).

X-ray crystallographic studies of E-selectin indicated its similarity to mannose binding protein (MBP) – another well-known and well-characterized lectin which requires Ca^{2+} for binding. Site directed mutagenesis studies indicated that [99] L-fucose possibly binds at a site similar to that required for D-mannose in MBP. Consequently, choice of the essential sugar residue for the synthesis of glycomimetics shifted from L-fucose to D-mannopyranose [99]. This strategy was extensively and

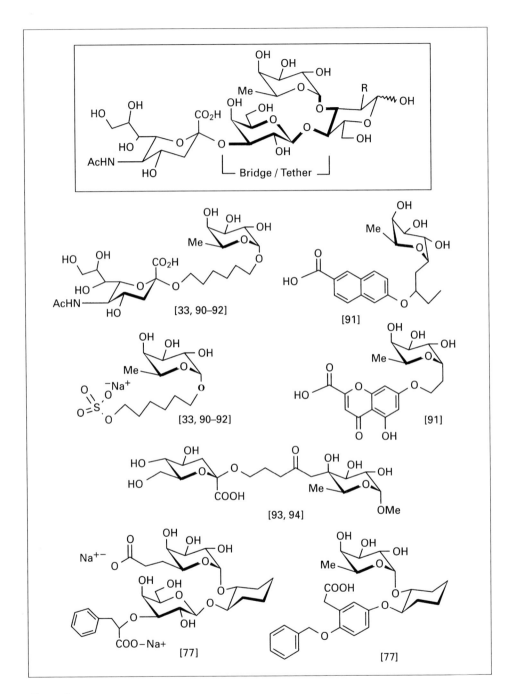

Figure 5
Tethered mimics of sialyl Lewis x (relevant references are shown in brackets).

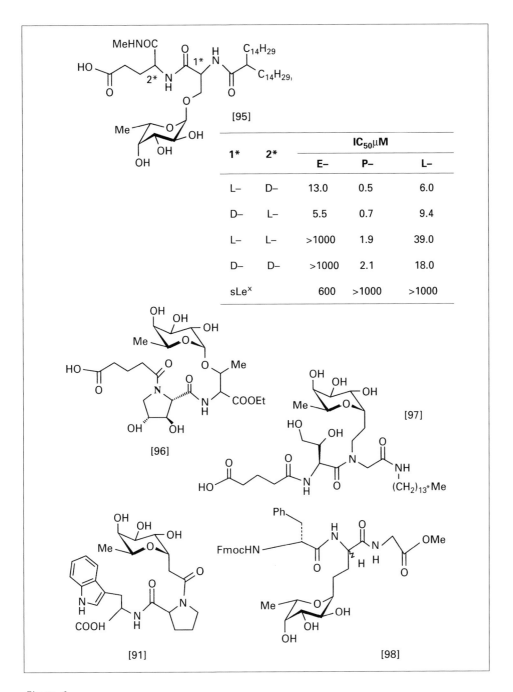

		IC$_{50}\mu$M		
1*	**2***	**E–**	**P–**	**L–**
L–	D–	13.0	0.5	6.0
D–	L–	5.5	0.7	9.4
L–	L–	>1000	1.9	39.0
D–	D–	>1000	2.1	18.0
sLe^x		600	>1000	>1000

Figure 6
Glycopeptides as sialyl Lewis x mimics (relevant references are shown in brackets).

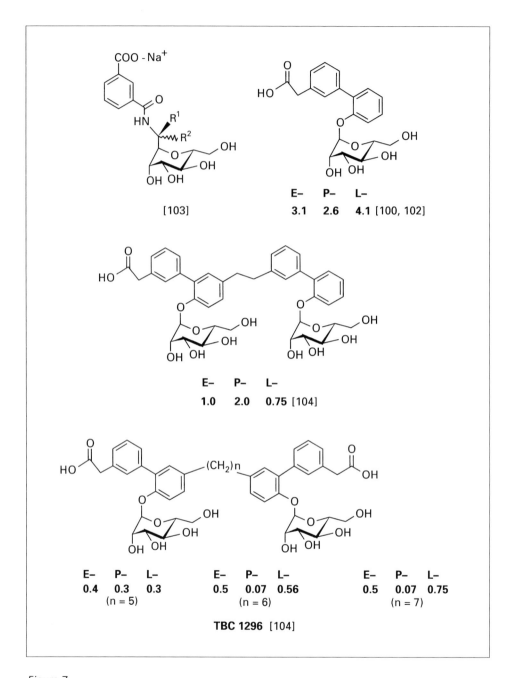

Figure 7
D-mannose instead of L-fucose in designing glycomimetics of sialyl Lewis x. IC_{50} values in mM (relevant references are shown in brackets).

Table 2 - Some of the companies targeting cell-adhesion based therapeutics

	Company name	Therapeutic areas
1.	Athena Neurosciences San Francisco, CA, USA	Multiple sclerosis, stroke, trauma
2.	Biogen Cambridge, MA, USA	Inflammatory diseases
3.	Cell Genesys Foster City, CA, USA	Reperfusion injury, acute respiratory distress syndrome
4.	COR Therapeutics South San Francisco, CA, USA	Arterial thrombosis, unstable angina, acute myocardial infarction
5.	Cytel San Diego, Califomia, USA	Reperfusion injury, trauma, chronic inflammatory disorders
6.	Genetics Institute Cambridge, MA, USA	Ischaemia/reperfusion injury, myocardial infarction, hemorrhagic shock
7.	Ibex Technology Montreal, Quebec, Canada	Reperfusion injury, restenosis
8.	Isis Pharmaceuticals Carlsbad, CA, USA	Psoriasis, rheumatoid arthritis, Crohn's disease, ulcerative colitis
9.	ICOS Bothel, WA, USA	Multiple sclerosis, cardiovascular diseases, asthma, hemorrhagic shock
10.	Oxford Glycosciences Oxford, United Kingdom	Inflammatory diseases
11.	Protein Design Labs. Mt. View, CA, USA	Inflammatory conditions
12.	Repligen Corporation Cambridge, MA, USA	Ischaemia, reperfusion injury
13.	Scios Nova Mt. View, CA, USA	Inflammatory disorders
14.	Texas Biotechnology Houston, TX, USA	Asthma, reperfusion injury, allergic rhinitis, rheumatoid arthritis, multiple sclerosis, metastatic cancer

methodically exploited to generate D-mannose-substituted glycopeptides and biphenyl derivatives with good inhibitory activities [100–104]. One such divalent compound (TBC 1269), from the Texas Biotechnology Corporation, exhibited very good *in vitro* activity that was at least ten times superior to the monomer [104]. TBC 1269 is currently being evaluated for treating asthma (Fig. 7).

Epilogue

It is clear from the above review of selectin antagonists that the work in this exciting area has just begun. Initial excitement of several biotech companies, which had expected quick success, have now given way to more objective, knowledge based views. It is evident that quite a few classes of compounds can be utilized as selectin-antagonists. Chemical methodologies as well as suitable technologies are now available for initiating combinatorial libraries of both peptidic as well as small molecular mimics of the active region of the ligand. The pharmacophore based approach [105] has not been fully exploited since its first use to identify glycyrrhizin and the C-fucoside analog of glycyrrhetinic acid as potent inhibitors of P-selectin (Fig. 4). The number of companies continuing to be attracted by the potentials of adhesion-based therapeutics have persistently increased [106]. Several compounds are presently being evaluated for therapeutic applications in such disorders as ischemia, ARDS, psoriasis, cancer metastasis, angiogenesis, asthma and several others (Tab. 2). Next among synthetic, small molecule analogues is TBC 1269 which has consistently shown activities in animal models that are reflective of its *in vitro* activity profile. However, the glycopeptides are also not too far behind and the extensive search for ideal antagonists, that will prove effective as therapeutic agents, is bound to bear sweet fruits of success in the near future.

Acknowledgements
I wish to thank Dr. Michael Kahn for the invitation to write this chapter. My special recognition to Dr. John C. Klock for getting me into Glycomed Inc. where I was inducted into this field.

References

1   Kornfeld S (1992) *Ann Rev Biochem* 61: 307–330
2   Drickemar K, Taylor ME (1993) *Ann Rev Cell Biol* 9: 237–264
3   Lowe JB (1994) In: M Fukuda and O Hindsgaul (eds): *Molecular glycobiology*. IRL Press, Oxford, 163–205
4   Varki A (1994) *Proc Natl Acad Sci USA* 91: 7390–7393
5   van den Eijnden DH, Joziasse V (1994) Animal lectins: Carbohydrate-recognizing molecules with important biological functions. *Carbohydrates in Europe* 11: 5–13
6   Varki A (1993) Biological role of oligosaccharides. *Glycobiology* 3: 97–130
7   Lemieux RU (1993) How proteins recognize and bind oligosaccharides. In: PJ Garegg and AA Lindberg (eds): *Carbohydrate antigens*, ACS Symposium Series Vol 519, Washington DC, 5–18

8   Bundle D (1994) The recognition of carbohydrate antigens by antibodies. *Carbohydrates in Europe* 11: 22–30

9   Elgavish S, Shaanan B (1997) Lectin-carbohydrate interaction: Different folds, common recognition principles. *Trends Biol Sci* 22 (Dec): 462–467

10   McEver RP (1994) Selectins. *Curr Opin Immunol* 6: 75–84

11   Bevilacqua MP, Stengelin S, Gimbrone MA, Seed B (1989) E-selectin is a cytokine induced, endothelial restricted selectin. *Science* 243: 1160–1165

12   Johnson GI, Cook RG, McEver RP (1989) P-selectin is detected on activated platelet. *Cell* 56: 1033–1044

13   Shanley TP, Warner RL, Ward PA (1995) The role of cytokines and adhesion molecules in the development of inflammatory injury. *Molecular Medicine Today*: 40–45

14   Bianchi E, Bender JR, Blasi F, Pardi R (1997) Through and beyond the walls: late steps in leukocyte transendothelial migration. *Immunology Today* 18: 586–589

15   Silber A, Newman W, Sasseville VG, Pauley D, Beall D, Walsh DG, Ringler DG (1994) Recruitment of lymphocytes in nonhuman primates is dependent on E-selectin and VCAM-1. *J Clin Invest* 93: 1554–1563

16   Labow MA, Norton CR, Rumberger JM, Lombart-Gillooly KM, Shuster DJ, Hubbard J, Bertko R, Knaack PA, Harbison ML et al (1994) E-selectin deficient mice: P-selectin adequate for neutrophil migration. *Immunity* 1: 709–720

17   Bosse R, Vestweber D (1994) Simultaneous blocking of the L- and P-selectin completely inhibits neutrophil migration. *Eur J Immunol* 24: 3019–3024

18   Paulson JC (1992) Selectin/carbohydrate mediated adhesion of Leukocytes. In: JM Harlan, DY Liu (eds): *Adhesion: Its role in inflammatory diseases*. WH Freeman & Co., New York, 19–42

19   Brandley BK, Sweidler S, Robbins P (1990) Carohydrate ligands for selectins. Cell 53: 861–863

20   Hakomori SI (1992) Lex and related structures as adhesion molecules. *Histochemical J* 24: 771–776

21   Feizi T (1993) Oligosaccharides that mediate mammalian cell adhesion. *Curr Opin Struct Biol* 3: 701–710

22   Foxall C, Watson S, Dowbenko D, Fennie C, Lasky L, Kiso M, Hasegawa A, Asa D, Brandley BK (1992) Three members of the selectin family recognise sLe^x. *J Cell Biol* 117: 895–902

23   Yuen C-T et al (1994) Sulfated blood group Le^a – A superior oligosaccharide ligand for human E-selectin. *J Biol Chem* 269: 1595–1598

24   Mulligan MS et al (1995) Anti-inflammatory effects of sulfatides in selectin-dependent acute lung injury. *Int Immunol* 7:1107–1113

25   Nair X, Todderud G, Davern L, Lee D, Aruffo A, Thamposch KM (1994) Inhibition of immune complex-induced inflammation by a small molecular weight selectin antagonist. *Mediators of Inflammation* 3: 459–463

26   Aruffo A, Kolanus W, Walz G, Fredman P, Seed B (1991) CD62/P-selectin recognition of myeloid and tumor cell sulfatides. *Cell* 67: 35–44

27   Grinnel GW, Herman RB, Yan SB (1994) Human protein C inhibits selectin-mediated cell adhesion. *Glycobiology* 4: 221–225

28   Renkonen O et al (1997) A polylactosarnine bearing sLe^x is a nanomolar L-selectin antagonist. *Glycobiology* 7: 453

29   Salminen H, Ashokas K, Niemela R, Penttila L, Maaheimo H, Helin J, Costello CE, Renkonen O (1997) Improved enzymatic synthesis of a highly potent oligosaccharide antagonist of L-selectin. *FEBS Lett* 419: 220–226

30   Cecconi O, Nelson RM, Roberts WG, Hanasaki K, Mannori G, Schultz C, Ulich TR, Aruffo A, Bevilacqua MP (1994) Inositol polyanions. Noncarbohydrate inhibitors of L- and P-selectins that block inflammation. *J Biol Chem* 269: 15060–15066

31   DeGrendele HC, Estess P, Picker LJ, Siegelman MH (1996) CD44 and its ligand hyaluronate mediate rolling under physiological flow: a novel lymphocyte-endothelial cell primary adhesion pathway. *J Exp Med* 183:1119–1130

32   Mousa SA (1998) Cell adhesion molecules and extracellular matrix proteins: potential therapeutic applications. *Exp Opin Invest Drugs* 7:1159–1171

33   Dasgupta F, Rao BNN (1994) Anti-adhesive therapeutics: a new class of anti-inflammatory agents. *Exp Opin Invest Drugs* 3: 709–724

34   Mulligan MS, Varani J, Dame MK, Lane CL, Smith CW, Anderson DC, Ward PA (1991) Anti-ELAM-1 Mab reduced neutrophil accumulation in inflamed peritonium and lung in the rats. *J Clin Invest* 88: 1396–1406

35   Gundel RM, Wegner CD, Torcellini CA, Clarke CC, Haynes N, Rothlein R, Smith CW, Letts LG (1991) Mabs to ELAM-1 inhibited neutrophil accumulation in the lung in a primate. *J Clin Invest* 88: 1407–1411

36   Mulligan MS, Polly MJ, Bayer RJ, Nunn MF, Paulson JC, Ward PA (1992) Neutrophil dependent acute lung injury: Requirement of P-selectin. *J Clin Invest* 90: 1600–1607

37   Stocks SC, Rerr MA (1993) *Biochem Biophvs Res Commun* 195: 468–473

38   Levinovitz A, Muhlhoff J, Isenmann S, Vestweber D (1993) *J Cell Biol* 121: 449–459

39   Moore KL, Stults NL, Diaz S, Smith DF, Cummings RD, Varki A, McEver RP (1992) *J Biol Chem* 118: 445–456

40   Cwirla SE, Peters EA, Barrett RW, Dower WJ (1990) *Proc Nat Acad Sci USA* 87: 6378–6382

41   Devlin JJ, Panganiban LC, Devlin PE (1990) *Science* 249: 404–406

42   Scott JK, Smith GP (1990) *Science* 249: 386–390

43   Cull MG, Miller JF, Schatz PJ (1992) *Proc Natl Acad Sci USA* 89: 1865–1869

44   Martens CL et al (1995) Peptides which bind to E-selectin and block neutrophil adhesion. *J Biol Chem* 270: 21129–21136

45   Moore KL, Patel KD, Bruehl RE, Fugang L, Johnson DA, Lichenstein HS, Cummings RD, Bainton DF, McEver RP (1995) P-selectin glycoprotein ligand-1 mediates rolling of human neutrophils on P-selectin. *J Cell Biol* 128: 661–671

46   Rozdzinski E, Burnette WN, Jones T, Tuomanen E (1993) Prokaryotic peptides that block leukocyte adherence to selectins. *J Exp Med* 178: 917–924

47 Hollenbaugh D, Bajorath J, Stenkamp R, Aruffo A (1993) Interaction of P-selectin (CD62) and its cellular ligand-analysis of critical residues. *Biochemistry* 32: 2960–2966

48 Geng J-G, Moore RL, Johnson AE, McKever RP (1991) Neutrophil recognition requires a Ca^{2+}-induced conformational change in the peptide domain fo GMP-140. *J Biol Chem* 266: 22313–22318

49 Geng J-G, Heavner GA, McEver RP (1992) Lectin domain peptides from selectins interact with both cell surface ligands and Ca^{2+} ions. *J Biol Chem* 267: 19846–19853

50 Erbe DV, Wolitzky BA, Presta LG, Norton CR, Ramos RJ, Burns DJK, Rumberger JM, Rao BNN, Foxall C, Brandley BK, Lasky LA (1992) Identification of a E-selectin region critical for carbohydrate recognition and cell adhesion. *J Cell Biol* 119: 215–227

51 Erbe DV, Watson SR, Presta LG, Wolitzky BA, Foxall C, Brandley BK, Lasky LA (1993) P- and E-selectin use common sites for carbohydrate ligand recognition and cell adhesion. *J Cell Biol* 120: 1227–1235

52 Briggs JB, Oda Y, Gilbert JH, Schaefer ME, Macher B (1995) Peptides inhibit selectin-mediated cell adhesion *in vitro* and neutrophil influx into inflammatory site *in vivo*. *Glycobiology* 5: 583–588

53 Briggs JB, Larsen RA, Harris RB, Sekar KVS, Macher B (1996) Structure/activity studies of anti-inflammatory peptides based on a conserved peptide region of the lectin domain of E-, P- and L-selectin. *Glycobiology* 6: 831–836

54 van Rees EP, Palmen MJHJ, van der Goot FRW, Macher B, Dieleman LA (1997) Leukocyte migration in inflammatory bowel disease. *Med of Inflamm* 6: 85–93

55 Lemieux RU (1978) Review of oligosaccharide synthesis. *Chem Soc Rev* 7: 423

56 Paulsen H (1984) Review of oligosaccharide synthesis. *Chem Soc Rev* 13: 15

57 Kunz H (1987) Glycosidation/oligosaccharide synthesis. *Chem Soc Rev* 26: 194

58 Schmidt RR (1989) Recent synthesis in the development of glycoconjugates. *Pure and Appl Chem* 61: 1257–1270

59 Paulsen H (1990) Review of oligosaccharide synthesis. *Chem Soc Rev* 29: 825

60 Nicolaou KC (1991) Chemical synthesis of glycosphingolipids. *Chemtracts-Organic Chemistry* 4: 181–198

61 Nicolaou KC (1993) Total synthesis of sulfated Le^x and Le^a-type oligosaccharide selectin ligands. *J Am Chem Soc* 115: 8843–8884

62 Ogawa T (1994) Experiments directed towards glycoconjugate synthesis. *Chem Soc Rev*: 397–407

63 Seeberger PH, Bilodeau MT, Danishefsky SJ (1997) Synthesis of biologically important oligosaccharides and other glycoconjugates. *Aldrichimica Acta* 30: 75–92

64 Hasegawa A, Kiso M (1996) Design and synthesis of cell adhesion carbohydrate ligands/inhibitors. In: ZI Witczak, KA Nieforth (eds): *Carbohydrates targets for drug design*. Marcel Dekker, Inc., New York. 137–155

65 Ichikawa Y, Lin Y-C, Dumas DP, Shen G-J, Williams G-JE, Bayer MA, Ketcham C, Walker LE, Paulson JC, Wong C-H (1992) *J Am Chem Soc* 114: 9283–9298

66 Wong C-H, Haynie SL, Whitesides GM (1982) *J Org Chem* 47: 5416–5418

67 DeLuca C, Lansing M, Martin I, Crescenzi F, Shen G-J, O'Regan M, Wong C-H (1995) *J Am Chem Soc* 117: 5869–5870

68 Tyrell D, James P, Rao BN, Foxall C, Abbas SA, Dasgupta F, Nashed MA, Hasegawa HA, Kiso M, Asa D, Kidd J, Brandley BK (1991) Structural requirements for the carbohydrate ligand of E-selectin. *Proc Natl Acad Sci USA* 88: 10372–10376

69 Ramphal JY, Zheng Z-L, Perez C, Walker L, DeFrees SA, Gaeta FCA (1994) *J Med Chem* 37: 3459–3463

70 Stahl W, Sprengard U, Kretzschmar G, Kunz H (1994) *Angew Chemie Int Ed Engl* 33: 2096–2098

71 Scheffler K, Ernst B, Katopodis A, Magnani JL, Wang WT, Weisemann R, Peters T (1995) Conformation of sLe^x bound to E-selectin. *Angew Chemie Intl Ed Engl* 34: 1841–1844

72 Hensley P, McDevitt PJ et al (1994) Conformation of sLe^x bound to E-selectin has been determined using NMR. *J Biol Chem* 269: 23949–23958

73 Lin Y-C, Hummel CW, Huang D-H, Ichikawa Y, Nicolaou KC, Wong C-H (1992) Conformation of sialyl Lewis^x in aqueous solution. *J Am Chem Soc* 114: 5452–5454

74 Nashed MA, Dasgupta F, Abbas SA, Musser SH, Darwin AS (1994) Substituted lactose and lactosamine derivatives as cell adhesion inhibitors. US Patent 5,326,752

75 Abbas SA, Dasgupta F, Asa D, Musser JH, Nashed MA (1997) Substituted lactose derivatives. US Patent 5,591,835

76 DeFrees SA, Gaeta FCA, Lin Y-C, Ichikawa Y, Wong C-H (1993) Ethylene glycol can replace the glucopyranose residue at the reducing end. *J Am Chem Soc* 115: 7549–7550

77 Liu A, Dillon K, Campbell RM, Cox DC, Huryn DM (1996) Tethered mimics of sLe^x. *Tetrahedron Lett* 37: 3785–3788

78 Kolb HC (1997) Design and synthesis of a macrocyclic E-selectin antagonist. *Bioorg Med Chem Lett* 7: 2629–2634

79 Welply JK, Abbas SZ, Scudder P et al (1994) Multivalent sLe^x: Potent inhibitors of E-selectin mediated cell adhesion. *Glycobiology* 4: 259–265

80 Lee RT, Lee YC (1994) Enhanced biochemical affinities of multivalent neoglycoconjugates. In: YC Lee, RT Lee (eds) Neoglycoconjugates: preparation and applications. Academic Press, San Diego, 23–50

81 Roy R, Park WKC, Srivastava 0, Foxall C (1996) Combined glycomimetic and multivalent strategies for the design of potent selectin antagonists. *Bioorg Med Chem Lett* 6: 1399–1402

82 Game SM et al (1998) Scintillation proximity assay for E-, P- and L-selectin utilizing polyacrylamide-based neoglycoconjugates as ligands. *Anal Biochem* 258: 127–135

83 Weitz-Schmidt G, Stockmaier D, Scheel G, Nifant'ev NE, Tuzikov AB, Bovin NV (1996) An E-selectin binding assay based on a polyacrylamide-type glycoconjugate. *Anal Biochem* 238: 184–190

84 Manning DD, Hu X, Beck P, Kiessling LL (1997) Synthesis of sulfated neoglycopolymers. selective P-selectin inhibitors. *J Am Chem Soc* 119: 3161–3162

85 Miyauchi H, Tanaka M, Koike H, Kawamura N, Hayashi M (1997) Synthesis and

inhibitory effects of a sLe^x-acrylamide homopolymer at preventing cell adhesion. *Bioorg Med Chem Lett* 7: 985–988

86   Roy R (1997) Sialoside mimetics and conjugates as antiinflammatory agents and inhibitors of flu virus infections. In: ZJ Witczak, KA Nieforth (eds): *Carbohydrates in drug design*. Mercel Dekker, New York, 83–135

87   Palcic M, Li H, Zanini D, Bhella RS, Roy R (1997) Chemoenzymatic synthesis of dendritic sLe^x. *Carbohydr Res* 305: 433–442

88   Spevak W, Foxall C, Charych DH, Dasgupta F, Nagy JO (1996) Carbohydrates in an acidic multivalent assembly: Nanomolar P-selectin inhibitors. *J Med Chem* 39: 1018–1020

89   Todderud G, Nair X, Lee D, Alford J, Davern L et al (1997) BMS-190394, a selectin inhibitor, prevents rat cutaneous inflammatory reactions. *J Pharmacol Exp Therap* 282: 1298–1304

90   Dasgupta F, Musser JH (1997) Sialic acid/fucose based assay reagents and assay methods. US Patent 5,660,992

91   Dasgupta F, Musser JH, Levy DE, Tang PC (1997) Sialic acid/fucose based medicaments. US Patent 5,658,880

92   Dasgupta F, Musser JH (1997) Sialic acid/fucose based medicaments. US Patent 5,679,321

93   Allanson NM, Davidson AH (1994) Disaccharide ligands. PCT no. WO 94117084

94   Allanson NM, Davidson AH, Floyd CD, Martin FM (1994) The synthesis of novel mimics of the sLex determinant. *Tetrahedron Asymmetry* 5: 2061–2076

95   Tsukida T, Hiramatsu Y, Tsujishita H et al (1997) Design synthesis and biological profile of sLex mimetics based on modified serine-glutamic acid dipeptides. *J Med Chem* 40: 3534–3541

96   Lin C-C, Shimazaki M, Heck M-P, Aoki S et al (1996) Synthesis and evaluation of N-(carboxy propyl amido)-3,4-dihydroxy prolyl-(O-α-L-fucopyranosyl)-threonyl ethyl ester and other glycopeptides as selectin antagonists. *J Am Chem Soc* 118: 6826–6840

97   Woltering T, Weitz-Schmidt G, Wong C-H (1996) C-Fucoside containing glycopeptides. *Tetrahedron Lett* 37: 9033–9036

98   Sutherlin DP, Todd MS, Hughes R, Armstrong RW (1996) Generation of C-glycoside peptide ligands for cell surface carbohydrate receptors using four-component condensation on solid support. *J Org Chem* 61: 8350–8354

99   Ng KK-S, Weiss WI (1997) Structure of selectin-like mutant of mannose-binding-protein complexed with sLe^x or sulfo Le^x oligosaccharides. *Biochemistry* 36: 979–988

100   Dupre B, Bui H, Scott IL, Market RV, Keller KM, Beck PJ, Kogan TP (1996) Glycomimetic selectin inhibitors: (α-D-mannopyranosyloxy)methylbiphenyls. *Bioorg Med Chem Lett* 6: 569–572

101   Kogan TP, Dupre B, Keller LKM et al (1995) Rational design and synthesis of small molecules. *J Med Chem* 38 : 4976–4984

102   Dupre B, Bui H, Scott IL, Market RV, Keller KM, Beck PJ, Kogan TP (1996) Glycomimetic selectin inhibitors. *Bioorg Med Chem Lett* 6: 569–572

103 Roche D, Banteli R, Winkler T, Casset F, Ernst B (1998) Synthesis of Benzylated (R)- and (S)-aminoethyl-C-α-D-mannopyranosides as conformationally restricted building blocks for the preparation of E- and P-selectin antagonists. *Tetrahedron Lett* 39: 2545–2548

104 Kogan TP, Dupre P, Bui H, McBee KL, Kassir JM, Scott IL, Hu X, Vanderslice P, Beck PJ, Dixon RF (1998) Novel synthetic inhibitors of selectin-mediated cell adhesion: Synthesis of 1,6-bis[3-(3-carboxymethylphenyl)-4-(2-α-D-mannopyranosyloxy)phenyl] hexane (TBC1269). *J Med Chem* 41: 1099–1111

105 Rao BNN, Anderson MA, Musser JH, Gilbert JH, Schaefer M, Foxall C, Brandley BK (1994) Sialyl Lewis x mimics derived from pharmacophore search are selectin inhibitors with anti-inflammatory activity. *J Biol Chem* 269: 19663–19666

106 Adhesion-based therapeutics (1997) *Genetic and Engineering News* 16: 12

Cell adhesion integrins as pharmaceutical targets

Kerry W. Fowler and David T. Crowe

ICOS Corporation, 22021 20th Avenue SE, Bothell WA 98021, USA

Introduction

The leukocyte integrins are transmembrane receptors expressed on circulating white blood cells that regulate their adhesion to other cells, the extracellular matrix, soluble proteins, and pathogens. Leukocyte adhesiveness is dynamically regulated in response to various cellular stimuli such as exposure to chemoattractants and cross-linking of B and T cell receptors. The capacity to modulate integrin adhesiveness prevents cells from non-specific attachment in the absence of specific inflammatory signals and allows them to detach from the blood vessel wall and migrate into the tissue.

Following ligand binding, integrins also transduce information into the interior of the cell. These signaling events regulate processes such as anchorage-dependent cell growth, intracellular pH, proliferation, and protein phosphorylation. Thus integrins serve as bidirectional conduits of information between the cell's interior and its environment. For a recent review of these signaling processes see Hughes' summary of integrin affinity modulation [1].

The adhesion of circulating leukocytes to the vascular endothelium is regulated in a multi-step process [2]. In response to various inflammatory stimuli, endothelial cells respond by up-regulating their expression of both E- and P-selectin. This facilitates the initial recruitment of leukocytes to sites of inflammation by promoting the initial attachment and subsequent rolling of circulating cells along the inner surface of the blood vessel. Selectins bind to the fucosylated, sialyl-Lewis X tetrasaccharide (sLe^x) on leukocytes. In turn, leukocytes expressing L-selectin bind to sLe^x on the sialylated endothelial glycoproteins GlyCAM-1 and CD34. A more detailed description of selectins can be found in the chapter by Dasgupta in this volume and will not be discussed here. Unexpectedly, the α4 integrins (α4β1 and α4β7) can also mediate rolling behavior [3]. The rolling of cells along the endothelial surface is thought to allow leukocytes to sample the local microenvironment for the presence of chemoattractants that decorate the endothelial cell surface.

Leukocytes express multiple G protein coupled receptors (GPCRs) on their surface which can bind chemoattractants and chemokines. These GPCRs initiate the second phase of the multi-step model that culminates in integrin activation. Here, a cascade of intracellular signaling events results in the rapid and transient up-regulation of integrin adhesiveness that promotes the stable attachment of leukocytes to the lumen of the blood vessel. The application of kinase and phosphatase inhibitors to the study of cell adhesion has been quite useful in identifying some of the components of the signal transduction cascade that leads to integrin activation. The up-regulation of integrin adhesiveness may be accomplished by either changes in integrin affinity and/or receptor clustering [4]. Following the stable arrest of leukocytes from the bloodstream, they begin a process known as extravasation, whereby cells transmigrate across the endothelium and the underlying basement membrane. Upon entering the tissue, leukocytes then migrate in response to the directional queues provided by gradients of chemoattractants. These gradients ultimately direct leukocytes to appropriate sites within the tissue where they carry out their specialized effector functions in the attempt to resolve the underlying inflammation.

Integrin structure

Integrins are α-β heterodimers of two transmembrane glycoprotein subunits that are noncovalently linked. Through the selective pairing of at least 16 α subunits and eight β subunits, at least 22 different integrins can be generated. The selective combinatorial pairing of α and β subunits allows cells to achieve a broad repertoire of ligand-binding activity through the expression of a limited number of proteins. Integrins also have the capacity to recognize multiple ligands. For example, the integrin $\alpha M\beta 2$ mediates leukocyte adhesion to numerous proteins including ICAM-1, ICAM-3, fibrinogen, iC3b, and factor X.

While the integrins can be identified by their constituent subunits (such as $\alpha 2\beta 2$), many are known by other names, some of which are listed in Table 1. The integrin $\alpha 1\beta 1$ is commonly known as VLA1 (very late activation antigen 1), for example. A convenient online summary of the naming of cell surface molecules is also available [5]. This web site from the National Center for Biotechnology Information also includes structure and function, and ligand information. Table 1 below summarizes some α and β subunit pairings for integrins related primarily to inflammation.

Integrin ligands

The integrin ligands currently known to mediate the stable attachment of leukocytes to the blood vessel wall are members of the immunoglobulin superfamily of cell adhesion molecules [6]. They include ICAM-1, ICAM-2, and ICAM-3, which are

Table 1 - Summary of integrins relevant to inflammation

	β1 (CD29)	β2 (CD18)	β7
α1 (CD49a)	VLA1		
α2 (CD49b)	VLA2		
α3 (CD49c)	VLA3		
α4 (CD49d)	VLA4		
			α4β7
αL (CD11a)		LFA-1	
αM (CD11b)		MAC-1	

ligands for the β2 integrins, VCAM-1 which is a ligand for α4β1 and α4β7, and MAdCAM-1 which binds to α4β7. These members of the IgSF share the immunoglobulin domain, composed of 90–100 amino acids arranged in a sandwich of two sheets of anti-parallel β strands. The crystal structure of the N-terminal two-domain fragment of these IgSF proteins has been determined for ICAM-1 [7], ICAM-2 [8], VCAM-1 [9], and MAdCAM-1 [10]. Numerous mutagenesis experiments have identified the primary integrin binding site on IgSF members to be primarily localized to a cluster of acidic amino acid residues located in the β turn between β strands C and D in domain 1. Alignment of these IgSF integrin-binding sites reveals a modest consensus structure: "small/Q-L/I-acidic-S/T-P/S"; most integrin ligands employ variants of either the RGD or LDV motif as the primary element of the integrin-binding site [11]. In fact cyclization of peptides containing the integrin binding site have modest inhibitory activity in *in vitro* cell-based adhesion assays [12]. These data suggest that the integrin binding site is both topographically constrained and primarily localized to a discrete site, although additional residues are known to contribute to integrin binding.

Scope of this review

This review will focus primarily on the description of antagonists for those integrins known to mediate leukocyte-endothelial interactions: the CD18 integrins (αLβ2 or LFA-1, αMβ2 or MAC-1, αDβ2, αXβ2), and CD49d integrins (α4β1 and α4β7). Perhaps the best studied integrin is αIIb-β3 (also known as GPIIb-IIIa), a receptor found on platelets for fibrinogen and other ligands, and a key player in the clotting cascade. In 1998, the first two small molecule RGD mimics were launched as drugs in the US: tirofiban HCl (Merck) and eptifibatide (Cor Therapeutics) [13]. More than a dozen other compounds are in Phase 1–3 clinical trials. This fruitful research is unfortunately beyond the scope of this review and the reader is referred to recent reviews [14–16]. Selectins are also essential determinants in leukocyte trafficking to sites of inflammation (see this volume and recent reviews [17, 18]) and will not be discussed here.

Integrins as pharmaceutical targets

The inflammatory process depends upon the recruitment and directed migration of leukocytes to the site of inflammation and there are multiple steps at which one could intervene. A successful anti-inflammatory drug could antagonize leukocyte adhesion, migration, or the leukocyte's functional properties. Integrins are clearly desirable pharmaceutical targets because of their pivotal role in nearly every step in the inflammatory process and their cell type specificity. There are also numerous animal models of chronic human diseases with an inflammatory component, e.g. EAE [19], inflammatory bowel disease [20], transplant rejection [21], rheumatoid arthritis [22], asthma [23], and ischemia-reperfusion injuries [24]. In these systems, anti-integrin antibodies have been tested for their therapeutic efficacy, and have shown utility in the treatment of these diseases. Certainly in acute settings, function blocking anti-integrin monoclonal antibodies may become the initial mode of treatment, and numerous clinical trials are underway which employ anti-integrin antibodies in many of these indications [25].

Challenges of integrins as drug targets

There are several hurdles to the development of a small molecule antagonist of integrin function. A successful integrin antagonist would display a high degree of receptor specificity, especially among those integrins sharing a common subunit. One could reasonably assume that an antagonist that binds to the common $\beta2$ subunit of $\alpha L\beta2$, $\alpha M\beta2$, $\alpha D\beta2$, and $\alpha X\beta2$ would exhibit greater immunosuppressive effects than an antagonist that binds to either a specific a subunit or a unique structure created by α-β dimerization. Immunosuppressive side effects might also be regulated by the biodistribution or half life of the drug since a compound with poor penetrance into tissue might be less immunosuppressive than one residing primarily in the bloodstream.

Two screening routes might be selected; cell-based static adhesion assays or recombinant protein-protein based ELISAs. Although protein-based screens display greater reproducibility and eliminate the numerous false positives that occur in cell-based screens due to cell toxicity, several problems remain. Specifically, do recombinant integrins and CAMs faithfully adopt the various activation states or conformational changes that the transmembrane receptors are thought to experience? A final concern relates to the potency of small molecule antagonists in protein-based screens versus cell-based screens. Most inhibitors identified in ELISA-based screens display a considerable reduction in potency when subsequently tested in cell-based assays. This is due to the difficulty in disrupting the highly avid nature of whole cells adhering to immobilized substrates.

New methods of drug discovery

In this decade, new technologies have made it possible to sample vast chemical space in ever shorter periods of time, giving us the opportunity to find better leads sooner. High throughput screening (HTS) and the synthesis of combinatorial libraries have changed the world of drug discovery and it is impossible to ignore their impact on the discovery process. The successes of LFA-1 and VLA-4 peptidomimetic antagonists (described below) show the growing influence of this approach.

Another new technology, a powerful spectroscopic technique known as "SAR by NMR" has been applied to the design of integrin inhibitors [26]. The method pioneered by Stephen Fesik of Abbott Laboratories [27] involves the screening of libraries of small fragment molecules in 2D protein NMR. Even molecules that bind with only micromolar affinities can induce readily observable changes in the 2D spectrum and indicate specific sites of binding. The tethering of two such ligands which bind to adjacent sites on a target can produce nanomolar inhibitors. The lack of discrete catalytic sites and 3D structures for integrins makes this technique particularly useful in detecting binding regions for small molecules.

Inhibitors of LFA-1/ICAM-1

The binding of LFA-1 with its counter receptor ICAM-1 is essential to both the initial adhesion and subsequent transmigration of leukocytes across the wall of blood vessels. Blockade of LFA-1/ICAM-1 engagement by monoclonal antibodies to LFA-1 is effective in several animal models of both acute and chronic inflammatory diseases. Unfortunately, monoclonal antibodies are not suitable for the treatment of chronic inflammatory diseases, justifying the considerable effort that has been placed on identifying a small molecule antagonist of LFA-1. Small molecule antagonists of LFA-1 function could in theory function by disrupting: 1) the signal transduction leading to LFA-1 activation, 2) LFA-1 expression, 3) the ligand binding site of LFA-1 for ICAM-1, or 4) the ability of LFA-1 to adopt an "activated" conformation.

Despite the variety of structures reported as LFA-1 inhibitors, the potencies are relatively low, particularly when compared with the nanomolar inhibitors of VLA-4 reported (see below). For example, researchers at R.W. Johnson [28] disclosed a series of 2-pyrazolylthiazoles as inhibitors of LFA-1-dependent adhesion of HL60

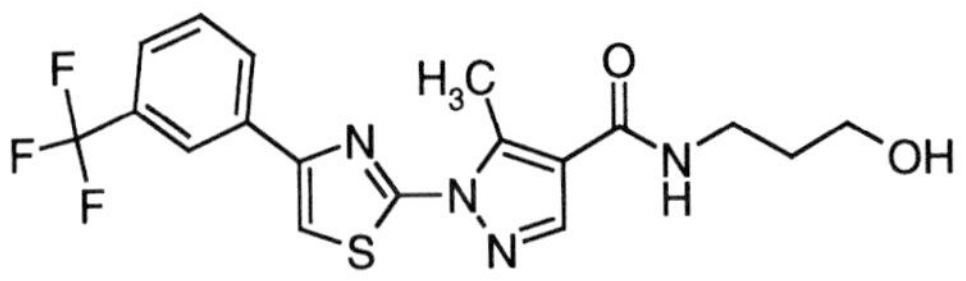

compound 1 (RWJ-50271)

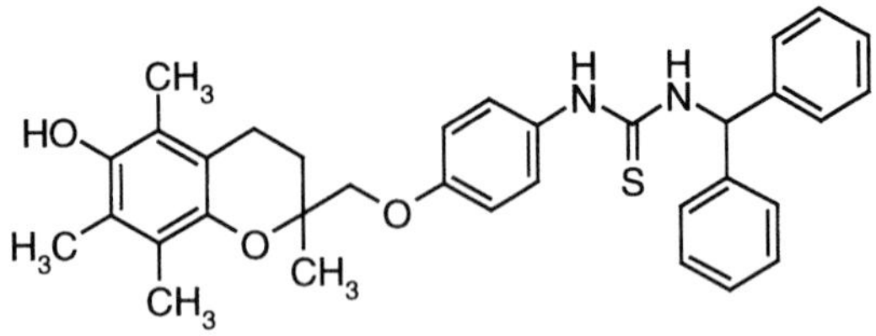

compound 2

cells binding to immobilized ICAM-1 (IC_{50} ~5 mM). Their experiments also showed that compound RWJ-50271 (**1**) did not affect Mac-1/ICAM-1, sLe^x/E-selectin, or VLA-4/VCAM-1 interactions and did not exhibit any cell toxicity up to a concentration of 20 µM. An oral dose of 50 milligrams per kilogram (mpk) 4 h post challenge also reduced foot pad swelling in mice tested in delayed-type hypersensitivity reaction (DTH) for T cell-mediated immunity.

Warner Lambert [29] has described a chroman derivative (**2**) as a mixed ICAM-1/VCAM-1 inhibitor with an IC_{50} of 23 µM.

Among the natural products discovered to inhibit integrin adhesion is an unusual peroxide derived from *Streptomyces* [30]. Adxanthromycin (**3**) inhibited the adhesion of SKW-3 leukemic T cells to soluble ICAM-1 at a concentration of 18.8 micrograms/mL (~ 23 µM). Another group of diterpenes [31] was isolated from the leaves of *Casearia guianensis* including **4** (casearinone B). Similar terpenes from the *Casearia* genus have reported antitumor properties [32].

Inhibition of the adhesion of cells expressing activated β2 integrin to recombinant ICAM-1 was accomplished by compound **5** (asperlin) [33], an *Aspergillus* metabolite (29% at 6.25 µg/mL, 94% at 50 µg/mL).

A group of lipophilic sulfonamides was reported in a patent to inhibit cell adhesion mediated by ICAM-1/LFA-1 [34]. The most potent compounds reported were submicromolar inhibitors, such as 0.5 µM for compound **6** shown below.

A series of compounds such as compound **7** are related to the quinolone antibiotics, and were shown to inhibit the expression of ICAM-1 in cultured HUVECs

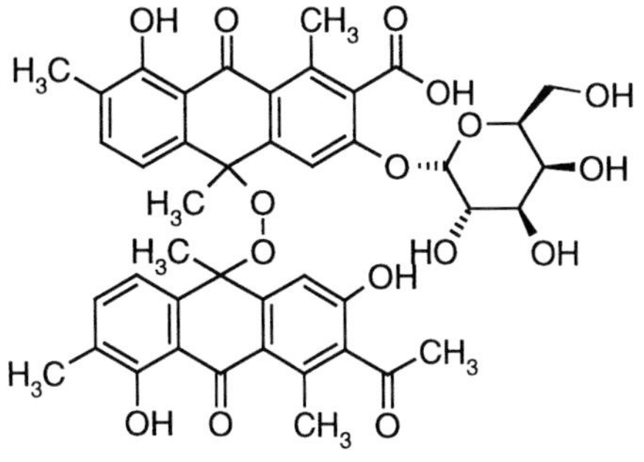

compound 3

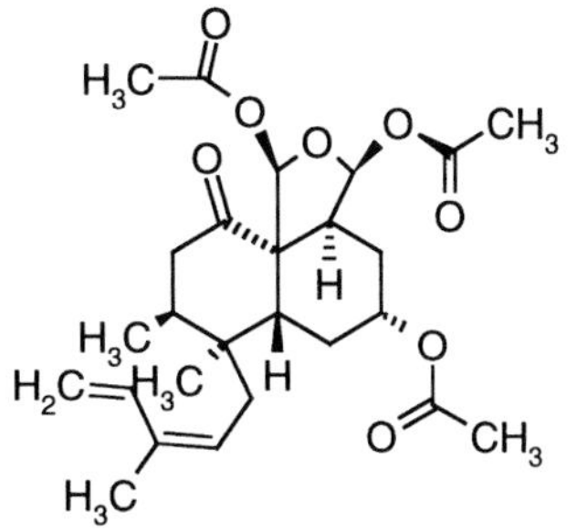

compound 4 (casearinone B)

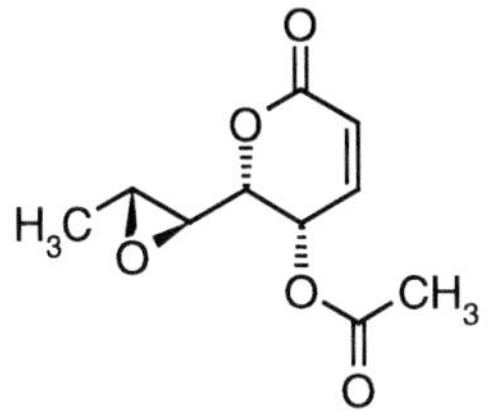

compound 5 (asperlin)

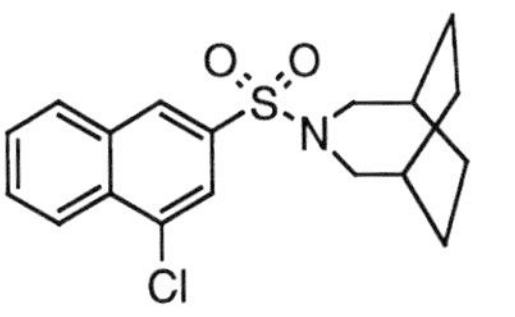

compound 6

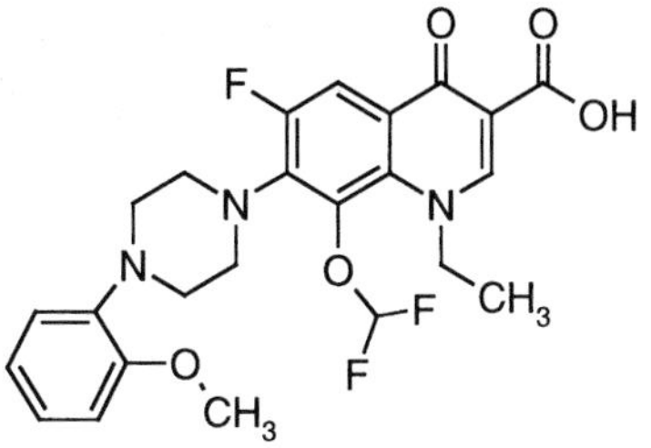

compound 7

(human umbilical vein endothelial cells) at 5 μg/mL (10 μM) in the presence of TNFα [35].

Inhibition of ICAM-1-dependent JY cell adhesion was reported [36] by isotetracenones such as compound 8 (AI-090) and compound 9 (AI-096). The former had an IC$_{50}$ of 10 μg/mL.

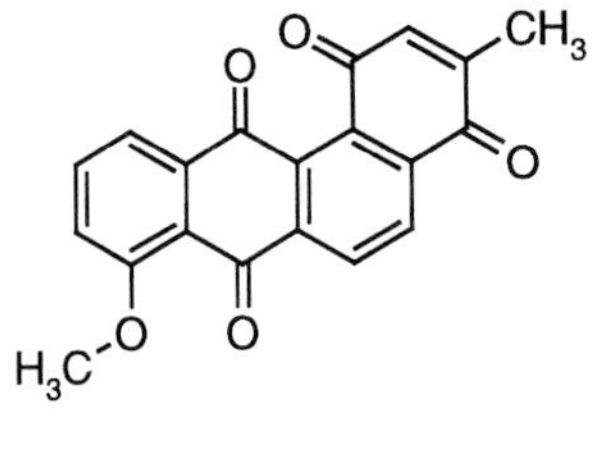

compound 8 (AI-090)

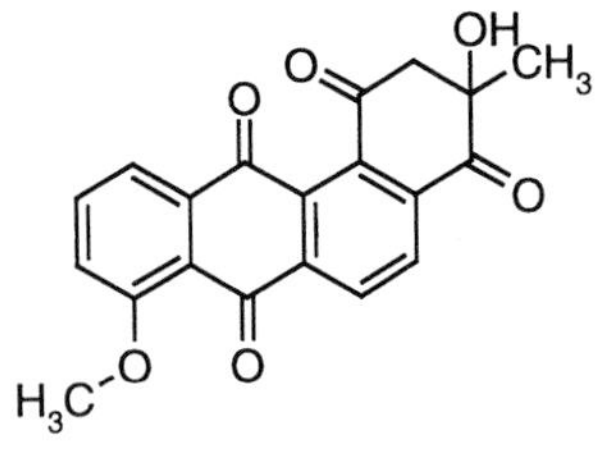

compound 9 (AI-096)

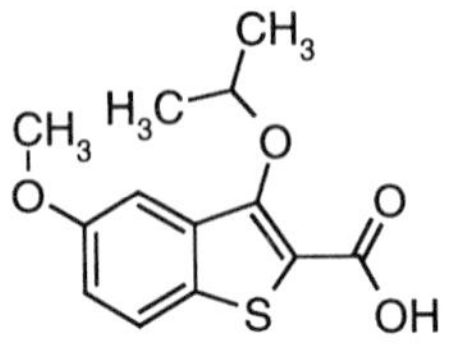

compound 10

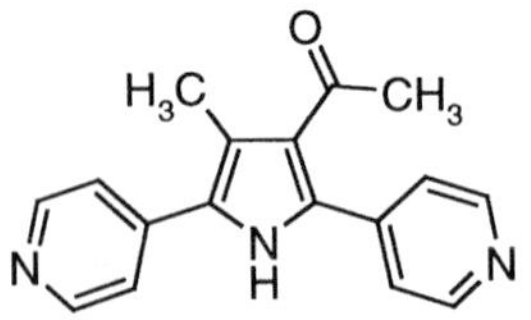

compound 11

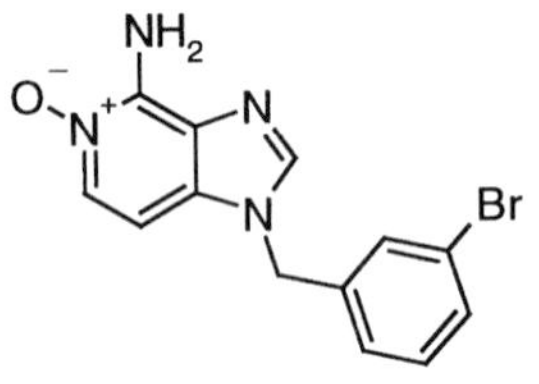

compound 12

Benzothiophenes such as compound **10** inhibited the expression of ICAM-1 in HUVECs with IC_{50} of 3.9 μM [37].

Two compounds reported [38, 39] to inhibit the expression of both ICAM-1 and E-selectin and adhesion of HL-60 cells to HUVECs are shown above (compounds **11** and **12**).

Some kinase inhibitors have also been reported to inhibit cell adhesion. For example, the protein kinase C inhibitor AG490 (**13**), a member of the class known as tyrphostins, was able to block the development of experimentally induced auto-encephalitis (EAE) in a murine model [40]. Leukocytes isolated from treated mice were also less adhesive to VCAM-1, and encephalogenic T cell lines treated with AG490 were less adherent to ICAM-1 and VCAM-1.

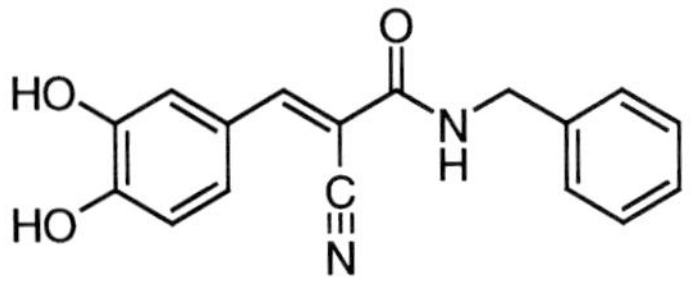

compound 13 (AG490)

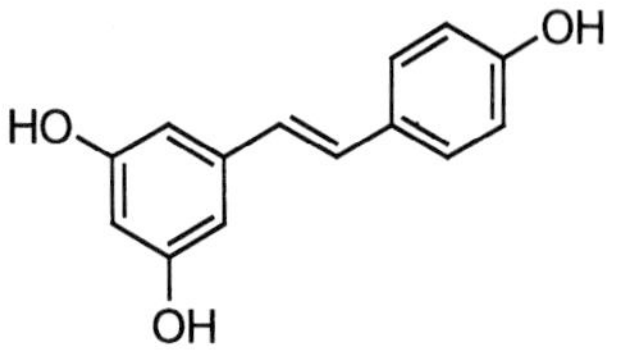

compound 14 (Resveratrol)

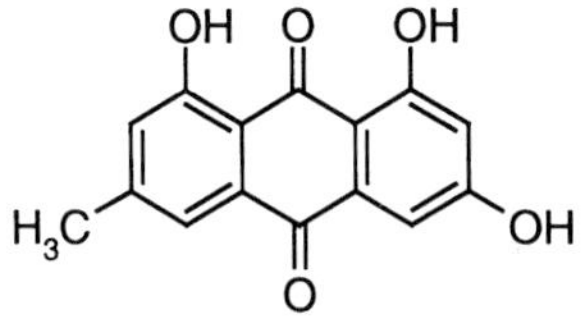

compound 15 (Emodin)

Compound **14** (Resveratrol) is found in red wine and attributed to the protection of LDL from peroxidative degradation. Because it is a potent tyrosine kinase inhibitor, Milanese researchers [41] postulated that like other such inhibitors it would inhibit cell adhesion. In fact, Resveratrol inhibited the expression of ICAM-1 and VCAM-1 in HSVECs (human saphenous vein endothelial cells) stimulated by TNFα at concentrations of 1 μmole/L and 0.1 μmole/L, respectively. It also inhibited U937 and neutrophil adhesion.

Compound **15** (Emodin) is another tyrosine kinase and protein kinase C inhibitor that is known to inhibit the growth of HER-2/neu-overexpressing tumors in mice and acts synergistically with paclitaxel [42]. Emodin inhibited monocyte adhesion to endothelial cells and blocked the expression of ICAM-1, VCAM-1, and ELAM-1 [43]. Its activity was attributed to the inhibition of the degradation of IκB, an inhibitory subunit of NFκB.

Inhibitors of VLA-4/VCAM-1

Like the RGD field, VLA-4 inhibitor design based upon peptide sequences has been productive. A 1998 review of VLA-4 antagonists from Biogen [44] describes inhibitors derived from the LDV sequence, the minimal recognition site for VLA-4 on the fibronectin CS-1 segment. Biogen incorporated rationally designed diaryl-ureas at the N-terminus of LDV analogues exploiting favorable hydrophobic inter-

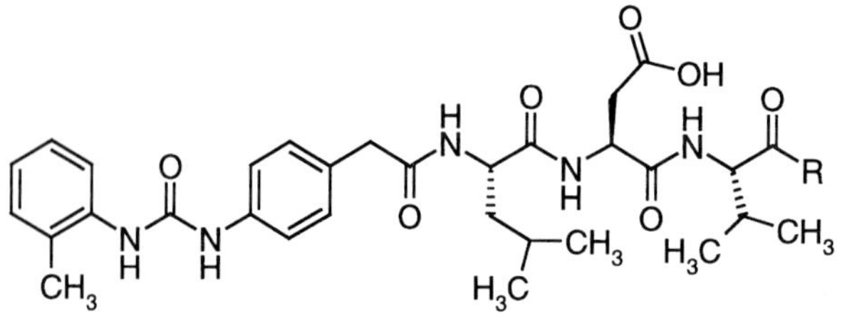

compound 16

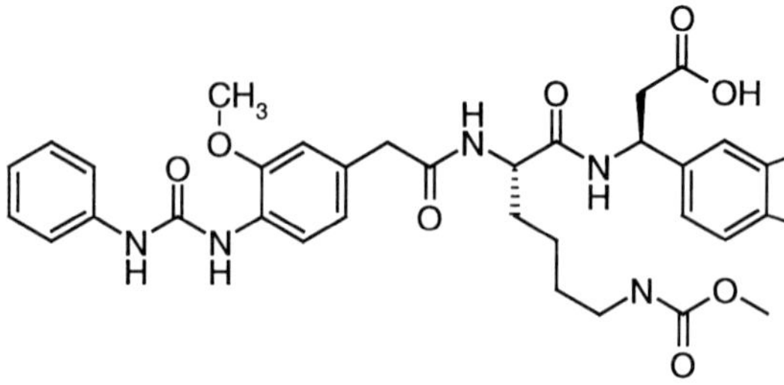

compound 17 (BIO-1272)

actions to arrive at very potent compounds. BIO 1211 (compound 16, R = proline) and the free acid (compound 16, R = OH) had IC_{50}s of 1 and 0.4 nM, respectively.

The most potent inhibitors reported by Biogen include peptidomimetics such as BIO1272 (17), with an IC_{50} of 0.3 nM [45].

Biogen has also applied for a patent on the design of VLA-4 inhibitors based upon the detailed description of a three-dimensional pharmacophore model [46]. The model consists of a NEG (negative) element and at least three features chosen from the seven groups including a hydrogen bond donor, a hydrogen bond acceptor, and a hydrophobic group (Tab. 2).

A Genentech group employed the peptide RCDPC derived from the VCAM-1 binding epitope. Beginning with 3.7 μM inhibitors, they eventually prepared inhibitors such as compound 18 (0.1 nM) with up to 1000 fold selectivity for VLA-4 over VLA-5 for one inhibitor [47].

Cyclic peptides from Zeneca inhibit the interaction of VLA-4 with VCAM-1 and fibronectin [48, 49] as well as α4β7/MAdCAM-1 interactions. The peptides are cyclo(MeFLCVDRDR), for example, and cyclo[ILDV(CH$_2$)$_5$CO]. The macrocyclic peptide derivative compound 19 was among those reported which inhibited the interaction of VLA-4 with ligands VCAM-1 or fibronectin [50]. It consists of two LDV sequences connected by piperazine linkers.

154

Table 2 - Pharmacophore elements describing VLA-4 inhibitors [46]

	Feature	X (Å)	Y (Å)	Z (Å)	Tolerance (Å)
N	NEG	−8.564	1.564	−0.236	1.702
1	HBA-1	−1.276	−1.259	−1.47	1.702
	HBA-2	−2.323	1.539	−1.35	1.702
2	HBD-1	6.693	1.988	−0.168	1.702
	HBD-2	7.217	0.939	2.630	1.702
3	HYD2	2.777	−1.061	−1.1501	1.702
4	HYD3	−3.803	−4.061	0.270	1.702
5	HYD4	9.337	2.219	1.050	1.702
6	HYD5	8.677	4.439	−1.330	1.702
7	HYD6	−9.123	−1.501	1.110	1.702

Where NEG is negative; HBA is hydrogen bond acceptor; HBD is hydrogen bond donor; HYD is hydrophobic

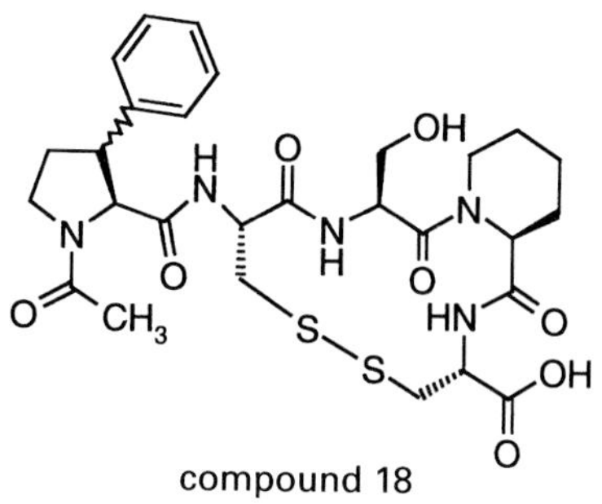

compound 18

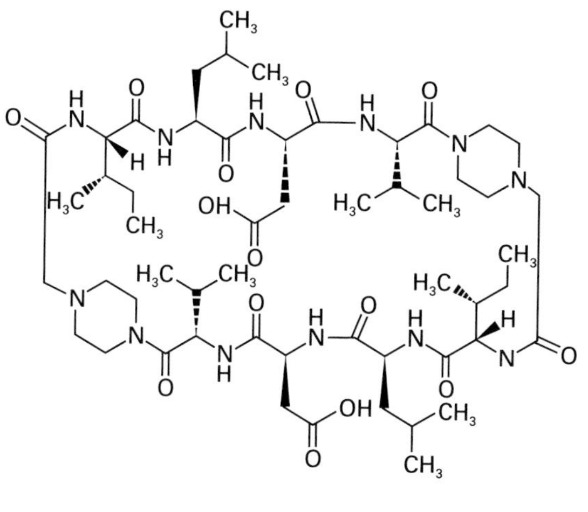

compound 19

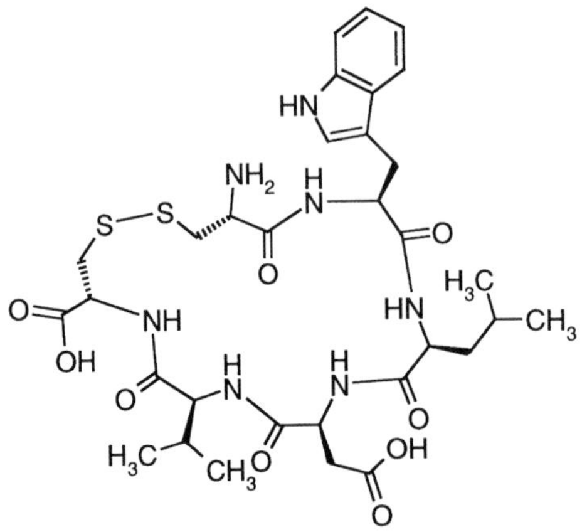

compound 20 (TBC722)

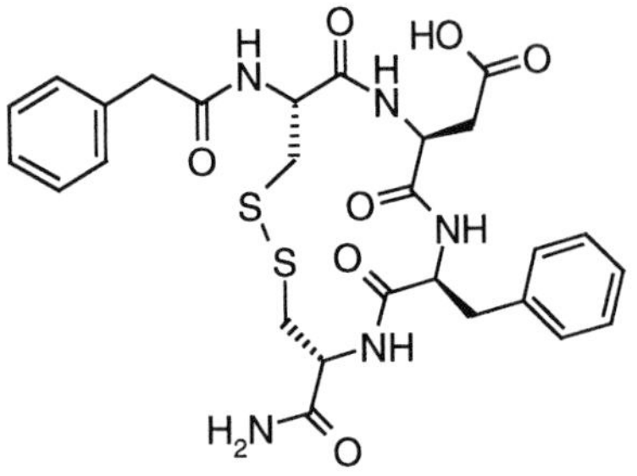

compound 21

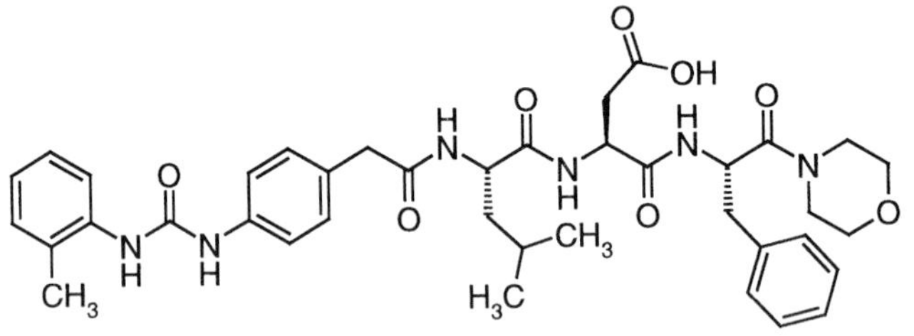

compound 22

Another series of cyclic peptide inhibitors was also based on the LDV sequence of the fibronectin splice variant containing connecting segment 1 (CS1). The most potent of these was compound 21 TBC722 which inhibited MnCl$_2$-stimulated lymphocytes with IC$_{50}$s of 0.4 mM for VCAM-1 and 0.05 mM for CS-1 [51]. Immunoprecipitation experiments showed that the peptide bound directly to $\alpha 4\beta 1$ and $\alpha 4\beta 7$. TBC722 (20) also inhibited the activation of T lymphocytes stimulated with VCAM-1 [52].

A Cytel patent [53] describes cyclic peptide inhibitors based upon the CS-1 sequence, the most preferred being disulfide N-phenylacetyl-C*DFC*NH$_2$ (compound 21).

Other Cytel compounds [54] bear substitutions on the phenylacetyl group. Compound 22, similar to the Biogen compound 16 is reported to have an IC$_{50}$ of 0.4 nM in a VLA-4 dependent Jurkat cell adhesion assay.

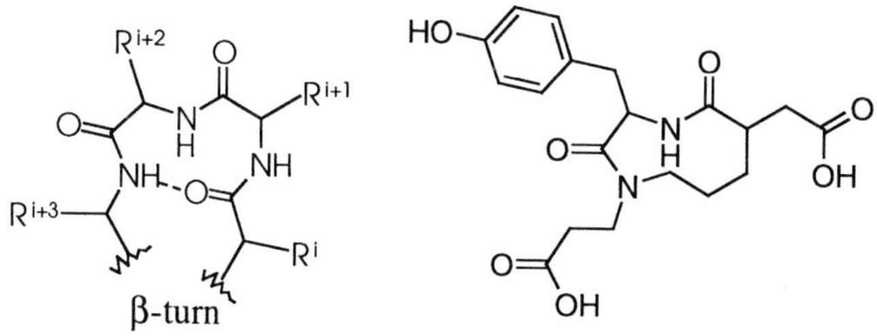

Figure 1

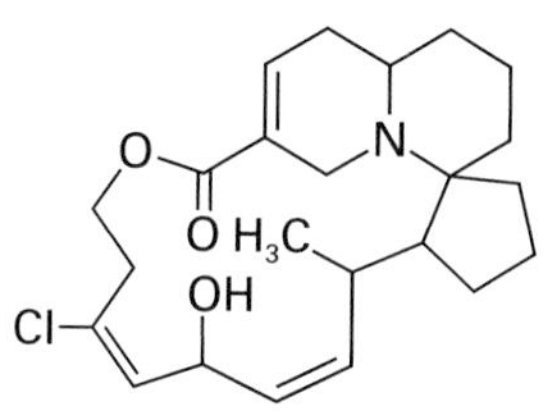

compound 23

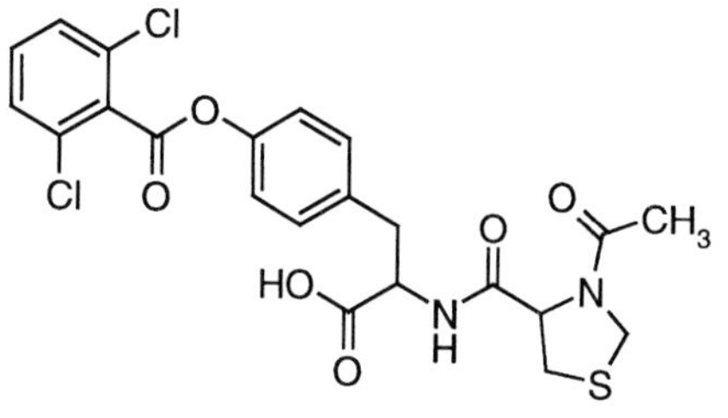

compound 24

An attempt to prepare nonpeptide antagonists based upon the LDV sequence led to the preparation on solid phase of a library of β-turn mimetics [55]. The scaffold in Figure 1 is shown next to a diagram of a β-turn for comparison. From a library of over 5500 compounds the authors chose 2304 which had the aspartic acid at one site and a diversity of residues at the others. The compounds were screened for their ability to inhibit the binding of fluorescently labeled cells to immobilized CS-1 peptide. Active compounds tended to possess an aspartate at the I+1 site and a hydrophobic group at I+2. The most potent compound shown here had an IC_{50} of 5 μM.

An extract of the sponge *Halicondria okadai* provided the macrocyclic lactone shown (23) which inhibits the expression of VCAM-1 on the surface of HUVECs induced by TNFα (IC_{50} 7 μg/mL) [56].

Submicromolar inhibitors of α4 integrin dependent adhesion were tyrosine derivatives [57]. They were selective for α4β1 and α4β7 (< 1 μM) compared with other integrins (> 50 μM) (24).

Hoechst researchers described heterocyclic derivatives such as the hydantoin shown as inhibitors [58–60] of the VLA-4 receptor (25).

Non-peptide natural product inhibitors of the α4β1 integrins include a macrocyclic ether from Sagami that inhibits binding VCAM-1 (26) [61].

The antibiotic bacitracin was reported to inhibit α4β7 and β1 dependent adhesion (IC_{50} ~1–2 mM), while having no effect on αvβ3 or αLβ2 mediated adhesion

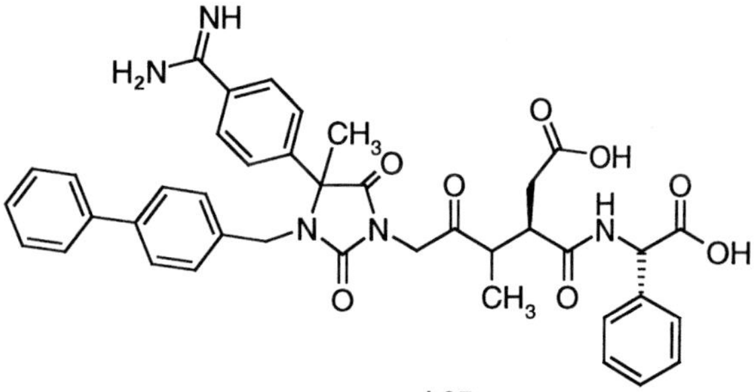

compound 25

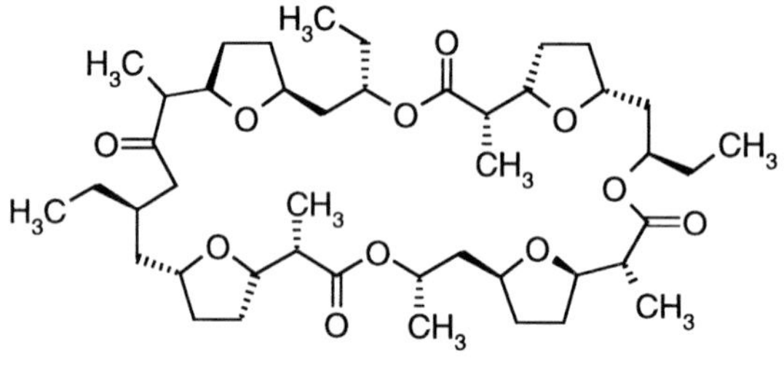

compound 26

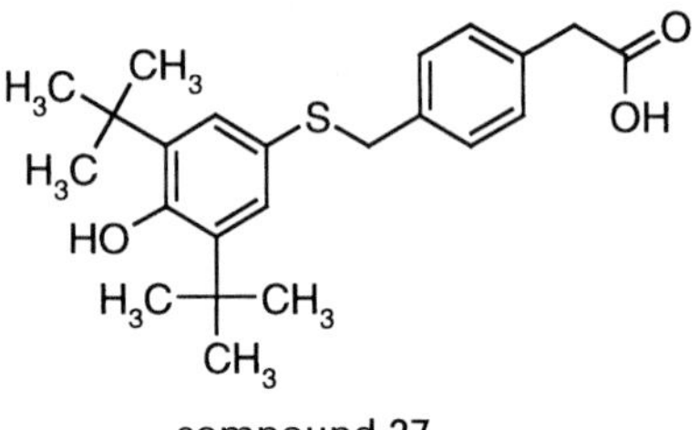

compound 27

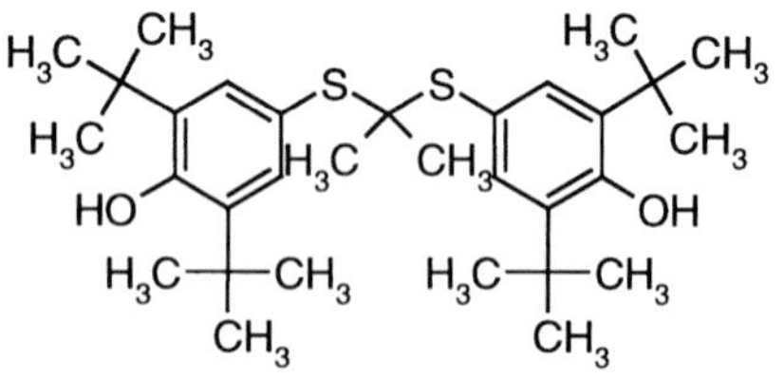

compound 28 (probucol)

[62]. Although bacitracin inhibits protein disulfide isomerase (PDI), several known PDI inhibitors failed to block lymphocyte adhesion. Their results therefore do not support a role of PDIs in the regulation of integrin function, but suggest that bacitracin is a selective inhibitor of β7 and β1 integrin function [63].

Antioxidative phenols such as compounds **27** and **28** (probucol) and their soluble monoesters have been reported to inhibit the expression of VCAM-1 by researchers at Atherogenics [63, 64]. Also reported were esters of the anticholesteremic drug compound **28** (probucol) [65].

Silicon-containing compounds similar to probucol developed by Hoechst Marion Roussel inhibited the expression of VCAM-1 on human aortic smooth muscle

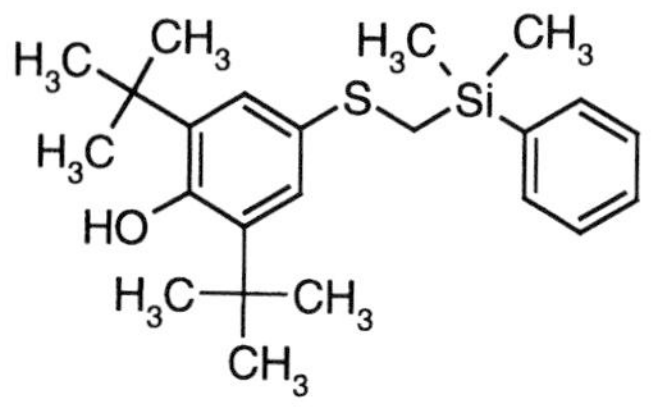

compound 29

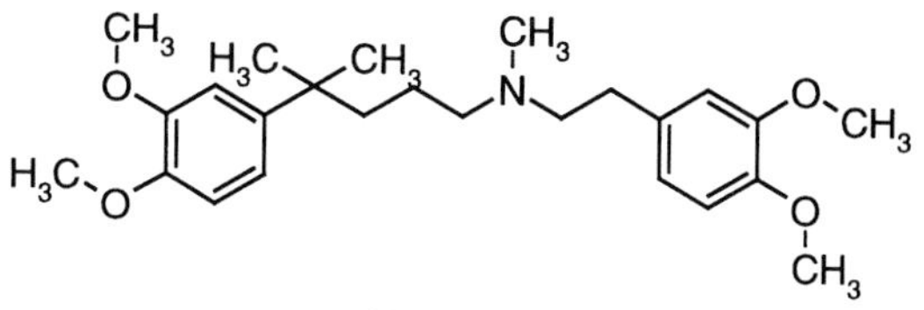

Verapamil

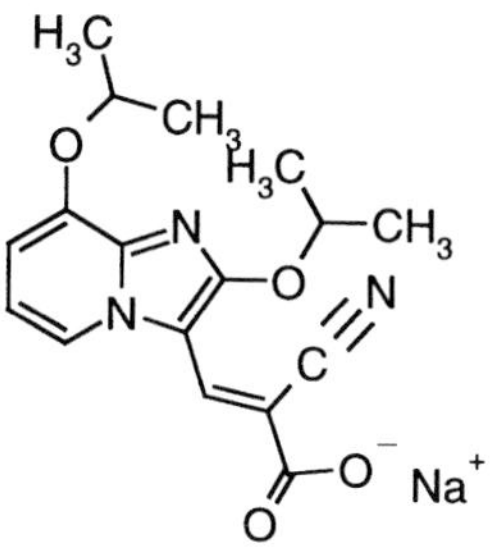

compound 30 (SJC13)

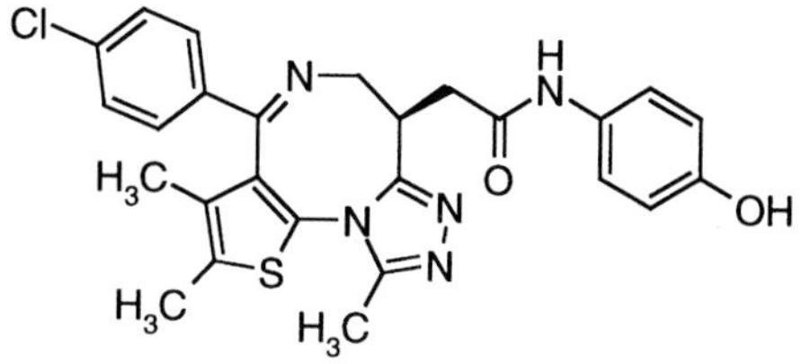

compound 31

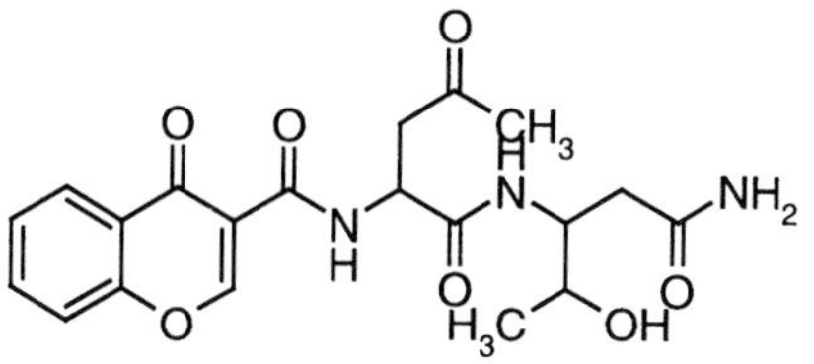

compound 32

cells incubated with IL-4 or HUVECs stimulated by TNFα (29) [66]. The highest potencies reported were in the 5–50 μM range. In some cases they also inhibited ICAM-1 expression.

The utility of calcium channel blockers in improving the success of transplantation and as immunosuppressants prompted a study of the effect of Verapamil on leukocyte adhesion and expression [67]. Verapamil reduced protein and mRNA levels of VCAM-1 and inhibited adhesion of endothelial cells stimulated by TNFα.

Compound 30 (SJC13) and compound 31 reportedly have mixed VCAM-1 and E-selectin inhibition.

α4β7/MAdCAM-1

Little research has appeared on inhibitors of α4β7 integrin. The LDTSL sequence of the CD loop of MAdCAM-1 is the likely site of recognition for α4β7 and this binding site is conserved in both murine and human proteins. Peptidomimetics [68] developed by LeukoSite based upon the LDT motif reduced the binding of the tripeptide from 250 μM to the low μM range. N-terminal acylation with aryl groups and C-terminal modification giving N-benzyl amides led to inhibitors down to 1 μM. Substitution of the amino acids with their D-enantiomers and β-analogues gave compounds such as the one shown below (32).

References

1   Hughes PE, Pfaff M (1998) Integrin affinity modulation. *Trends Cell Biol* 8 (9): 359–364

2   Springer TA (1994) Traffic signals for lymphocyte recirculation and leukocyte emigration: the multistep paradigm. *Cell* 76 (2): 301–314

3   Berlin C, Bargatze RF, Campbell JJ, von Andrian UH, Szabo MC, Hasslen SR, Nelson RD, Berg EL, Erlandsen SL, Butcher EC (1995) Alpha 4 integrins mediate lymphocyte attachment and rolling under physiologic flow. *Cell* 80 (3): 413–422

4   Diamond MS, Springer TA (1994) The dynamic regulation of integrin adhesiveness. *Curr Biol* 4 (6): 506–517

5   http://www.ncbi.nlm.nih.gov/prow/cd/index_molecule.htm

6   Wang J, Springer TA (1998) Structural specializations of immunoglobulin superfamily members for adhesion to integrins and viruses. *Immunol Rev* 163: 197–215

7   Casasnovas JM, Stehle T, Liu JH, Wang JH, Springer TA (1998) A dimeric crystal structure for the N-terminal two domains of intercellular adhesion molecule-1. *Proc Natl Acad Sci USA* 95 (8): 4134–4139

8   Casasnovas JM, Springer TA, Liu JH, Harrison SC, Wang JH (1997) Crystal structure of ICAM-2 reveals a distinctive integrin recognition surface. *Nature* 387 (6630): 312–315

9   Jones EY, Harlos K, Bottomley MJ, Robinson RC, Driscoll PC, Edwards RM, Clements JM, Dudgeon TJ, Stuart DI (1995) Crystal structure of an integrin-binding fragment of vascular cell adhesion molecule-1 at 1.8 Å resolution. *Nature* 373 (6514): 539–544

10   Tan K, Casasnovas JM, Liu JH, Briskin MJ, Springer TA, Wang JH (1998) The structure of immunoglobulin superfamily domains 1 and 2 of MAdCAM-1 reveals novel features important for integrin recognition. *Structure* 6 (6): 793–801

11   Newham P, Craig SE, Seddon GN, Schofield NR, Rees A, Edwards RM, Jones EY, Humphries MJ (1997) Alpha4 integrin binding interfaces on VCAM-1 and MAdCAM-1. Integrin binding footprints identify accessory binding sites that play a role in integrin specificity. *J Biol Chem* 272 (31): 19429–19440

12 Cardarelli PM, Cobb RR, Nowlin DM, Scholz W, Gorcsan F, Moscinski M, Yasuhara M, Chiang SL, Lobl TJ (1994) Cyclic RGD peptide inhibits alpha 4 beta 1 interaction with connecting segment 1 and vascular cell adhesion molecule. *J Biol Chem* 269 (28): 18668–18673

13 *Prous Science Daily Essentials*, "Spotlight update: fibrinogen (gpIIb/IIIa) receptor antagonists", March 1, 1999

14 Topol EJ, Byzova TV, Plow EF (1999) Platelet GPIIb-IIIa blockers. *Lancet* 353 (9148): 227–231

15 Hoekstra WJ, Poulter BL (1998) Combinatorial chemistry techniques applied to non-peptide integrin antagonists. *Curr Med Chem* 5 (3): 195–204

16 Ojima I, Chakravarty S, Dong Q (1995) Antithrombotic agents: from RGD to peptide mimetics. *Bioorg Med Chem* 3 (4): 337–360

17 Simanek EE, McGarvey GJ, Jablonowski JA, Wong C-H (1998) Selectin-carbohydrate interactions: from natural ligands to designed mimics. *Chem Rev* 98: 833–862

18 Levy DE, Tang PC, Musser JH (1994) Cell adhesion and carbohydrates. *Annual Reports in Medicinal Chemistry* 29: 215–224

19 Rose LM, Richards TL, Peterson J, Petersen R, Alvord EC Jr (1997) Resolution of CNS lesions following treatment of experimental allergic encephalomyelitis in macaques with monoclonal antibody to the CD18 leukocyte integrin. *Mult Scler* 2 (6): 259–266

20 Hesterberg PE, Winsor-Hines D, Briskin MJ, Soler-Ferran D, Merrill C, Mackay CR, Newman W, Ringler DJ (1996) Rapid resolution of chronic colitis in the cotton-top tamarin with an antibody to a gut-homing integrin alpha 4 beta 7. *Gastroenterology* 111 (5): 1373–1380

21 Jendrisak M, Jendrisak G, Gamero J, Mohanakumar T (1993) Prolongation in murine cardiac allograft survival with monoclonal antibodies to LFA-1, ICAM-1, and CD4. *Transplant Proc* (1 Pt 1): 825–827

22 Zeidler A, Brauer R, Thoss K, Bahnsen J, Heinrichs V, Jablonski-Westrich D, Wroblewski M, Rebstock S, Hamann A (1995) Therapeutic effects of antibodies against adhesion molecules in murine collagen type II-induced arthritis. *Autoimmunity* 21 (4): 245–252

23 Schleimer RP, Bochner BS (1998) The role of adhesion molecules in allergic inflammation and their suitability as targets of antiallergic therapy. *Clin Exp Allergy* 28 (3): 15–23

24 Thiagarajan RR, Winn RK, Harlan JM (1997) The role of leukocyte and endothelial adhesion molecules in ischemia-reperfusion injury. *Thromb Haemost* 78 (1): 310–314

25 Adgey AA (1998) An overview of the results of clinical trials with glycoprotein IIb/IIIa inhibitors. *Am Heart J* 135 (4): S43–S55

26 ICOS and Abbott Expand Collaboration. *ICOS Corporation press release*, September 7, 1997

27 Shuker SB, Hajduk PJ, Meadows RP, Fesik SW (1996) Discovering high-affinity ligands for proteins: SAR by NMR. *Science* 274 (5292): 1531–1534

28 Sanfilippo PJ, Jetter MC, Cordova R, Noe RA, Chourmouzis E, Lau CY, Wang E (1995)

Novel thiazole based heterocycles as inhibitors of LFA-1/ICAM-1 mediated cell adhesion. *J Med Chem* 38 (7): 1057–1059

29 US 5747528

30 Koiwa T, Nakano T, Takahashi S, Koshino H, Yamazaki M, Takashi T, Nakagawa A (1999) Adxanthromycin: a new inhibitor of ICAM-1/LFA-1 mediated cell adhesion from Streptomyces sp. NA-148. *J Antibiot (Tokyo)* 52 (2): 198

31 Hunter MS, Corley DG, Carron CP, Rowold E, Kilpatrick BF, Durley RC (1997) Four new clerodane diterpenes from the leaves of Casearia guianensis which inhibit the interaction of leukocyte function antigen 1 with intercellular adhesion molecule 1. *J Nat Prod* 60 (9): 894–899

32 Itokawa H, Totsuka N, Morita H, Takeya K, Iitaka Y, Schenkel EP, Motidome M (1990) New antitumor principles, casearins A-F, for *Casearia sylvestris* Sw. (Flacourtiaceae). *Chem Pharm Bull (Tokyo)* 38 (12): 3384–3388

33 WO 9807432

34 US 5,707,985

35 JP 98042887

36 JP 10042887

37 JP 10175970

38 WO 9802430

39 JP 98231297

40 Constantin G, Laudanna C, Brocke S, Butcher EC (1999) Inhibition of experimental autoimmune encephalomyelitis by a tyrosine kinase inhibitor. *J Immunol* 162 (2): 1144–1149

41 Ferrero ME, Bertelli AE, Fulgenzi A, Pellegatta F, Corsi MM, Bonfrate M, Ferrara F, De Caterina R, Giovannini L, Bertelli A (1998) Activity *in vitro* of resveratrol on granulocyte and monocyte adhesion to endothelium. *Am J Clin Nutr* 68 (6): 1208–1214

42 Zhang L, Lau YK, Xia W, Hortobagyi GN, Hung MC (1999) Tyrosine kinase inhibitor emodin suppresses growth of HER-2/neu-overexpressing breast cancer cells in athymic mice and sensitizes these cells to the inhibitory effect of paclitaxel. *Clin Cancer Res* 5 (2): 343–353

43 Kumar A, Dhawan S, Aggarwal BB (1998) Emodin (3-methyl-1,6,8-trihydroxyanthraquinone) inhibits TNF-induced NF-kappaB activation, IkappaB degradation, and expression of cell surface adhesion proteins in human vascular endothelial cells.*Oncogene* 17 (7): 913–918

44 Lin K-C, Castro AC (1998) Very late antigen 4 (VLA4) antagonists as anti-inflammatory agents. *Curr Opin Chem Biol* 2 (4): 453–457

45 213th ACS National Meeting, April 13–17, San Francisco 1997

46 WO 9804913

47 Jackson DY, Quan C, Artis DR, Rawson T, Blackburn B, Struble M, Fitzgerald G, Chan K, Mullins S, Burnier JP et al (1997) Potent alpha 4 beta 1 peptide antagonists as potential anti-inflammatory agents. *J Med Chem* 40 (21): 3359–3368

48 WO 9749731

49 WO 9620216

50 WO 9702289

51 Vanderslice P, Ren K, Revelle JK, Kim DC, Scott D, Bjercke RJ, Yeh ET, Beck PJ, Kogan TP (1997) A cyclic hexapeptide is a potent antagonist of alpha 4 integrins. *J Immunol* 158 (4): 1710–1718

52 McIntyre BW, Woodside DG, Caruso DA, Wooten DK, Simon SI, Neelamegham S, Revelle JK, Vanderslice P (1997) Regulation of human T lymphocyte coactivation with an alpha4 integrin antagonist peptide. *J Immunol* 158 (9): 4180–4186

53 US 5869448

54 WO9842656

55 Souers AJ, Virgilio AA, Schurer SS, Ellman JA, Kogan TP, West HE, Ankener W, Vanderslice P (1998) Novel inhibitors of alpha 4 beta 1 integrin receptor interactions through library synthesis and screening. *Bioorg Med Chem Lett* 8 (17): 2297–2302

56 JP 97208588

57 WO 9854207

58 DE 19647382

59 DE 19647381

60 DE 19647380

61 JP 96198752

62 WO 9851662

63 Mou Y, Ni H, Wilkins JA (1998) The selective inhibition of beta 1 and beta 7 integrin-mediated lymphocyte adhesion by bacitracin. *J Immunol* 161 (11): 6323–6329

64 WO 9851662

65 WO 9851289

66 US 5795876

67 Yamaguchi M, Suwa H, Miyasaka M, Kumada K (1997) Selective inhibition of vascular cell adhesion molecule-1 expression by verapamil in human vascular endothelial cells. *Transplantation* 63 (5): 759–764

68 Shroff HN, Schwender CF, Baxter AD, Brookfield F, Payne LJ, Cochran NA, Gallant DL, Briskin MJ (1998) Novel modified tripeptide inhibitors of alpha 4 beta 7 mediated lymphoid cell adhesion to MAdCAM-1. *Bioorg Med Chem Lett* 8 (13): 1601–1606

Inhibitors of the MAPK pathway

Brion W. Murray, Yoshitaka Satoh and Bernd Stein

Signal Pharmaceuticals Inc., 5555 Oberlin Drive, San Diego, CA 92121, USA

Introduction

The mitogen-activated protein kinase (MAPK) family of protein kinases is a series of three highly conserved protein kinases arrayed in a cascade. Members of this family are proline-directed serine/threonine kinases that are activated by dual-phosphorylation. MAPK belong to the rapidly growing family of mammalian protein kinases. Less than 200 mammalian protein kinases were known in 1994. As of 1998, more than 700 distinct mammalian protein kinases have been identified by genomic technologies and estimates are that the human genome encodes around 2000 protein kinases. MAPK impact many cellular processes such as proliferation, oncogenesis, development and differentiation, cell cycle and cell death [1–4]. Selective inhibition of signal transduction processes has been considered by many pharmaceutical companies as an approach to disease management [5]. Two of the best-characterized anti-inflammatory drugs in patients, rapamycin and cyclosporin, act by directly affecting protein phosphorylation. Multiple clinical trials are underway with specific kinase inhibitors, in particular PKC and tyrosine kinase inhibitors. Therefore, targeting MAPK with therapeutics may be an effective way for treating a large number of diseases. This chapter will review the current field of biological and small molecule inhibitors of MAPKs. The authors recommend as starting point the following reviews on inhibitors of protein kinases [6–15].

Three major MAPK cascades have been identified in mammalian cells, the JNK, p38 and ERK cascades. The basic structure of each of these cascades is very similar. A MAPK activates by phosphorylation its substrate(s), which in most cases is either a transcription factor or another protein kinase. MAPKs are activated by dual phosphorylation at the motif Threonine-X-Tyrosine by a MAPKK, which themselves are activated by a MAPKKK at two conserved serine residues. This cascade of events provides specificity and signal amplification (Fig. 1).

The catalytic domains of protein kinases are highly conserved making them amenable to structure-based drug discovery approaches [16]. Interestingly, despite the similarity of this critical domain, drug specificity can be achieved with as little

High Throughput Screening for Novel Anti-Inflammatories, edited by M. Kahn
© 2000 Birkhäuser Verlag Basel/Switzerland

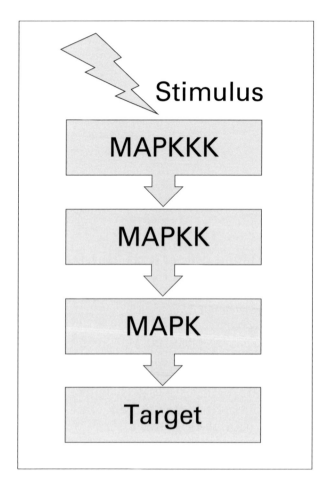

Figure 1
Schematic drawing of MAPK cascades

as one amino acid difference [17]. The crystal structures for several MAPKs, e.g. ERK2 [18], p38 [19, 20] and JNK3 [21] have been identified. These reports helped greatly to understand how the conformation of a kinase changes with the activation states [22] and how small molecule inhibitors compete for ATP binding [23, 24]. Kinases have multiple regions which can be effectively targeted for the discovery of small molecule inhibitors, including the active site, the substrate binding cleft, the phosphorylation loop involved in kinase activation and distinct sites involved in kinase interactions with its substrate or regulator proteins (e.g. an upstream kinase). Therefore, a major focus of many pharmaceutical companies is the rational drug (lead) design by taking advantage of crystallographic data available from these protein kinases. These kinase-directed compound libraries can be used in high-through-put screening technologies using recombinant MAPK.

We will introduce each MAPK cascade and then summarize the status of bio-logical inhibitors (e.g. dominant negative mutants, anti-sense nucleotides, gene tar-geting constructs) and small molecule compounds.

The JNK Pathway

Background

The c-Jun N-terminal kinase (JNK) subgroup (also known as stress-activated pro-tein kinases; SAPK) is composed of three MAPKs (JNK1, 2, 3), two MAPKKs (JNKK1 and JNKK2/MKK7; [25–28]), and MAPKKKs (MEKK1, 2, 4 and Tpl-2; [29–32]). Each of these kinases exists in several isoforms whose distinct function is currently not known. The JNK cascade is potently activated by pro-inflammatory cytokines, environmental stress such as heat and osmotic shocks, and UV [33–38]. Interestingly, while JNK1 and JNK2 are widely expressed in many tissues, JNK3 expression is restricted to brain, heart and testis with highest expression found in the brain [4, 39]. Several laboratories have generated mice with knockout of the JNK genes [4, 40]. Knockout mice may aid in the better understanding of the phys-iological role of some of these kinases. The examination of JNK-deficient mice sug-gests that JNK1 and JNK2 play different roles in the control of T cell growth, dif-ferentiation and death [40, 41]. Mice with a knockout of the JNK3 gene are resis-tant to the excitotoxic stress response caused by kainic acid [4]. Therefore, JNK3 inhibitors may be useful in treating neurodegenerative diseases such as stroke and epilepsy.

Biological JNK inhibitors

A murine cytoplasmic JNK inhibitor, JNK interacting protein-1 (JIP-1), was shown to specifically bind to JNK, cause cytoplasmic retention of JNK, and inhibit JNK-regulated gene expression [42]. However, JIP-1 does not seem to discriminate between the three JNK family members described so far. Further studies showed that JIP-1 acts as a scaffold-like protein which also binds a mixed-lineage group MAP-KKK, MKK7 (JNKK2) [43].

Epidermal growth factor (EGF) plays a stimulatory role in non-small cell lung cancer cell autocrine growth and EGF induces JNK activity in A549 lung carcino-ma cells. A549 cells stably expressing a JNK substrate that can no longer be phos-phorylated, c-Jun(S63A, S73A), no longer responded to EGF-stimulated prolifera-tion but still showed basal proliferation [44]. In addition, antisense oligonucleotides targeted to JNK1 and JNK2 blocked EGF-stimulated but not basal growth of A549 lung carcinoma cells [44]. A patent has been filed for an antisense approach to vascular injury inhibition via JNK inhibition [45].

JNKs, p38 kinases and ERKs are activated in IMCD-3 renal cells in response to extracellular hypertonicity. A mutant of JNK2 that can no longer be activated by upstream signals (dominant-negative) inhibited hypertonicity-induced c-Jun phosphorylation by 40–70% while the dominant-negative JNK1 had no significant effects [46].

Protein p21WAF/CIP I/Sdil is a DNA-damage-inducible cell-cycle inhibitor, which acts as an inhibitor of Jun kinases [47]. p21 inhibited JNK-mediated cJun phosphorylation *in vitro* with a K_i = 75 nM. Binding studies showed direct interaction of p21 with JNK. Transient transfection studies in HEK 293 cells showed that p21 inhibited JNK activity from both UV-stimulated cells and cells cotransfected with MEKK1/MKK4.

Small molecule JNK inhibitors

The development of pharmacologically active JNK inhibitors is significantly less advanced compared to the related MAPK p38 (see below). Potent, selective JNK inhibitors with pharmaceutical properties have yet to be identified but the development of such compounds has been accelerated by the development of inhibitors of p38. Testing such inhibitors on JNK should allow the development of a structure-activity-relationship (SAR) which will aid in the development of JNK-selective inhibitors. In addition, peptide inhibitors and generic inhibitors (dexamethasone, nitric oxide) have been reported to block JNK activity. The JNK3 crystal structure co-crystallized with an ATP analog has recently been published [21]. This information will allow computer-modeling studies to determine the best fit of an ATP-competitive small molecule agent and will certainly speed up the drug discovery process. The structures of the JNK inhibitors discussed in this chapter are shown in Figure 2.

Known protein kinase inhibitors

A panel of protein kinase inhibitors was assembled to contain ATP-competitive Ser/Thr kinase inhibitors, ATP-competitive tyrosine kinase inhibitors, MAPK inhibitors, and generic protein kinase inhibitors (Tab. 1) (B. W. Murray, unpublished results). These compounds were tested for inhibition of JNK activity. The profiled ATP-competitive protein kinase inhibitors displayed marked differences in JNK inhibition, which demonstrates that ATP-competitive inhibitors can provide Ser/Thr kinase selective inhibitors (#1–7, Tab. 1). Similar results have been reported for tyrosine kinases [48]. Most of the tested protein kinase inhibitors did not significantly or selectively inhibit JNK except for the pyridinylimidazole compounds

Table 1 - Inhibitor potencies of known protein kinase inhibitors with JNK1/2/3. Assays were performed at an equal level of JNK (7 nM) with 15 µM ATP and 2.5 µM GST-cJun(1-79).

	Inhibitor	IC_{50} (µM) JNK1	JNK2	JNK3
1	SB202190	8.5 ± 0.8	0.35 ± 0.02	2.2 ± 0.1
2	SB203580	6.3 ± 0.5	0.43 ± 0.04	2.1 ± 0.1
3	Staurosporine	0.53 ± 0.03	2.2 ± 0.2	0.91 ± 0.14
4	Olomoucine	> 30	> 30	> 30
5	Bisindolylmaleimide I	> 30	20.6 ± 4.2	> 30
6	Isoquinoline sulfonamide H-89	> 30	> 30	> 30
7	Tyrphostin A47	1.4 ± 0.1	3.7 ± 0.4	ND*
9	Apigenin	14.9 ± 2.5	10.6 ± 2.3	21.8 ± 6.0
10	Calphostin C	7.3 ± 2.1	> 30	ND*
11	Wortmannin	> 30	> 30	> 30
12	Tyrphostin AG126	> 30	> 30	> 30
13	PD98059	> 30	> 30	> 30

Not determined

(SB203580, SB202190), that were originally described to be p38-specific [49, 50]. The ATP-competitive inhibitors staurosporine and tyrphostin A47 inhibited JNK1 and JNK2 at low micromolar concentrations (Tab. 1). Staurosporine is a weak inhibitor of JNK (IC_{50} = 0.5–2.2 µM) but a nanomolar inhibitor of PKA [51]. JNK enzymes were not significantly inhibited by potent ATP-competitive inhibitors of PKA and PKC, such as calphostin C, bisindolylmaleimide I, and H-89. Non-ATP-competitive protein kinase inhibitors showed modest to no JNK inhibition (#1, 2 in Tab. 1). Although tyrphostin A47 was a modest inhibitor of JNK enzymes, this inhibition may be due to the known nonspecific protein binding properties of tyrphostins [52]. In summary, the panel of inhibitors listed in Table 1 should probe kinase and isoform selectivity issues.

Pyridinylimidazole Inhibitors

Controversy exists in the literature on the specificity of the pyridinylimidazole class of p38 protein kinase inhibitor [53–55]. Early studies of SB203580 reported only p38 and not JNK inhibition [54]. No significant effect on JNK1 by pyridinylimidazole inhibitors was observed [56]. Immunoprecipitation studies of JNK family members from cardiac cells indicated that SB203580 did not inhibit JNK1 isoforms but inhibited total JNK activity with an IC_{50} of 3–10 µM [57]. The IC_{50} values of

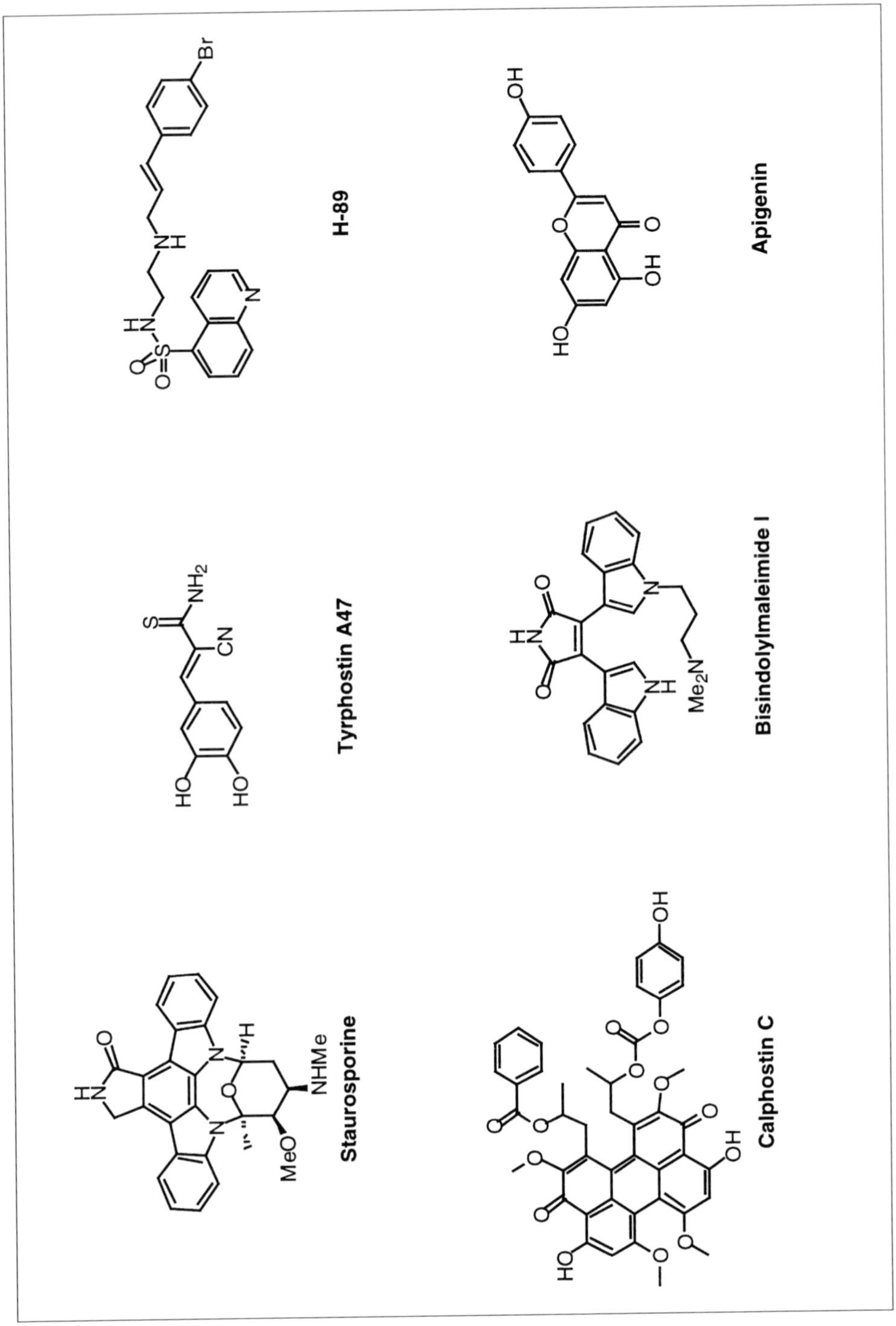

H-89

Tyrphostin A47

Staurosporine

Apigenin

Bisindolylmaleimide I

Calphostin C

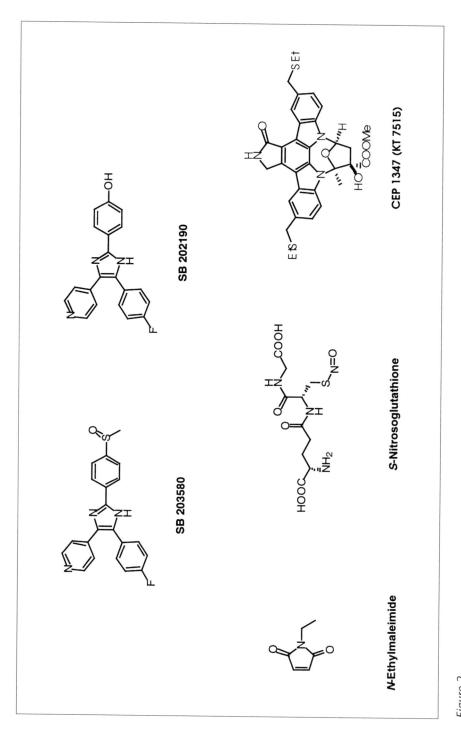

SB 202190

SB 203580

CEP 1347 (KT 7515)

S-Nitrosoglutathione

N-Ethylmaleimide

Figure 2
JNK inhibitors

SB203580 and SB202190 for inhibition of JNK were determined (Tab. 1). Isoform selective inhibition by pyridinylimidazole inhibitors has been observed. By double reciprocal analysis, inhibition by JNK2 by SB203580 has been shown to be ATP-competitive with a $K_i = 0.11$ μM and non-competitive with respect to ($K_{is} = 0.40$ μM, $K_{ii} = 0.45$ μM) (B.W. Murray, unpublished results). This finding is consistent with the mechanism of action with respect to p38, and was recently confirmed in independent studies [24, 53]. By comparison of the inhibition constants, SB203580 was selective for p38 (K_i = 21–24 nM [58, 59]), compared to JNK2 (K_i = 110 nM) (B.W. Murray, unpublished results). From analysis of the crystal structures of p38 co-crystallized with pyridinylimidazole inhibitors, the kinase selectivity of this class of inhibitors was attributed to interactions between the compound and Thr106 of p38 [23, 24] which is a methionine in JNKs. Further studies of 23 active site mutations of p38 were used to demonstrate that MAPK selectivity was based on three amino acid residues (Thr106, Met109, Ala157) near the hinge of the ATP pocket [56]. Nonetheless, pyridinylimidazole inhibitors are ATP-competitive, isoform-selective inhibitors of JNK.

Miscellaneous JNK inhibitors

JNK2 is sensitive to cysteine modifying agents such as N-ethylmaleimide, in a site protected by the substrate c-Jun (B.W. Murray, unpublished results). JNK2 activity is suppressed in a concentration and time-dependent manner *in vitro* by S-nitrosylation through S-nitrosoglutathione, a nitric oxide donor [60]. Thus, a natural strategy for JNK inhibition may be via modifying a critical cysteine residue.

JNK pathway inhibitors

Several small molecule reagents have been described that block JNK activity *in vivo* without blocking JNK directly. These compounds are thought to affect signaling molecules upstream in the JNK cascade. Inherently these upstream blockers may not be specific for JNK at all.

Both a kinase-inactive JNK and the glucocorticoid dexamethasone were shown to inhibit TNFα production in LPS-stimulated RAW 264.7 cells. This effect was overcome with the overexpression of wild-type JNK [61]. Dexamethasone specifically blocked LPS stimulation of JNK but not that of p38, ERK1, ERK2, MEK3, MEK4, or MEK6. Further, dexamethasone blocked sorbitol but not anisomycin stimulation of JNK. This observation indicates that the dexamethasone mechanism-of-inhibition is upstream of JNK and that inhibitors of JNK activity will modulate the cellular level of the pro-inflammatory cytokine, TNFα.

The CEP-1347 is an analog of the indolocarbazole staurosporine, which has been shown to block activation of JNK1 in cultured cells [62] and *in vivo* [63]. The inhibition of the JNK signaling pathway promoted long term-survival of cultured chick embryonic dorsal root ganglion, sympathetic, ciliary, and motor neurons [62]. CEP-1347 blocked neuronal programmed cell death and injury-induced dedifferentiation *in vivo* [63]. The activity of CEP-1347 was specific for the JNK1 activation pathway compared to the ERK1 activation pathway but JNK1 is clearly not the molecular target [64]. The IC_{50} of CEP-1347 for JNK1 inhibition was the same as the EC_{50} of motoneuron survival [64].

Curcumin is known to suppress tumor initiation/promotion and potently inhibits activation of AP-1 and NF-κB. Activation of JNK by various agonists (PMA/ionomycin, anisomycin, UV-C, gamma irradiation, TNFα, sodium vanadate) was inhibited with an IC_{50} between 5–10 μM while inhibition of ERK activation had an IC_{50} of 20 μM. Curcumin inhibited JNK activated by co-transfection of TAK1, GCK, or HPK1. However, curcumin did not directly inhibit JNK, JNKK1, MEKK1 or HPK1 activity. The authors propose a mechanism of inhibition via a MAPKKK [65].

The immunosuppressant rapamycin inhibited the basal activity of JNK in the murine T lymphoblastoid cell line S49, which was reversed by the addition of FK506. Thus, rapamycin inhibited JNK activity in lymphocytes, which enhanced apoptosis [66]. JNK and p38 but not ERK pathways were shown to contribute to IL-2 gene expression in T lymphocytes in a cyclosporin A-sensitive manner [67]. All-trans retinoic acid inhibits JNK dependent signaling pathways and the ERK pathway to a lesser extent in normal human bronchial epithelial cells [68].

2-deoxyglucose inhibited anticancer drug (etoposide, camptothecin, mitomycin)-induced but not TNFα-induced apoptosis in human monocytic leukemia U937 cells. This effect was correlated with cancer drug-induced JNK1 activation [69].

Inhibition of UV-C irradiation induced AP-1 activity by aspirin is through inhibition of the JNK pathway but not ERK or p38 MAPK pathway in JB6 cells [70, 71]. It should be noted that O'Neill and coworkers report that 80% of protein kinase activity in non-stimulated proliferating Jurkat T cells could be inhibited by aspirin [72].

The JB6 mouse epidermal cell line was used as an *in vitro* model for tumor promotions studies. Tea polyphenols (–)-epigallocatechin gallate (EGCG) and theaflavins inhibited EGF- or PMA-induced cell transformation and inhibited AP-1-dependent transcriptional activity and DNA binding. Inhibition of AP-1 activation occurred through inhibition of JNK but not ERK pathways.

The p38 pathway

Background

The p38 pathway is composed of four MAPKs (p38α, p38-2(p38β), p38γ, p38δ) [55, 73–77], two MAPKKs (MKK3, MEK6) [78–82], and several MAPKKKs (MEKK1, MLK-3, DLK and others) [83–87].

The p38 cascade was originally identified by homology of one of its members, p38α (p38, CSBP1/2), with the yeast HOG1 protein kinase. Like the JNK cascade, p38 family members are activated by pro-inflammatory cytokines, environmental stress and UV. Among the substrates identified for p38 are transcription factors (e.g. ATF2, CHOP-1, Elk1, MEF2-C) and protein kinases (e.g. MAPKAP K2/3, MNK1, PRAK). An important role of p38 in many physiological processes was established early on due to the availability of a relatively specific inhibitor, the pyridinylimidazole derivative SB203580 (see below).

Biological p38 inhibitors

Several laboratories are in the process of generating knockout mice for the individual p38 family members. This should greatly help in understanding the redundancy and specificity of these proteins. Further, constitutive active and dominant negative versions of MEK6 have been generated. Constitutively active MEK6 is a strong stimulator of IL-1α and IL-6 production in HeLa cells and of IL-1α and TNFα in THP-1 cells (B. Stein et al., unpublished results).

Small molecule p38 inhibitors

It has been long known that certain anti-inflammatory agents reduce production of cytokines such as TNFα and interleukins *in vitro* and *in vivo* [88]. This class of compounds was therefore named as CSAIDs (cytokine-suppressive anti-inflammatory drugs). In 1994, with the aid of a radiolabeled cytokine suppressor, a group at SmithKline Beecham reported isolation of a binding protein (cytokine-suppressor binding proteins, CSBPs) for this class of drugs, and established that it was essentially identical to the yeast HOG1 protein and the at the same time cloned murine p38 [49]. SB203580 [50], a pyridinylimidazole, emerged as a potent, orally active inhibitor of p38α which showed a spectrum of anti-inflammatory activity in animal pharmacology models (*vide infra*), and remains the most extensively studied inhibitor of p38 (Fig. 3). Many patent applications for SB203580-like inhibitors with templates other than imidazoles have appeared and were reviewed elsewhere [89].

Enzymology studies showed that SB203580 is a reversible inhibitor with a K_i value of 21 nM, and is ATP-competitive [59]. In the CSBP/p38 binding assay using ^{3}H-SB202190 as the radioligand, SB203580 has an IC_{50} value of 42 nM [90]. The X-ray crystallography studies [23] of a close analog of SB203580 bound to p38 clearly indicates that the nitrogen atom of the 4-pyridyl group of SB203580 forms an essential interaction with Met[109] while the fluorophenyl group provides a critical hydrophobic binding in a lipophilic pocket in the active site. The crystal structure of a similar p38 inhibitor, VK-19911, was also published [24]. In the cellular systems, SB203580 inhibited LPS stimulated production of IL-1α and TNFα at 0.05 and 0.1 μM, respectively, in human monocytes. Although SB203580 did not affect the TNFα induced activation of p38, phosphorylation and activation of the p38 substrate MAPKAP kinase-2 was clearly demonstrated. SB203580 inhibited TNFα induced IL-6, GM-CSF production in murine L929 cells, human U937 cells, and HeLa cells. No effect of SB203580 on the TNFα-induced NF-κB DNA binding in L929 was observed. SB203580 inhibited IL-1 stimulated p38 kinase activity in bovine cartilage-derived chondrocytes, an *in vitro* model of rheumatoid arthritis, with an IC_{50} value of about 1 μM.

SB203580 was extensively evaluated in a series of animal pharmacology models of inflammation [91]. SB203580 was shown to be a potent inhibitor of cytokine production in mice and rats at ED_{50} of 15–25 mg/kg, and had therapeutic activity in collagen-induced arthritis at 50 mg/kg in DBA/LACJ mice. In the adjuvant-induced arthritis models in Lewis rats when administrated p.o. at 30 and 60 mg/kg, improvement in bone mineral density and histological scores were observed. SB203580 reduced mortality in a murine model of endotoxin-induced shock in a dose dependent manner at 25–100 mg/kg p.o. In order to determine whether chronic administration of CSAIDs leads to immunosuppression, ovalbumin-sensitized BALB/c mice were treated for 2 weeks with SB203580 at 60 mg/kg i.p. and subsequently evaluated. Although the ovalbumin antibody titer was suppressed to some extent, *ex vivo* lymphocytic responses were unaffected.

Increased liver weight and significant elevations of hepatic P450 enzymes by SB203580 in the rat 10-day dose-ranging toxicological studies were attributed to potent inhibition of cytochrome P450s by this pyridine-based compound. A search for a surrogate functionality for the pyridine group yielded potent p38 inhibitors based on 2-aminopyrimidines such as SB220025 [92], SB216385 [93], which inhibited p38 with IC_{50} values of 0.060, and 0.48 μM, respectively. These compounds showed much less affinity toward a variety of P450 isozymes, and therefore presumed to be more suitable for clinical development. SB220025, at 30 mg/kg b.i.d. p.o., inhibited the inflammatory angiogenesis by 40% in the murine air pouch granuloma model. SB220025 reduced the LPS-induced TNFα production with an ED_{50} value of 7.5 mg/kg p.o. in mice. In the murine collagen-induced arthritis model, SB220025 inhibited the progression of arthritis. SB226882 showed inhibition of LPS-induced TNFα production at 3.0 and 5.7 mg/kg p.o. in the mice and rat, and was effective in the rat adjuvant- and mice collagen-induced arthritis model.

A number of 1-(4-pyridyl)-2-arylheterocycles were identified to be potent inhibitors of p38 MAPK. L-167,307 [94], a pyrrole analog of SB203580, was shown to inhibit p38α and p38β with the IC_{50} values of 5.0 and 8.1 nM, respectively. This compound is also a modest inhibitor of Raf Kinase (0.47 μM). LPS-induced TNFα release is also inhibited by L-167,307 in human monocytes at 65 nM. It is interesting to note that L-167,307, upon i.v. or p.o. administration to

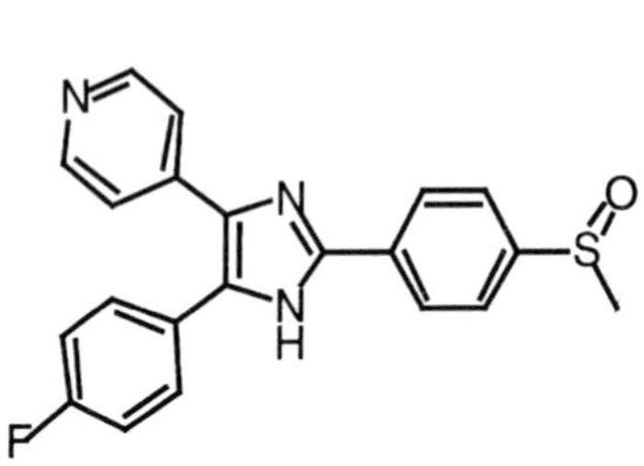

SB 203580

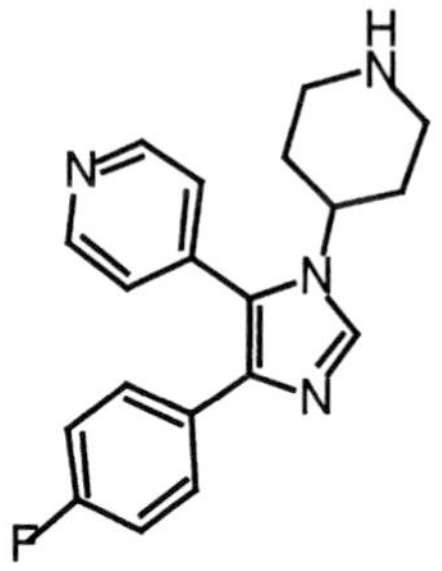

VK -19911

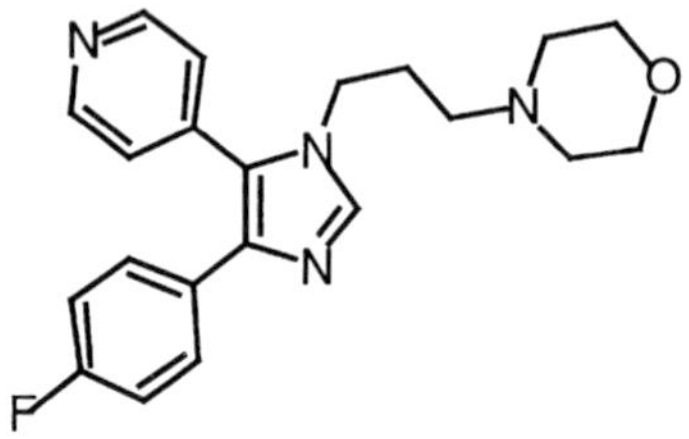

SB 210313

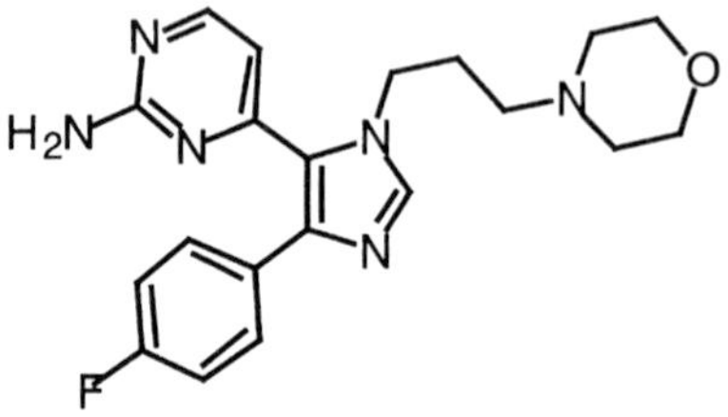

SB 216385

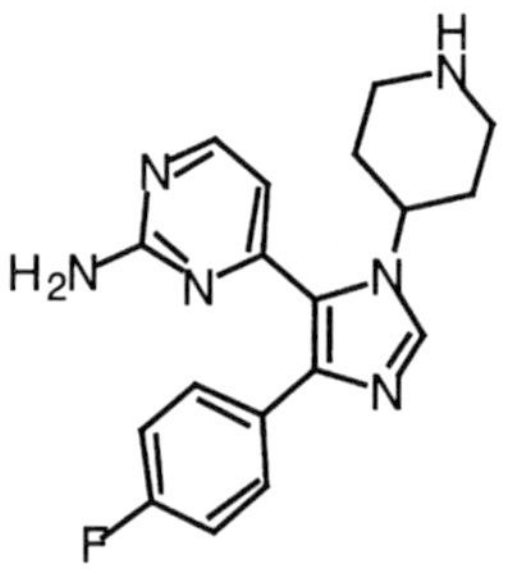

SB-220025

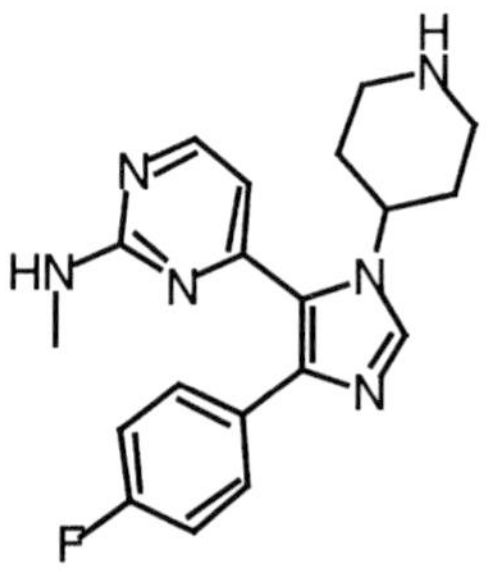

SB-226882

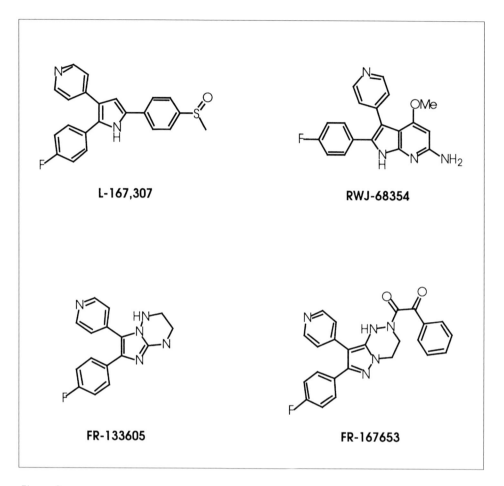

L-167,307

RWJ-68354

FR-133605

FR-167653

Figure 3
p38 inhibitors

the rat, is readily metabolized to the corresponding sulfone which, in turn, shows a much longer half-life than the sulfoxide precursor. L-167,307 reduced paw edema in the rat adjuvant arthritis model with the ED_{50} value of 7.4 mg/kg/b.i.d. p.o. At the 20 mg/kg/b.i.d. dose, radiographic examination of the hind paw joints showed a reduced degree of destruction.

Investigation of indole and pyrrolopyridine templates yielded a series of CSAIDs/ p38 inhibitors [95, 96]. RWJ-68354 [97, 98] inhibits p38 immunoprecipitated from human monocytes at 150 nM, and suppresses the LPS-induced production of TNFα and IL-1α at 6.3 and 26 nM, respectively, and *Staphylococcus* enterotoxin B-induced TNFα generation at 23 nM, in the human PBM. In female BALB/c mice and male Lewis rats, RWJ-68354 prevented LPS-induced TNFα production in a dose dependent manner upon oral administration. In the adjuvant arthritis model in male Lewis rats, RWJ-68354 reduced the size of hind paw edema by 50% at 5 mg/kg/day.

The following two Fujisawa CSAIDs, FR-133605 and FR-167653, have structural features very similar to the pyridinylimidazole p38 inhibitors, although no information on their MAPK inhibitory activity is currently available. These compounds are worth mentioning since rather extensive pharmacological studies were performed which may help understand the role of CSAID/p38 inhibitors in a variety of disease states. FR-133605 [99] showed inhibition of LPS-induced IL-1 and TNFα production at 0.52 and 1.0 μM in human monocytes, and reduced the production of LPS-stimulated serum IL-1 and TNFα at the ED_{50} of 4.3 and 2.0 mg/kg in the mice. In the adjuvant arthritis model in rats, FR-133605 reduced paw swelling and destruction of bone and cartilage.

In *in vitro* cytokine production assays, FR-167653 [100] inhibited IL-1α, IL-1β, and TNFα at 0.84, 0.088, and 1.1 μM, respectively, in LPS-treated human monocytes, and TNFα at 0.072 μM in lymphocytes stimulated with phytohemaglutinin-M. In the LPS-induced disseminated intravascular coagulation model in the rat, FR-167653 upon i.v. infusion markedly improved thrombocytopenia and plasma coagulation. Suppression of IL-1 and TNFα production by 100 and 89% was observed. In the rabbit model of septic shock, FR-167653 reduced mortality, attenuated the hypotensive response and nearly normalized mean arterial blood pressure upon LPS challenge [101]. In the dog model of liver resection with ischemia, FR-167653 improved liver function and survival [102]. Most interestingly, FR-167653 dose-dependently reduced the size of myocardial infarct size in the rat model of ischemia-reperfusion [103]. The mRNA levels of TNFα and IL-1α were also reduced in the FR-167653-treated animals.

As of today all small molecule p38 inhibitors described fall into a class of compounds that blocks p38α and p38-2 but not p38γ and p38δ. Although most of the published p38 inhibitors are based on the SB203580 template, there are recent patent disclosures of inhibitors of highly distinct structural classes such as indol-3-carboxamides [104], pyrimidinopyridazinones [105], guanylhydrazone [106], and N-substituted ureas [107]. The structures of the p38 inhibitors discussed in this chapter are shown in Figure 3.

In summary, dramatic progress has been made in terms of identifying potent, orally active inhibitors of p38 in the past five years. The pharmacological effects of such inhibitors are actively being investigated and profiled in a variety of animal models of diseases such as acute and chronic inflammatory diseases, septic shock, bone loss, ischemia-reperfusion, and cancer. Human clinical trial data, which will undoubtedly become available in the near future, will shed further light on the full therapeutic potential of p38 inhibitors.

The ERK pathway

Background

The ERK pathway is composed of two MAPKs (ERK1, 2) [108-110], two MAP-KKs (MEK1, 2), and several MAPKKKs including Raf-1, B-Raf, c-Mos, MEKK3 and Tpl-2 [31, 32, 111, 112]. The ERK cascade was the first MAPK cascade identified and since then has been widely studied. In addition, ERK2 was the first MAPK to be analyzed by crystallography [18]. ERK2 is activated by dual phosphorylation on Tyr^{185} and Thr^{183}. Both of these amino acids lie in a phosphorylation lip at the mouth of the catalytic site. Activation of the kinase result in conformational changes that are associated with a refolding of this lip structure. In contrast to JNKs and p38s, ERKs are predominantly activated by phorbol esters and growth factors.

Biological ERK inhibitors

Recombinant glial maturation factor (GMF) is a 17 kDa brain protein which inhibits the activity of ERK1 and ERK2 in an *in vitro* kinase assay. Pre-phosphorylation of GMF by PKA increases the inhibitor potency 600-fold (IC_{50} 2.7 versus 1800 nM). The potency of GMF is comparable to the inhibition of PKA by PKI (K_i = 2 nM) [113]. Immunoprecipitation studies in C6 rat glioma cells suggest that GMF physically associates with ERK1/2 [114]. GMF does not inhibit the proline-directed kinases cdc2, MEK, or MAPKAP2.

Two examples of inhibition of the ERK pathway have been shown operative by inhibition of MEK/ERK protein-protein interactions. (1) Anthrax toxin is a lethal factor, which is a metalloprotease that cleaves the amino terminus of MEK1 and MEK2. These truncated forms inhibit the ERK signal transduction pathway [115]. (2) A 15 amino-acid peptide derived from the αC helix of human ERK1 is a competitive inhibitor of ERK1-MEK binding with a dissociation constant K_i = 0.84 μM. Circular dichroism spectroscopic studies indicated that the peptide has little secondary structure in aqueous buffer but readily adopts an α-helical structure in aprotic solvents. The synthetic peptide also inhibits p38 and ERK phosphorylation by MKK3. However, JNK1 activation by JNKK is at least three-fold less potently inhibited by the peptide, which suggests that the αC helix is not the sole determinant of activator selectivity [116].

The ERK pathway is critical to infection and as such, targeted by bacteria such as *Yersinia enterocolitica*. *Yersinia enterocolitica*-induced suppression of TNFα release by infected macrophages is caused by the YopP protein. This event correlates with inhibition of endogenous ERK1/2 and p38 activities. Knockout *Yersinia* mutants and complementation studies were used to identify the YopP protein as crit-

Table 2 - Inhibitors of ERK.

| Inhibitor | IC$_{50}$ (μM) | | Reference |
	ERK1	ERK2	
Roscovitine	34	14	[120]
Olomoucine	50	40	[120]
Staurosporine	1.5		[119]
Glia maturation factor	0.0029		[114]

ical to the suppression of TNFα release [117]. Raf-1 kinase activity was also inhibited by YopP viral infection which lead the authors to speculate that YopP was acting at the MAPKKK level [117].

Small molecule ERK inhibitors

Although potent biological inhibitors of ERK have been identified, none of them is very selective. ERK1/2 is susceptible to inhibition by ATP-competitive inhibitors (Tab. 2). ERK1 was inhibited by staurosporine in an ATP-competitive mode and a non-competitive mode with respect to phosphoacceptor (K_i = 1.0 μM) [118]. The purine analog olomoucine inhibited ERK1 *in vitro* (IC$_{50}$ = 25 μM) while 35 other highly purified kinases were not significantly inhibited [119]. Roscovitine, another purine analog (2-(1-ethyl-2-hydroxyethylamino)-6-benzylamino-9-isopropylpurine) was profiled against a panel of 25 protein kinases and shown to be a potent and selective inhibitor of cyclin-dependent kinases cdc2, cdk2, and cdk5. Although most other protein kinases were not inhibited by roscovitine (IC$_{50}$ >100 μM) it modestly inhibited ERK1 (IC$_{50}$ = 34 μM) and ERK2 (IC$_{50}$ = 14 μM) [120]. The structures of the ERK inhibitors discussed in this chapter are shown in Figure 4.

Small molecule MEK inhibitors

PD98059 inhibits MEK at low micromolar concentrations without significant effects on ERK1/2 [121]. This inhibition was shown to prevent downstream activation of ERK and subsequent phosphorylation of ERK substrates *in vitro*. PD98059 prevented stimulation of cell growth and reversed the phenotype of ras-transformed mouse 3T3 fibroblast cells and rat kidney cells. PD98059 appears to bind preferentially to the non-phosphorylated form of MEK, and is highly selective among relat-

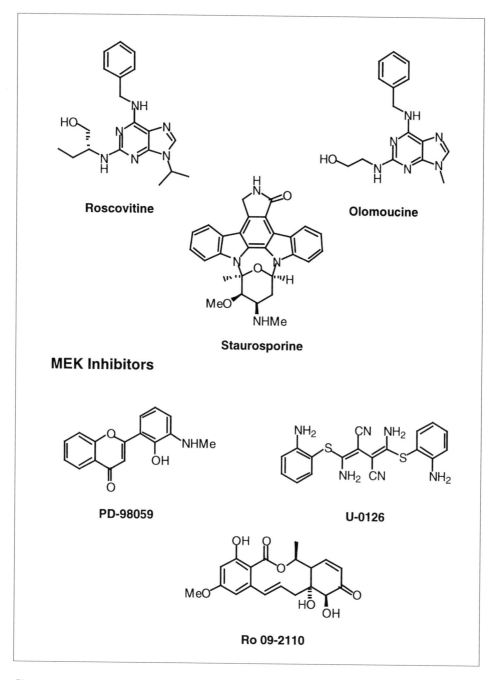

Roscovitine

Olomoucine

Staurosporine

MEK Inhibitors

PD-98059

U-0126

Ro 09-2110

Figure 4
ERK inhibitors

ed Ser/Thr kinases [122]. Since its discovery, PD98059 has been extensively used as a research tool to identify the biological role of the MEK cascade.

U-0126 is a dual inhibitor of MEK1/2 with IC_{50} values of 72 and 58 nM, respectively, and selectivity against other closely related kinases [123]. The inhibition is reversible and non-competitive with respect to ATP and ERK. This compound prevents T cell proliferation induced by concanavalin A and anti-CD3 crosslinking and blocks PMA/ionomycin-stimulated upregulation of IL-2 mRNA in peripheral blood leukocytes [124].

Screening of fermentation broth for inhibitors of T-cell activation yielded Ro 09-2210 [125], a macrocyclic lactam from *Curvularia sp.* Ro 09-2110 inhibits anti-CD3- and ionomycin-induced T-cell activation with an IC_{50} of 58–139 nM, and anti-CD3-stimulated IL-2 release in Jurkat T cells at 16 nM. Rabbit skeletal muscle MEK and human recombinant MEK1 were potently inhibited by Ro 09-2110 at 59 and 140 nM, respectively, while no or little inhibition was observed with MAPK, PKC, ZAP-70 and p56[lck]. In contrast to PD98057, Ro 09-2110 is also able to inhibit activated MEK.

Conclusion

Substantial progress has been made over the past few years to understand how MAPK regulate gene expression. New family members and isoforms have been cloned and a complicated network of signaling cascades has emerged. These studies are supported by the generation of knockout mice with interesting disease-related phenotypes. The convergence of this knowledge with modern drug discovery technologies make MAPK an opportune drug target for the next millennium.

In parallel, extensive efforts in the pharmaceutical industry led to the identification of small molecule MAPK inhibitors. While some of them are not suitable for development as drugs, they still serve as valuable tools for understanding how MAPKs affect cellular processes. These compounds also clearly demonstrated that kinase-selective inhibition can be achieved with ATP-competitive molecules. In addition, it is very likely that inhibitors of the substrate binding site will be found.

While most progress has been made in developing MAPK inhibitors for p38, in particular p38α/p38β, we anticipate that inhibitors of p38γ/p38δ will be found soon. Inhibition of individual p38 family members will be an exciting opportunity based on emerging data that these four family members have different functional roles. Additionally, data from gene knockout animals, e.g. the JNK3 knockout, revealed interesting disease-related phenotypes. We anticipate a strong interest in selective inhibitors of the JNK family for the treatment of a variety of diseases.

The value of intervention of a MAPK cascade at the MAPKK level has been demonstrated by the development of a small molecule inhibitor of MEK in the ERK pathway. Extension of this work to the MAPKK MEK6 in the p38 pathway should provide an alternative mechanism to downregulate the p38 pathway with a different therapeutic output. Many other MAPKK targets are also available as drug targets. There is strong belief that inhibitors of each step of the MAPK cascade may provide a different selectivity profile.

In summary, this review demonstrates that protein kinases at multiple levels in the MAPK cascade are fruitful targets for small molecule drugs that have the potential to treat a variety of different diseases. In addition, it is anticipated that the majority of MAPK yet to be explored will also be excellent drug targets for treatment of multiple major diseases.

References

1   Hunter T, Karin M (1992) The regulation of transcription by phosphorylation. *Cell* 70: 375–387

2   Hunter T (1995) Protein kinases and phosphatases: The Yin and Yang of protein phosphorylation and signaling. *Cell* 80: 225–236

3   Karin M, Hunter T (1995) Transcriptional control by protein phosphorylation: signal transmission from the cell surface to the nucleus. *Curr Biology* 5: 747–757

4   Yang DD, Kuan CY, Whitmarsh AJ, Rincon M, Zheng TS, Davis RJ, Rakic P, Flavell RA (1997) Absence of excitotoxicity-induced apoptosis in the hippocampus of mice lacking the Jnk3 gene. *Nature* 389: 865–870

5   Levitzki A (1994) Signal transduction interception as a novel approach to disease management. *Ann NY Acad Sci* 766: 363–368.

6   Stein B, Anderson D (1996) The MAP kinase family: new "MAPs" for signal transduction pathways and novel targets for drug discovery. In: JA Bristol (ed): *Annual Reports in Medicinal Chemistry*. Academic Press, San Diego, 289–298

7   Clarke PR (1994) Switching off MAP kinases. *Curr Opin* 4: 647–650

8   Lee JC, Adams JL (1995) Inhibitors of serine/threonine kinases. *Curr Opin Biotech* 6: 657–661

9   Taylor SS, Radzio-Andzelm E (1997) Protein kinase inhibition: natural and synthetic variation on a theme. *Curr Opin Chem Biol* 1: 219–226

10 Hemmings HCJ (1997) Protein kinase and phosphatase inhibitors: applications in neuroscience. *Neuromethods* 30: 112–218

11 Seger R, Krebs EG (1995) The MAPK signaling cascade. *FASEB J* 9: 726–735

12 Cooper JA (1994) Straight and narrow or tortuos and intersecting? *Curr Biology* 4: 1118–1121

13 Cano E, Mahadevan LC (1995) Parallel signal processing among mammalian MAPKs. *Trends Biochem* 20: 117–122

14 McMahon G, Sun L, Liang C, Tang C (1998) Protein kinase inhibitors: structural determinants for target specificity. *Current Opinion in Drug Discovery & Development* 1: 131–146

15 Bhagwat S, Manning A, Hoekstra MF, Lewis A (1999) Gene regulating protein kinases as important anti-inflammatory targets. *Drug Disc Today; in press*

16 Hanks SK, Quinn AM (1991) Protein kinase catalytic domain sequence database: Identification of conserved features of primary structure and classification of family members. *Methods Enzym* 200: 38–62

17 Cohen P, Goedert M (1998) Engineering protein kinases with distinct nucleotide specificities and inhibitor sensitivities by mutation o fa single amino acid. *Chem & Biol* 5: R161–164

18 Zhang F, Strand A, Robbins D, Cobb MH, Goldsmith EJ (1994) Atomic structure of the MAP kinase ERK2 at 2.3 Å resolution. *Nature* 367: 704–711

19 Wang Z, Harkins PC, Ulevitch RJ, Han J, Cobb MH, Goldsmith EJ (1997) The structure of mitogen-activated protein kinase p38 at 2.1-Å resolution. *Proc Natl Acad Sci USA* 94: 2327–2332

20 Wilson KP, Fitzgibbon MJ, Caron PR, Griffith JP, Chen W, McCaffrey PG, Chambers SP, Su MS-S (1996) Crystal structure of p38 mitogen-activated protein kinase. *J Biol Chem* 271: 27696–27700

21 Xie X, Gu Y, Fox T, Coll JT, Fleming MA, Markland W, Caron PR, Wilson KP, Su MS-S (1998) Crystal structure of JNK3: a kinase implicated in neuronal apoptosis. *Structure* 6: 983–991

22 Cobb MH, Goldsmith EJ (1995) How MAP kinases are regulated. *J Biol Chem* 270: 14843–14846

23 Tong L, Pav S, White DM, Rogers S, Crane KM, Cywin CL, Brown ML, Pargellis CA (1997) A highly specific inhibitor of human p38 MAP kinase binds in the ATP pocket. *Nat Struct Biol* 4: 311–316

24 Wilson KP et al (1997) The structural basis for the specificity of pyridinylimidazole inhibitors of p38 MAP kinase. *Chem Biol* 4: 423–431

25 Sánchez I, Hughes RT, Mayer BJ, Yee K, Woodgett JR, Avruch J, Kyriakis JM, Zon LI (1994) Role of SAPK/ERK kinase-1 in the stress-activated pathway regulating transcription factor c-Jun. *Nature* 372: 794–798

26 Yashar BM, Kelley C, Yee K, Errede B, Zon LI (1993) Novel members of the mitogen-activated protein kinase activator family in *Xenopus laevis*. *Mol Cell Biol* 13: 5738–5748

27 Dérijard B, Raingeaud J, Barrett T, Wu I-H, Han J, Ulevitch RJ, Davis RJ (1995) Independent human MAP kinase signal transduction pathways defined by MEK and MKK isoforms. *Science* 267: 682–685

28 Lin A, Minden A, Martinetto H, Claret F-X, Lange-Carter C, Mercurio F, Johnson GL, Karin M (1995) Identification of a dual specificity kinase that activates the Jun kinases and p38-Mpk2. *Science* 268: 286–290

29 Lange-Carter CA, Pleiman CM, Gardner AM, Blumer KJ, Johnson GL (1993) A divergence in the MAP kinase regulatory network defined by MEK kinase and Raf. *Science* 260: 315–319

30 Yan M, Dai T, Deak JC, Kyriakis JM, Zon LI, Woodgett JR, Templeton DJ (1994) Acti-

vation of stress-activated protein kinase by MEKK1 phosphorylation of its activator SEK1. *Nature* 372: 798–800

31 Blank JL, Gerwins P, Elliott EM, Sather S, Johnson GL (1996) Molecular cloning of mitogen-activated protein/ERK kinase kinases (MEKK) 2 and 3. *J Biol Chem* 271: 5361–5368

32 Salmerón A, Ahmad TB, Carlile GW, Pappin D, Narsimhan RP, Ley SC (1996) Activation of MEK-1 and SEK-1 by Tpl-2 proto-oncoprotein, a novel MAP kinase kinase kinase. *EMBO J* 15: 817–826

33 Dérijard B, Hibi M, Wu I-H, Barrett T, Su B, Deng T, Karin M, Davis RJ (1994) JNK1: A protein kinase stimulated by UV light and Ha-Ras that binds and phosphorylates the c-Jun activation domain. *Cell* 76: 1025–1037

34 Kyriakis JM, Banerjee P, Nikolakaki E, Dai T, Rubie EA, Ahmad MF, Avruch J, Woodgett JR (1994) The stress-activated protein kinase subfamily of c-Jun kinases. *Nature* 369: 156–160

35 Minden A, Lin A, Smeal T, Dérijard B, Cobb M, Davis R, Karin M (1994) c-Jun N-terminal phosphorylation correlates with activation of the JNK subgroup but not the ERK subgroup of mitogen-activated protein kinases. *Mol Cell Biol* 14: 6683–6688

36 Adler V, Schaffer A, Kim J, Dolan L, Ronai Z (1995) UV irradiation and heat shock mediate JNK activation via alternate pathways. *J Biol Chem* 270: 26071–26077

37 Cano E, Hazzalin CA, Mahadevan LC (1994) Anisomycin-activated protein kinases p45 and p55 but not mitogen-activated protein kinases ERK-1 and -2 are implicated in the induction of c-fos and c-jun. *Mol Cell Biol* 14: 7352–7362

38 Westwick JK, Weitzel C, Minden A, Karin M, Brenner DA (1994) Tumor necrosis factor α stimulates AP-1 activity through prolonged activation of the c-Jun kinase. *J Biol Chem* 269: 26396–26401

39 Mohit AA, Martin JH, Miller CA (1995) p493F12 kinase: A novel MAP kinase expressed in a subset of neurons in the human nervous system. *Neuron* 14: 67–78

40 Dong C, Yang DD, Wysk M, Whitmarsh AJ, Davis RJ, Flavell RA (1998) Defective T cell differentiation in the absence of Jnk1. *Science* 282: 2092–2095

41 Yang DD, Conze D, Whitmarsh AJ, Barrett T, Davis RJ, Rincon M, Flavell RA (1998) Differentiation of CD4+ T cells to Th1 cells requires MAP kinase JNK2. *Immunity* 9: 575–585

42 Dickens M, Rogers JS, Cavanagh J, Taitano A, Xia Z, Halpern JR, Greenberg ME, Sawyers CL, Davis RJ (1997) A cytoplasmic inhibitor of the JNK signal tranduction pathway. *Science* 277: 693–696

43 Whitmarsh AJ, Cavanagh J, Tournier C, Yasuda J, Davis RJ (1998) A mammalian scaffold complex that selectively mediates MAP kinase activation. *Science* 281: 1671–1674

44 Bost F, McKay R, Dean N, Mercola D (1997) The Jun kinase/stress-activated protein kinase pathway is required for epidermal growth factor stimulation of growth of human A549 lung carcinoma cells. *J Biol Chem* 272: 33422–33429

45 Chien S, Shyy JY-J (1997) Therapeutic methods for vascular injury using inhibition of the Ras signal transduction pathways. USA patent WO 97-US20404

46   Wojtaszek PA, Heasley LE, Siriwardana G, Berl T (1998) Dominant-negative c-Jun NH2-terminal kinase 2 sensitizes renal inner medullary collecting duct cells to hypertonicity-induced lethality independent of organic osmolyte transport. *J Biol Chem* 273: 800–804

47   Shim J, Lee H, Park K, Kim H, Choi E-J (1996) A non-enzymatic p21 protein inhibitor of stress-activated protein kinases. *Nature* 381: 804–807

48   Levitzki A, Gazit A (1995) Tyrosine kinase inhibition: an approach to drug development. *Science* 267: 1782–1788

49   Lee JC et al (1994) A protein kinase involved in the regulation of inflammatory cytokine biosynthesis. *Nature* 372: 739–746

50   Gallagher TF et al (1997) Regulation of stress-induced cytokine production by pyridinylimidazoles; inhibition of CSBP kinase. *Bioorg Med Chem* 5: 49–64

51   Herbert JM, Sedan E, Maffrand JP (1990) Characterization of specific binding sites for [^{3}H]-staurosporine on various protein kinases. *Biochem Biophys Res Commun* 171: 189–195

52   Hoffman R, Dennis IF, Donaldson J (1995) Protein binding modulates inhibition of the epidermal growth factor recptor kinase and DNA synthesis by tyrphosptins. *Cancer Chemother Pharmacol* 36: 316–324

53   Whitmarsh AJ, Yang H-H, Su MS-S, Sharrocks AD, Davis RJ (1997) Role of p38 and JNK mitogen-activated protein kinases in the activation of ternary complex factors. *Mol Cell Biol* 17: 2360–2371

54   Cuenda A, Touse J, Doza YN, Meier R, Cohen P, Gallagher TF, Young PR, Lee JC (1995) SB203580 is a specific inhibitor of a MAP kinase homologue which is stimulated by cellular stresses and interleukin-1. *FEBS Lett* 364: 229–233

55   Jiang Y, Chen C, Li Z, Guo W, Gegner JA, Lin S, Han J (1996) Characterization of the structure and function of a new mitogen-activated protein kinase (p38β). *J Biol Chem* 271: 17920–17926

56   Gum RJ et al (1998) Acquisition of sensitivity of stress-activated protein kinases to the p38 inhibitor, SB203580 by alteration of one or more amino acids within the ATP binding pocket. *J Biol Chem* 273: 15605–15610

57   Clerk A, Sugden PH (1998) The p38-MAPK inhibitor SB203580, inhibits cardiac stress-activated protein kinases/c-Jun N-terminal kinases (SAPKs/JNKs). *FEBS Lett* 426: 93–96

58   LoGrasso PV, Frantz B, Rolando AM, O'Keefe SJ, Hermes JD, O'Neill EA (1997) Kinetic mechanism for p38 MAP kinase. *Biochemistry* 36: 10422–10427

59   Young PR et al (1997) Pyridinyl imidazole inhibitors of p38 mitogen-activated protein kinase bind in the ATP site. *J Biol Chem* 272: 12116–12121

60   So HS, Park RK, Kim HS, Lee SR, Jung BH, Chung SY, Jun CD, Chung HT (1998) Nitric oxide inhibits c-Jun N-terminal kinase 2 (JNK2) bia S-nitrosylation. *Biochem Biophys Res Commun* 247: 809–813

61   Swantek JL, Cobb MH, Geppert TD (1997) Jun N-terminal kinases/stress-activated protein kinases (JNK/SAPK) is required for lipopolysaccharide stimulation of tumor necro-

sis factor a (TNF-a) translation: glucocorticoids inhibit TNF-a transation by blocking JNK/SAPK. *Mol Cell Biol* 17: 6274–6282

62 Borasio GD, Horstmann S, Anneser JMH, Neff NT, Glicksman MA (1998) CEP-1347/KT7515, A JNK pathway inhibitor, supports the *in vitro* survival of chick embryonic neurons. *NeuroReport* 9: 1435–1439

63 Glicksman MA et al (1998) CEP-1347/KT7515 prevents motor neuronal programmed cell death and injury-induced dedifferentiation *in vivo. J Neurobiol* 35: 361–370

64 Maroney AC et al (1998) Motoneuron apoptosis is blocked by CEP-1347 (KT 7515), a novel inhibitor of the JNK signaling pathway. *J Neurosci* 18: 104–111

65 Chen Y-R, Tan T-H (1998) Inhibition of the cJun N-terminal kinase (JNK) signaling pathway by curcumin. *Oncogene* 17: 173–178

66 Ishizuka T, Sakata N, Johnson GL, Gelfand EW, Terada N (1997) Rapamycin potentiates dexamethasone-induced apoptosis and inhibits JNK activity in lymphoblastoid cells. *Biochem Biophys Res Commun* 230: 386–391

67 Matsuda S, Moriguchi T, Koyasu S, Nishida E (1998) T lymphocyte activation signals for interleukin-2 production involve activation of MKK6-p38 and MKK7-SAPK/JNK signaling pathways sensitive to cyclosporin A. *J Biol Chem* 273: 12378–12382

68 Lee H-Y, Walsh GL, Dawson MI, Hong WK, Kurie HM (1998) All-trans retinoic acid inhibits Jun N-terminal kinase-dependent signaling pathways. *J Biol Chem* 273: 7066–7071

69 Haga N, Naito M, Seimiya H, Tomida A, Dong J, Tsuruo T (1998) 2-Deoxyglucose inhibits chemotherapeutic drug-induced apoptosis in human monocytic leukemia U937 cells with inhibition of c-Jun N-terminal kinase 1/stress-activated protein kinase activation. *Int J Cancer* 76: 86–90

70 Dong Z, Huang C, Brown RE, Ma W-Y (1997) Inhibition of activator protein 1 activity and neoplastic transformation by aspirin. *J Biol Chem* 272: 9962–9970

71 Ma W-Y, Huang C, Dong Z (1998) Inhibition of ultraviolet C irradiation-induced AP-1 activity by aspirin is through inhibition of JNKs but not Erks or p38 MAP kinase. *Int J Oncol* 12: 565–568

72 Frantz B, O'Neill EA (1995) The effect of sodium salicylate and aspirin on NF-kB. *Science* 270: 2017–2018

73 Han J, Richter B, Li Z, Kravchenko V, Ulevitch RJ (1995) Molecular cloning of human p38 MAP kinase. *Biochim Biophys Acta* 1265: 224–227

74 Cuenda A, Alonso G, Morrice N, Jones M, Meier R, Cohen P, Nebreda AR (1996) Purification and cDNA cloning of SAPKK3, the major activator of RK/p38 in stress- and cytokine-stimulated monocytes and epithelial cells. *EMBO J* 15: 4156–4164

75 Stein B, Yang MX, Young DB, Janknecht R, Hunter T, Murray BW, Barbosa MS (1997) p38-2, a novel mitogen-activated protein kinase with distinct properties. *J Biol Chem* 272: 19509–19517

76 Wang XS et al (1997) Molecular cloning and characterization of a novel p38 mitogen-activated protein kinase. *J Biol Chem* 272: 23668–23674

77 Lechner C, Zahalka MA, Giot J-F, Møller NPH, Ullrich A (1996) ERK6, a mitogen-acti-

vated protein kinase involved in C2C12 myoblast differentiation. *Proc Natl Acad Sci USA* 93: 4355–4359

78 Stein B, Brady H, Yang MX, Young DB, Barbosa MS (1996) Cloning and characterization of MEK6, a novel member of the MAP kinase kinase cascade. *J Biol Chem* 271: 11427–11433

79 Goedert M, Cuenda A, Craxton M, Jakes R, Cohen P (1997) Activation of the novel stress-activated protein kinase SAPK4 by cytokines and cellular stresses is mediated by SKK3 (MKK6); comparison of its substrate specificity with that of other SAP kinases. *EMBO J* 16: 3563–3571

80 Han J, Lee J-D, Jiang Y, Li Z, Feng L, Ulevitch RJ (1996) Characterization of the structure and function of a novel MAP kinase kinase (MKK6). *J Biol Chem* 271: 2886–2891

81 Moriguchi T et al (1996) A novel kinase cascade mediated by mitogen-activated protein kinase kinase 6 and MKK3. *J Biol Chem* 271: 13675–13679

82 Enslen H, Raingeaud J, Davis RJ (1998) Selective activation of p38 mitogen-activated protein (MAP) kinase isoforms by the MAP kinase kinases MKK3 and MKK6. *J Biol Chem* 273: 1741–1748

83 Tibbles LA, Ing YL, Kiefer F, Chan J, Iscove N, Woodgett JR, Lassam NJ (1996) MLK-3 activates the SAPK/JNK and p38/RK pathways via SEK1 and MKK3/6. *EMBO J* 15: 7026–7035

84 Fan G, Merritt SE, Kortenjann M, Shaw PE, Holzman LB (1996) Dual leucine zipper-bearing kinase (DLK) activates p46 SAPK and p38 MAPK but not ERK2. *J Biol Chem* 271: 24788–24793

85 Guan Z, Buckman SY, Pentland AP, Templeton DJ, Morrison AR (1998) Induction of cyclooxygenase-2 by the activated MEKK1 → SEK1/MKK4 → p38 mitogen-activated protein kinase pathway. *J Biol Chem* 273: 12901–12908

86 Ichijo H et al (1997) Induction of apoptosis by ASK1, a mammalian MAPKKK that activates SAPK/JNK and p38 signaling pathways. *Science* 275: 90–94

87 Zhang S, Han J, Sells MA, Chernoff J, Knaus UG, Ulevitch RJ, Bokoch GM (1995) Rho family GTPases regulate p38 mitogen-activated protein kinase through the downstream mediator Pak1. *J Biol Chem* 270: 23934–23936

88 Lee JC, Badger AM, Griswold DE, Dunnington D, Truneh A, Votta B, White JR, Young PR, Bender PE (1993) Bicyclic imidazoles as a novel class of cytokine biosynthesis inhibitors. *Ann NY Acad Sci* 696: 149–170

89 Hanson GJ, Gunner J (1997) Inhibitors of p38 kinase. *Expert Opinion in Therapeutic Patents* 7: 729–733

90 Boehm JC et al (1996) 1-substituted 4-aryl-5-pyridinylimidazoles: a new class of cytokine suppressive drugs with low 5-lipoxygenase and cyclooxygenase inhibitory potency. *J Med Chem* 39: 3929–3937

91 Badger AM, Bradbeer JN, Votta B, Lee JC, Adams JL, Griswold DE (1996) Pharmacological profile of SB 203580, a selective inhibitor of cytokine suppressive binding protein/p38 kinase, in animal models of arthritis, bone resorption, endotoxin shock and immune function. *J Pharmacol Exp Ther* 279: 1453–1461

92 Jackson JR, Bolognese B, Hillegass L, Kassis S, Adams J, Griswold DE, Winkler JD (1998) Pharmacological effects of SB 220025, a selective inhibitor of P38 mitogen-activated protein kinase, in angiogenesis and chronic inflammatory disease models. *J Pharmacol Exp Ther* 284: 687–692

93 Adams JL et al (1998) Pyrimidinylimidazole inhibitors of CSBP/p38 kinase demonstrating decreased inhibition of hepatic cytochrome P450 enzymes. *Bioorg Med Chem Lett* 8: 3111–3116

94 de Laszlo SE et al (1998) Pyrroles and other heterocycles as inhibitors of p38 kinase. *Bioorg Med Chem Lett* 8: 2689–2694

95 Zablocki J, Tarlton E Jr, Rizzi J, Mantlo N (1998) Aryl and heteroaryl substituted fused pyrrole antiinflammatory agents. Patent WO 9822457

96 Dodd JH, Henry JR, Rupert K (1998) Preparation of substituted pyrrolopyridines for the treatment of inflammatory diseases. Patent WO 9847899

97 Henry JR et al (1998) 6-Amino-2-(4-fluorophenyl)-4-methoxy-3-(4-pyridyl)-1H-pyrrolo[2, 3-b]pyridine (RWJ 68354): a potent and selective p38 kinase inhibitor. *J Med Chem* 41: 4196–4198

98 Henry JR, Rupert KC, Dodd JH, Turchi IJ, Wadsworth SA, Cavender DE, Schafer PH, Siekierka JJ (1998) Potent inhibitors of the MAP kinase p38. *Bioorg Med Chem Lett* 8: 3335–3340

99 Yamamoto N, Sakai F, Yamazaki H, Kawai Y, Nakahara K, Okuhara M (1996) Effect of FR133605, a novel cytokine suppressive agent, on bone and cartilage destruction in adjuvant arthritic rats. *J Rheumatol* 23: 1778–1783

100 Yamamoto N, Sakai F, Yamazaki H, Nakahara K, Okuhara M (1996) Effect of FR167653, a cytokine suppressive agent, on endotoxin-induced disseminated intravascular coagulation. *Eur J Pharmacol* 314: 137–142

101 Yamamoto N, Sakai F, Yamazaki H, Sato N, Nakahara K, Okuhara M (1997) FR167653, a dual inhibitor of interleukin-1 and tumor necrosis factor-alpha, ameliorates endotoxin-induced shock. *Eur J Pharmacol* 327: 169–174

102 Kobayshi J, Takeyoshi I, Ohwada S, Iwanami K, Matsumoto K, Muramoto M, Morishita Y (1998) The effects of FR167653 in extended liver resection with ischemia in dogs. *Hepatology* (Philadelphia) 28: 459–465

103 Hoshida SY N, Tanouchi J, Yamada Y, Kuzuya T, Hori M (1998) The effect of FR-167653 in an extended liver resection with ischemia. *J Am Coll Cardiol* 31: 279A

104 Boehm JC, Chan GW (1998) Preparation of indole-3-carbonyl piperidides and analogs as proinflammatory cytokine inhibitors. Patent WO 9828292

105 Bemis G, Salituro F, Duffy JP, Cochran JE, Harrington EM, Murcko M, Su M, Galullo VP (1998) Preparation of annelated pyrimidinones and analogs as p38 kinase inhibitors. Patent WO 9827098

106 Tracey K, Cohen P, Bukrinsky M, Schmidtmayerova H (1998) Guanylhydrazones useful for treating diseases associated with T-cell activation. Patent WO 9820868

107 Ranges G et al (1998) Inhibition of p38 kinase activity by aryl ureas. Patent WO 9852558

108 Boulton TG et al (1991) ERKs: a family of protein-serine/threonine kinases that are activated and tyrosine phosphorylated in response to insulin and NGF. *Cell* 65: 663–675

109 Cobb MH, Robbins DJ, Boulton TG (1991) ERKs, extracellular signal-regulated MAP-2 kinases. *Curr Opin Cell Biol* 3: 1025–1032

110 Haycock JW, Ahn NG, Cobb MH, Krebs EG (1992) ERK1 and ERK2, two microtubule-associated protein 2 kinases, mediate the phosphorylation of tyrosine hydroxylase at serine-31 in situ. *Proc Natl Acad Sci USA* 89: 2365–2369

111 Catling AD, Schaeffer H-J, Reuter CWM, Reddy GR, Weber MJ (1995) A proline-rich sequence unique to MEK1 and MEK2 is required for Raf binding and regulates MEK function. *Mol Cell Biol* 15: 5214–5225

112 Wu X, Noh SJ, Zhou G, Dixon JE, Guan K-L (1996) Selective activation of MEK1 but not MEK2 by A-Raf from epidermal growth factor-stimulated HeLa cells. *J Biol Chem* 271: 3265–3271

113 Glass DB, Cheng HC, Mende-Mueller L, Reed J, Walsh DA (1989) Primary structural determinants essential for potent inhibition of cAMP-dependent protein kinase by inhibitory peptides corresponding to the active portion of the heat-stable inhibitor protein. *J Biol Chem* 264: 8802–8810

114 Zaheer A, Lim R (1996) *In vitro* inhibition of MAP kinase (ERK1/ERK3) activity by phosphorylated glia maturation factor (GMF). *Biochem* 35: 6283–6288

115 Duesbery NS et al (1998) Proteolytic inactivation of MAP-kinase-kinase by anthrax lethal factor. *Science* 280: 734–737

116 Horiuchi KY, Scherle PA, Trzaskos JM, Copeland RA (1998) Competitive inhibition of MAP Kinase Activation by a Peptide Representing the aC Helix of ERK. *Biochem* 37: 8879–8885

117 Boland A, Cornelis GR (1998) Role of YopP in suppression of tumor necrosis factor alpha release by macophages during *Yersinia* infection. *Infect Immun* 66: 1878–1884

118 Meggio F et al (1995) Different susceptibility of protein kinases to staurosporine inhibition. Kinetic studies and molecular bases for the resistance of protein kinase CK2. *Eur J Biochem* 234: 317–322

119 Vesely J et al (1994) Inhibition of cyclin-dependent kinases by purine analogs. *Eur J Biochem* 224: 771–786

120 Meijer L, Borgne A, Mulner O, Chong JPJ, Blow JJ, Inagaki N, Inagaki M, Delcros JG, Moulinoux JP (1997) Biochemical and cellular effects of roscovitine, a poten and selective inhibitor of the cyclin-dependent kinases cdc2, cdk2, and cdk5. *Eur J Biochem* 243: 527–536

121 Dudley DT, Pang L, Decker SJ, Bridges AJ, Saltiel AR (1995) A synthetic inhibitor of the mitogen-activated protein kinase cascade. *Proc Natl Acad Sci USA* 92: 7686–7689

122 Alessi DR, Cuenda A, Cohen P, Dudley DT, Saltiel AR (1995) PD 098059 is a specific inhibitor of the activation of mitogen-activated protein kinase kinase *in vitro* and *in vivo*. *J Biol Chem* 270: 27489–27494

123 Favata MF et al (1998) Identification of a novel inhibitor of mitogen-activated protein kinase kinase. *J Biol Chem* 273: 18623–18632

124 DeSilva DR, Jones EA, Favata MF, Jaffee BD, Magolda RL, Trzaskos JM, Scherle PA (1998) Inhibition of mitogen-activated protein kinase kinase blocks T cell proliferation but does not induce or prevent anergy. *J Immunol* 160: 4175–4181

125 Williams DH, Wilkinson SE, Purton T, Lamont A, Flotow H, Murray EJ (1998) Ro 09-2210 exhibits potent anti-proliferative effects on activated T cells by selectively blocking MKK activity. *Biochemistry* 37: 9579–9585

Inhibition of NF-κB

Mark J. Suto[1] and Anthony M. Manning[2]

[1]DuPont Pharmaceuticals Research Labs, 4570 Executive Drive, Suite 400, San Diego, CA 92121, USA; [2]Signal Pharmaceuticals, Inc., 5555 Oberlin Drive, San Diego, CA 92121, USA

Introduction

The use of high-throughput screening has revolutionized the drug discovery process. Recently, biotechnology companies focused on assay detection methodologies, automation capabilities, miniaturization of assays and microfluidics have emerged. Many of these companies and their associated technology are geared toward the generation of thousands of data points, across a variety of screening platforms (cell-based, biochemical, receptors), quickly and at minimal cost. Nonetheless, the screening of hundreds of thousands of samples can be an expensive endeavor and much of the work wasted if a well established screening strategy is not in place.

It is often believed that increased screening capacity will automatically result in a shortened discovery pipeline. However, if adequate resources and a definitive decision network are not established, the use of HTS may in fact have the opposite effect. To increase the chances of success when establishing a high-throughput drug discovery program, several important points should be considered. These include (a) the selection of a validated target or pathway, (b) establishing relevant primary and secondary assays and (c) access to a diverse library of compounds. In addition, hits identified in any HTS program will require sufficient medicinal chemistry and lead optimization resources at an early stage.

For example, if a library of 500,000 samples is screened in a validated biochemical assay and a "hit" criteria to obtain a primary hit rate of 1% is established, 5000 samples would be identified and require follow-up analysis. Typically, a library of this size would be screened over several months, and access to the 5000 samples needed for confirmation would require "cherry picking" of individual samples from over 6200, 96-well microtiter plates. These samples would of course be needed to perform dose-response analysis in the primary screen, specificity against related biochemical targets and some type of functional or cell-based determination of activity, which will require resources in addition to those directly involved in the screening operation. In addition, chemistry resources will be needed to perform initial profiling of the structures for prioritization of compounds and follow-up. This process if not managed properly will result in a great deal of wasted effort and most importantly, time.

To circumvent several of these bottlenecks, Signal has established a pathway for lead discovery for each drug discovery program (Fig. 1). The pathway consists of "criteria" to prioritize compounds and move them forward in a quick and efficient manner (decision points) were instituted. Ideally, as much information as possible about a potential lead or hit should be obtained at each stage including the primary screen. For example, as part of Signal's kinase inhibitor strategy including the NF-κB program, a library is simultaneously evaluated against several kinase targets such as JNK1, JNK2, p38-2 and the desired IκB kinase. This approach addresses the activity of a screening sample against the target of interest (IκB), and its specificity with respect to other kinases. The assays are performed on a Zymark robotics system capable of running several kinases simultaneously and performing dose-response analysis as well. The system is capable of running a library against four different kinases, examining the primary single point data (based upon predefined internal criteria) and then performing a dose response analysis on those compounds that meet the hit criteria. The result is that in a single "run" a sample's ability to inhibit a kinase of interest, the IC_{50} of inhibition and the specificity across related kinases is determined. This procedure identifies a smaller number of "hit or lead compounds", but they are usually of higher quality.

Another important HTS consideration is the diversity of the compound library and whether it is available in a suitable format for the type of assays running. Registration, storage and retrieval of a large library are very resource dependent and should not be overlooked. Although the size of the library is important, the diversity or variety of samples in the library is key to a successful hit rate. Over several years, Signal has established a rather diverse library consisting of compounds from multiple commercial vendors, natural product extracts, combinatorial libraries from collaborators and focused kinase libraries generated internally. In total, Signal has approximately 350,000 samples available for screening against each target.

NF-κB pathway

Many autoimmune diseases or chronic inflammatory states result in self-perpetuating destruction of normal tissues or organs. This is caused by the induction of adhesion molecules, chemotaxis of leukocytes, activation of leukocytes and the production of mediators of inflammation [1]. All of these events are regulated at the level of transcription for the production of new proteins such as growth factors, interleukins, proteinases and cytokines. Inducible transcription of and eventual protein production, is controlled by a family of proteins known as transcription factors (TFs) [2]. These TFs bind to specific regions on DNA when activated and act as molecular switches or messengers to induce or upregulate gene expression. The activa-

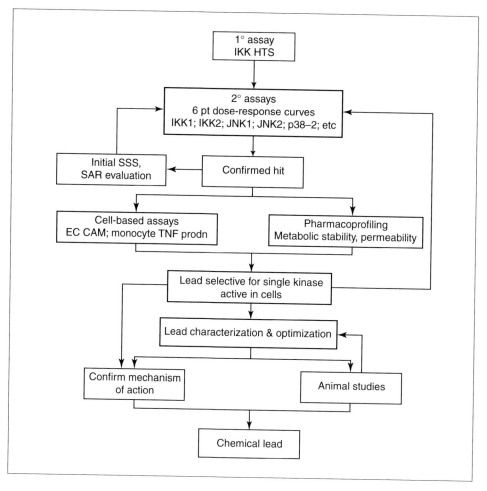

Figure 1

Prototypical lead discovery pathway for IκB kinase inhibitors: A series of successive assays is established to characterize and prioritize novel compounds in biochemical and cellular assays, and animal models of human disease. Compounds identified as active in a primary (1°) IKK HTS assay are tested for potency and selectivity in a panel of secondary (2°) kinase assays. Confirmed hits are prioritized for initial chemical evaluation using sub-structure searches and structure-activity relationships (SAR). Selected compounds are tested in cell-based models of NF-κB-dependent gene expression and their pharmacologic properties (e.g. metabolic stability, GI permeability) assessed using in vitro assays. Selected compounds with suitable activities are then subjected to an extensive chemistry lead optimization effort. Advanced compounds are then tested for efficacy in animal models of disease and detailed studied to confirm the molecular mechanism of action of lead compounds are performed. These studies lead to the selection of a chemical lead for detailed pharmacologic evaluation.

tion of these TFs is caused by a variety of external signals including physiological stress, infectious agents and other bioregulatory molecules [3]. Once the plasma membrane receptors are activated, a cascade of protein kinases and second messengers are induced which, in turn, result in the stimulation of transcription [4]. The end result is the production of proteins which can alter the function of the cell or of other cells nearby [5]. This system displays a high level of specificity, responding to defined stimuli and activating discrete TFs.

TFs are the central control points in gene activation and as such are found at the terminus of signaling pathways. They and their enzymatic activators are highly regulated, affording multiple strategies for selectively intervening in disease processes by controlling TF function. It is possible to inhibit or augment TF function with agents that act upon the TF itself or on its regulatory proteins. These regulatory proteins are enzymes which, historically, have been ideal targets for small molecule intervention and, as such, make excellent targets for Signal's drug discovery programs.

For example, a specific set of external signals could result in the activation of a single transcription factor which can induce many pathogenic proteins responsible for a given disease [5]. Therefore, regulating this process by disrupting the production of activated TF(s) has the potential to attenuate the production of the associated pathological proteins, thereby halting or reversing the course of the disease.

NF-κB is a transcription factor that was first identified as a lymphoid specific protein that binds to a decameric motif present in the κ-light chain intronic enhancer [6]. Functional NF-κB binding sites were subsequently found in the promoters/enhancer regions of many genes, including IL-2, IL-6, IL-8, GM-CSF, ICAM-1 and class I MHC [7]. Rapidly it became clear that NF-κB played a central role in various responses leading to host defense and immune function, activating a program of gene expression.

NF-κB and human disease

The therapeutic utility of inhibitors of NF-κB is quite broad. For example, the inappropriate activation of NF-κB and its dependent genes have been associated with various pathological conditions including toxic/septic shock, graft versus host reaction, acute-phase response, radiation damage, atherosclerosis, viral replication, and cancer [8]. The role of NF-κB in arthritis is documented by the observation of activated NF-κB in human inflamed synovial tissue [9, 10]. The activation of NF-κB in vascular endothelium and type A synovial lining cells, detected by immunohistochemical staining, was shown to be a feature of synovial tissue from both RA and osteoarthritis (OA) patients [11].

Septic shock is a systemic inflammatory response that develops when microbial products such as LPS stimulate expression of various inflammatory cytokines. Several animal studies have demonstrated that the inhibition of NF-κB activation in in vivo models of septic shock correlates with suppression of TNFα formation, reduced ICAM-1 gene expression and protection against endotoxin induced tissue injury [12–14].

NF-κB may also be involved in the pathogenesis of atherosclerosis. Using immunofluorescence and immunohistochemical techniques, activated NF-κB was detected in smooth muscle cells, endothelial cells, and macrophages from the fibrotic-thickened intima/media and artheromatous areas of an atherosclerotic lesion [15, 16]. Little expression was detected in vessels lacking atherosclerosis [15]. Furthermore, angiotensin converting enzyme inhibition was shown to prevent NF-κB activation, monocyte chemoattractant protein-1 (MCP-1) expression, and macrophage infiltration in a rabbit model of early accelerated atherosclerosis [17]. In similar studies, treatment with anti-sense RelA oligonucleotides was shown to inhibit the thrombin-stimulated growth of vascular smooth muscle cells *in vitro* [18]. Taken together, these results implicate NF-κB activation in the chronic inflammation and proliferative processes involved in atherosclerosis.

NF-κB as a drug discovery target

NF-κB can be activated in cells by a wide variety of stimuli associated with stress, injury and inflammation. Potent inducers of NF-κB include: cytokines such as interleukin 1β (IL-1β) and tumor necrosis factor α (TNFα); bacterial and viral products such as lipopolysaccharide (LPS), sphingomyelinase, double-stranded RNA and the Tax protein from human T cell leukemia virus 1 (HTLV-1); and pro-apoptotic and necrotic stimuli such as oxygen free radicals, UV light and γ-irradiation [19]. This diversity of inducers highlights an intriguing aspect of NF-κB regulation, namely the ability of many different signal transduction pathways emanating from a wide variety of induction mechanisms to converge on a single target: the cytosolic NF-κB:IκB complex. The recent discovery of several key enzyme components of the NF-κB activation pathway suggests a molecular basis for signal integration in this pathway.

NF-κB exists in the cytoplasm in an inactive form associated with inhibitory proteins termed IκB's, of which the most important may be IκBα, IκBβ and IκBγ [20, 21]. The activation of NF-κB is achieved through the signal-induced proteolytic degradation of IκB in the cytoplasm (Fig. 2). Extracellular stimuli initiate a signaling cascade leading to activation of two IκB kinases, IKK-1 (IKKα) and IKK-2 (IKKβ), which phosphorylate IκB at specific N-terminal serine residues (S32 and S36 for IκBα, S19 and S23 for IκBβ) [22–29]. Phosphorylated IκB is then selectively ubiquitinated, presumably by an E3 ubiquitin ligase, the terminal member of a cascade of ubiquitin-conjugating enzymes [30, 31]. In the last step of this signaling cascade, phosphorylated and ubiquitinated IκB, which is still associated with NF-κB

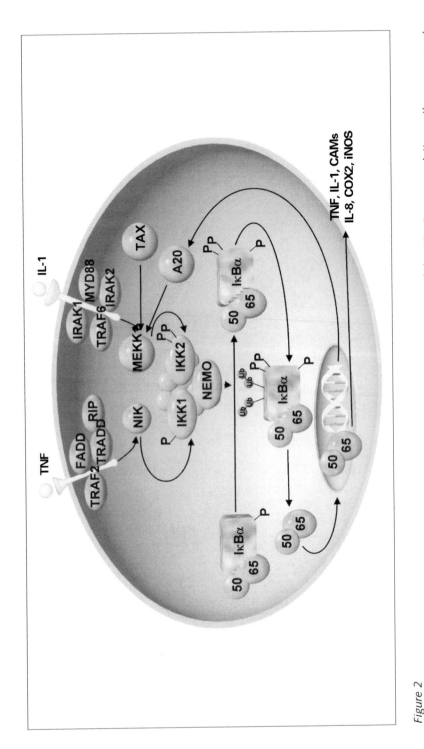

Figure 2

TNF and IL-1 activate the NF-κB gene regulation pathway: Molecular components of the NF-κB gene regulation pathway represent attractive targets for drug discovery. TNF, tumor necrosis factor; IL-1, interleukin 1; TRAF, TNF receptor associated factor; IRAK, IL-1-receptor associated kinase; RIP, receptor-interacting protein; TRADD, TNF receptor-associated death domain; NIK, NF-κB inducing kinase; IKK, IκB kinase; NEMO, NF-κB essential modulator; CAMs, cell adhesion molecules; COX2, cyclooxygenase 2; iNOS, inducible nitric oxide synthase; IL-8, interleukin 8.

in the cytoplasm, is selectively degraded by the 26S proteasome [32]. This process exposes the NLS, thereby freeing NF-κB to interact with the nuclear import machinery and translocate to the nucleus [33], where it binds its target genes to initiate transcription. Thus the NF-κB pathway contains many potential targets or points of intervention for small molecule drugs.

IκB phosphorylation serves as a molecular tag leading to rapid ubiquitination and degradation of IκB by components of the ubiquitin-proteasome system. Using peptides as substrate mimics, it was established that IκBα phosphorylation generates a binding site for the specific ubiquitin ligase(s) responsible for conjugation of ubiquitin to IκBα, and that microinjection of these phosphopeptides into cells could interfere with NF-κB activation [31]. These results emphasize the importance of the ubiquitin ligase system in IkB degradation. The IκB-specific E3 ligase was recently identified [34].

The IκB kinases IKK1 and IKK2, their upstream activating kinases MEKK and NIK, and their downstream effector, the putative E3 ligase, all represent attractive targets for the discovery of drugs which selectively regulate NF-κB function. These proteins may all be part of a large 600–800 kDa protein complex, the IKK signalsome [25].

The basic drug discovery strategy is to prevent the activation of NF-κB, and the associated production of proinflammatory proteins. As shown in Figure 2, there are several approaches that could be considered as viable targets including, blocking cell surface receptors, interfering with intracellular targets or mobilization, modulating key kinases and preventing localization of proteins. Many of the upstream approaches that have been attempted thus far, such as antibodies to cytokines and blocking cell surface receptors are too non-specific to be useful for drug discovery, although several drugs have advanced into Phase 2 or Phase 3 clinical trials following these approaches.

Several groups including Signal have identified compounds that prevent the degradation of IκBα by the 26S proteosome [35]. These compounds blocked NF-κB activation, but they also had an effect on several other biological processes including the transcription factor, AP-1 [36].

In summary, a wide variety of compounds have been shown to block NF-κB activation, including several different classes of antioxidants. Although effective these compounds lack the selectivity to be developed into a therapeutic agent. More recently, the IκB-specific E3 ligase was identified and shown to be inhibited by small peptides encompassing the IκB binding site for the E3 ligase. However, assays to identify inhibitors by these methods thus far have not been adapted to the type of high throughput format needed for a successful drug discovery program.

In 1993, Signal developed a cell based assay for identifying inhibitors of the NF-κB pathway. A stably transfected Jurkat T cell line was generated that contained a NF-κB binding site driving luciferase. The cells were stimulated with PMA/PHA and luciferase activity measured. Using this cell line and a Zymark robotics system, approximately 12,000 samples could be evaluated in a week. In addition, dose response analysis and cytokine determinations could be performed using the same cell line. Hit compounds were identified and then optimized using a combination of parallel synthesis and classical medicinal chemistry. Several leads were derived that were active in animal models of inflammation and transplantation [37]. However, the exact molecular target of these dual-inhibitors of AP-1 and NF-κB has yet to be fully elucidated, illustrating one of he potential problems with this particular cell-based approach.

IκB kinase high throughput screening

As described, phosphorylation of the NF-κB/IκB heterodimer by IκB kinase is one of the key steps in the activation of NF-κB and represents a viable drug discovery target for several reasons. These include: (a) the IκB kinases represent a known molecular target for drug discovery and performing structure-activity studies, (b) it can be adapted to an automated format and (c) potentially could be used as part of a rational drug discovery strategy, if the structure of the protein is solved.

Signal's initial approach to the identification of novel inhibitors of the NF-κB pathway focused on one of the IκB kinases, IKK2. Initially, an assay was established that consisted of ^{32}P (ATP) and GST-IκBα as the substrate. Recombinant IKK2 was purified from SF9 cells using affinity chromatography techniques and found to be active. Although this initial assay was of sufficient throughput, the use of ^{32}P presented problems regarding radiation exposure and contamination of equipment. Therefore the assay was converted to a non-radioactive format similar to that we had used with the mitogen-activated protein kinases [38]. The method of choice was time-resolved fluorescence, which was easily implemented and readily adaptable to a robotics system.

The assay consists of a 96-well microtiter plate coated with GST IκBα, the IKK2 described and antibodies to the phosphorylated IκBα. The antibodies were purified and labeled with europium chelates (DELFIA, WALLAC) and the assay optimized using different concentrations of ATP (Km level ATP = 0.5 μM). Samples to be tested are dissolved in DMSO and diluted with buffer to the appropriate screening concentrations. As shown in Figure 3, screening samples are incubated with IKK2 in GST IκBα plates. The plates were washed after one hour and the extent of phosphorylation measured using the europium labeled antiphospho IκB antibody. Compounds blocking the phosphorylation of the substrate via IKK2 result in a decreased signal. Compounds meeting a preset activity criteria are then run in a dose response analysis to generate IC_{50} values.

The assay has been adapted to operate on a Zymark robotics system capable of performing four different kinases simultaneously. Therefore, a specific library of

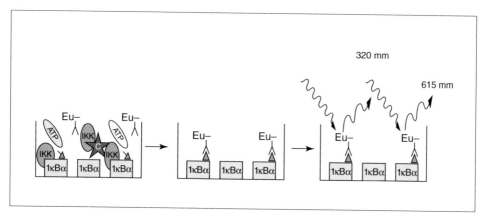

Figure 3

compounds is evaluated not only against the target of interest, but against related kinases as well. Compounds identified under this format have been profiled for activity and specificity and if they meet the criteria established, move through the decision tree outlined in Figure 1.

Also it is critical to have established the appropriate secondary assays. Therefore, the cytotoxicity of the compounds (MTT assay), their effect on cytokine gene transcription, NF-κB activation and IκB phosphorylation in a range of cells is examined. In addition, assays to address metabolism, cell penetration, and bioavailability are used routinely to examine potential hits.

Conclusions

The HTS system established at Signal has resulted in the identification of potent and selective inhibitors of the IκB kinase, a key target in the NF-κB pathway, as well as inhibitors of several different mitogen activated kinases. Secondary assays of sufficient throughput to address cytotoxicity, cell activity and penetration have been established and are critical to the program. In addition relevant and predictive animal models of disease are needed particularly when dealing with a potential new therapeutic approach such as inhibiting NF-κB.

It is important to realize that a successful high throughput screening system is not capable of standing alone and requires support and resources from several different functional areas. Also, when establishing an HTS system the earlier the other functional groups are involved and understand their role the greater the chance for success.

References

1   Ben-Baruch A, Michiel D, Oppenheim J (1995) Signals and receptors involved in recruitment of inflammatory cells. *J Biol Chem* 270: 11703–11706

2   Manning A (1996) Transcription Factors: A new frontier for drug discovery. *Drug Disc Today* 1: 151–160

3   Cahill M, Janknecht R, Nordheim A (1996) Signaling pathways: Jack of all cascades. *Current Biology* 1: 16–19

4   Hill C, Treisman R (1995) Transcriptional regulation by extracellular signals: Mechanisms and specificity. *Cell* 80: 199–211

5   Warren J (1993) Inflammation. *Drug News and Persp* 6: 450–455

6   Sen R, Baltimore D (1986) Multiple nuclear factors interact with the immunoglobulin enhance sequences. *Cell* 46: 705–710

7   Baldwin A (1996) The NF-κB and IκB proteins: New discoveries and insights. *Annu Rev Immunol* 14: 649–681

8   Siebenlist U, Franzo G, Brown K (1994) Structure, regulation and function of NF-κB. *Annu Rev Cell Biol* 10: 405–455

9   Asahara H, Asanuma M, Ogawa N, Nishibayashi S, Inoue H (1995) High DNA binding activity of transcription factor NF-κB in synovial membranes of patients with rheumatoid arthritis. *Biochem Mol Biol Int* 37: 827

10   Marok P, Winyard, P, Columbe A, Kus M, Gaffney K, Blades S, Mapp P, Morris C, Blake D, Kaltschmidt C, Baeuerle P (1996) Activation of the transcription factor nuclear factor-κB in human inflamed synovial tissue. *Arthritis Rheum* 39: 583–591

11   Handel M, McMorrow L, Gravallese E, (1995) Nuclear factor-κB in rheumatoid synovium. Localization of p50 and p65. *Arthritis Rheum* 38: 1762–1770

12   Essani N, Fisher M, Jaeschke H (1997) Inhibition of NF-κB activation by dimethyl sulfoxide correlates with suppression of TNF-alpha formation, reduced ICAM-1 gene transcription, and protection against endotoxin-induced injury. *Shock* 7: 90–96

13   Schow S, Joly A (1997) N-Acetyl-leucinyl-leucinyl-norleucinal inhibits lippopolysaccharide-induced NF-κB activation and prevents TNF and IL-6 synthesis *in vivo*. *Cell Immunol* 175: 199–202

14   Sprong R, Aarsman C, van Oirschot J, van Asbeck B (1997) Dimethylthiourea protects rats against gram-negative sepsis and decreases tumor-necrosis factor and nuclear factor κB activity. *J Clin Med* 129: 470–481

15   Brand K, Page S, Rogler G, Bartsch A, Brand R, Knuechel R, Page M, Kaltschmidt C, Baeuerle P, Neumeier D (1996) Activated transcription factor nuclear factor-κB is present in the artherosclerotic lesion. *J Clin Invest* 97: 1715–1722

16   Brand K, Page S, Walli A, Neumeier D, Baeuerle P (1997) Role of nuclear factor-κB in atherogeneis. *Exp Physiol* 82: 297–304

17   Hernandez-Presa M, Bustos C, Ortego M, Tunon J, Renedo G, Ruiz-Ortega M, Egido J (1997) Angiotensin-converting enzyme inhibition prevents arterial nuclear factor κB

activation, monocyte chemoattractant protein-1 expression, and macrophage infiltration in a rabbit model of early accelerated atherosclerosis. *Circulation* 95: 1532–1541

18 Maruyama I, Shigeta, K, Miyahara H, Nakajima T, Shin H, Ide S, Kitajima I (1997) Thrombin activates NF-κB through thrombin receptor and results in proliferation of vascular smooth muscle cells: Role of thrombin in artherosclerosis and restonosis. *Ann NY Acad Sci* 811: 429–436

19 Bauerle P, Baichwal V (1997) NF-κB as a frequent target for immunosuppressive and anti-inflammatory molecules. *Adv Immunol* 65: 111–136

20 Baeuerle P, Baltimore D (1996) NF-κB: Ten years after. *Cell* 87: 13–20

21 Whiteside S, Epinat J, Rice N, Israel A (1997) IκB epsilon, a novel member of the IκB family, controls RelA and cRel NF-κB activity. *EMBO J* 16: 1413–1426

22 Regnier C, Song H, Gao H, Goeddel D, Cao Z, Rothe M (1997) Identification and characterization of an IκB kinase. *Cell* 90: 373–383

23 DiDonato J, Hayakawa M, Rothwarf D, Zandi E, Karin M (1997) A cytokine-responsive IκB kinase that activates the transcription factor NF-κB. *Nature* 388: 548–554

24 Zandi E, Rothwarf D, Delhasse M, Hayakawa M, Karin M (1997) The IκB kinase complex (IKK) contains two kinase subunits, IKKα and IKKβ, necessary for IκB phosphorylation and NF-κB activation. *Cell* 91: 243–252

25 Mercurio F, Zhu H, Murray B, Shevchenko A, Bennett B, Li J, Young D, Barbosa M, Mann M, Manning A, Rao A (1997) IKK-1 and IKK-2: Cytokine-activated IκB kinases essential for NF-κB activation. *Science* 278: 860–866

26 Woronicz J, Gao X, Cao Z, Rothe M, Goeddel D (1997) IκB kinase-β: NF-κB activation and complex formation with IκB kinase-α and NIK. *Science* 278: 866–869

27 Stancovski I, Baltimore D (1997) NF-κB activation: the IκB kinase revealed. *Cell* 91: 299–302

28 Maniatis T (1997) Catalysis by a multiprotein IκB kinase complex. *Science* 278: 818–819

29 Verma I, Stevenson J (1997) IκB kinase: beginning, not end. *Proc Nat Acad Sci USA* 94: 11758–11760

30 Alkalay I, Yaron A, Hatzubai A, Orian A, Ciechanover A, Ben-Neriah Y (1995) Stimulation-dependent IκBα phosphorylation marks the NF-κB inhibitor for degradation via the ubiquitin-proteasome pathway. *Proc Natl Acad Sci USA* 92: 10599–10603

31 Yaron A, Alkalay I, Hatzubai A et al (1997) Inhibition of NF-κB cellular function via specific targeting of the IκB ubiquitin ligase. *EMBO J* 16: 101–107

32 Chen Z, Hagler J, Palombella VJ, Melandri F, Scherer D, Ballard D, Maniatis T (1995) Signal-induced site-specific phosphorylation targets IκB-α to the ubiquitin-proteasome pathway. *Genes Dev* 9: 1586–1597

33 Henkel T, Zabel U, Van Zee K, Muller JM, Fanning E, Baeuerle P (1992) Intramolecular masking of the nuclear location signal and dimerization domain in the precursor for the p50 NF-κB subunit. *Cell* 68:1121–1133

34 Yaron A, Hatzubai A, Davis M, Lavon I, Amit S, Manning AM, Andersen JS, Mann M,

Mercurio F, Ben-Neriah Y (1998) Identification of the receptor component of the IκBα-ubiquitin ligase. *Nature* 396: 590–594

35 Suto M, Sullivan R, Ransone L (1996) Peptide inhibitors of IkB protease: modification of the C-termini of Z-LLFCHO. *Bio and Med Chem Lett* 2965–2930

36 Suto M, Ransone L (1997) Novel approaches for the treatment of inflammatory diseases: Identification of inhibitors of NF-κB/AP-1. *Current Pharmaceutical Design* 3: 505–518

37 Sullivan R, Bigam C, Erdman, P, Palanki M, Anderson D,Goldman M, Ransone L, Suto M (1998) 2-Chloro-4-(trifluoromethyl)pyrimidine-5-N-(3',5'-bis(trifluoromethyl) phenyl)-carboxamide: A potent inhibitor of NF-κB- and AP-1-mediated gene expression identified using solution-phase combinatorial chemistry. *J Med Chem* 41: 413–419

38 Gaarde W, Hunter T, Brady H, Murray B, Goldman M (1997) Development of a non-radioactive, time-resolved fluorescence assay for the measurement of Jun N-terminal kinase activity. *J Biomol Screening* 2: 213–223

IL-1 antagonist discovery

Terry L. Bowlin[1], Stephen D. Yanofsky[2] and Herman Schreuder[3]

[1]BioChem Pharma, 275 Armand-Frappier Blvd., Laval, Quebec, Canada H7V 4A7; [2]Affymax Research Institute, Palo Alto, CA 94304; [3]Hoechst Marion Roussel, 65926 Frankfurt, Germany

Introduction

Interleukin 1 (IL-1) is a pivotal pro-inflammatory cytokine involved in many types of inflammatory and autoimmune diseases [1]. IL-1 production whether initiated by infection or host antigen, initiates an inflammatory cascade which includes the induction of other mediators (e.g. IL-6, IL-8), upregulation of adhesion molecules (e.g. ICAM-1, E-selectin) and potent synergistic activity with other macrophage, proinflammatory cytokines (e.g. tumor necrosis factor) [2, 3]. The IL-1 family consists of three structurally related naturally occurring ligands: two agonists, IL-1α, and IL-1β; and one antagonist, the IL-1 receptor antagonist (IL-1RA) [4–6]. IL-1 is the only cytokine known to have a naturally occurring receptor antagonist. Two distinct cell membrane receptors have been characterized: The type I, IL-1 receptor (IL-1RtI) responsible for biological responses; and the type II receptor (IL-1RtII), which is shed, and acts as a decoy to modulate IL-1 activity [7–11]. The existence of a naturally occurring antagonist and a decoy receptor further illustrates the importance and need for the tight regulation of IL-1 activity and its critical role in inflammation.

IL-1RA and the soluble IL-1RtI have been shown to have therapeutic value in preclinical animal studies and clinical studies [1–3, 12]. However, although these molecules may provide effective IL-1 antagonism, since they are rather large proteins, their therapeutic potential may be limited. Our objective was to identify a low molecular weight interleukin-1 receptor antagonist, which could be produced synthetically and delivered locally at much higher concentrations. Utilizing recombinant peptide display libraries, we identified several peptide families which antagonize IL-1 *in vitro* and *in vivo* [13, 14]. Furthermore, our crystallographic studies on IL-1RA bound to the ILIRtI, identified a critical core motif required for antagonist binding [15] and present in our peptide antagonists, as described below.

Identification of IL-1RtI binding peptides

The extracellular domain of the Type I IL-1R was cloned from HepG2 cell RNA using PCR primers with homology to the Type I IL-1R sequence [16] and additional sequences encoding the kemptide epitope LRRASLG [17] and PIG linkage. Stably transfected G418 resistant CHO cell lines were stained with FITC-labeled IL-1α, analyzed by FACS for high level expression of IL-1RtI, and individual clones were examined for binding of ^{125}I labeled IL-1α. A soluble form of the IL-1RtI extracellular domain was prepared by PIPLC treatment of clone 1C2 cells following their harvest from a 36 liter bioreactor [16]. The extracellular portion of the Type I IL-1R was purified by passing this material over an MBP-IL-1RA sepharose column. Non-blocking monoclonal antibodies to the IL-1RtI were generated [13]. For screening purposes, monoclonal antibody (Ab79) was coated onto wells of a microtitre plate and used to capture soluble IL-1RtI [13].

Libraries of peptides expressed on the surface of bacteriophage fd represent an enormous degree of structural diversity, and therefore serve as ideal sources for the identification of high affinity receptor-binding compounds. In fact, such libraries have been used to identify high affinity ligands for the Type I IL-1R [13], E-selectin [18], the TPO-R [19] and EPO-R [20]. A number of peptide display libraries were constructed as shown in Table 1. An NNK motif was used to encode random amino acids. The random peptide libraries ranged in size from 10^8–10^{11} recombinants and expressed random peptides on the N-terminus of fd phage pIII [21], on the N-terminus of fd phage pVIII [18] or at the C-terminus of the lac repressor [22].

The phage libraries described above were screened against the Type I IL-1R immobilized on Ab79 in microtitre wells in the following manner. Approximately 10^{11} PFU/ml were incubated in wells containing immobilized receptor for 2 h. Wells were washed with PBS and bound phage eluted with acid. E. coli were infected with eluted phage and grown overnight to amplify the culture to about 10^{12} PFU/ml. After three cycles of this panning protocol, individual phage clones were isolated and tested for receptor-specificity in an ELISA format [23]. Detection was accomplished using a polyclonal rabbit anti-phage antibody and an alkaline phosphatase conjugated goat anti-rabbit antibody. Binding of phage to IL-1RtI immobilized on Ab79 was compared to binding to wells coated with Ab79 alone. DNA was prepared and sequenced for receptor-specific phage, and the indicated peptide sequences are listed in Table 2. The peptides on plasmids Lac I library were panned for three rounds essentially as described [22]. Individual clones after three rounds of panning were tested by ELISA as described [22]. DNA was sequenced for those exhibiting receptor-specificity and representative sequences are shown in Table 2.

Receptor-specific peptides were identified from all of the primary libraries that were screened. The recovered sequences were related, all containing the consensus sequence WxxxGLW. To determine whether these peptides were competitive with IL-1, the peptide RB16 (WWTDDGLWASGS-NH$_2$) was synthesized. This peptide

Table 1 - Peptide libraries screened against the Type I IL-IR

Name	Vector	Sequence	Spacer	Size
ON141	pIII	$(X)_8$	ASGSA	2×10^9
ON159	pIII	$(X)_{12}$	GG	3×10^8
ON644	pVIII phagemid	$(X)_{10}$	$(GGGGS)_3$	6×10^9
R12	LacI	$(X)_{12}$	GADGGA	6.0×10^9
ON2158	pVIII phagemid	$(X)_{11}$	$(GGGGS)_3$	1.1×10^{11}

Table 2 - Peptides specific for the Type I IL-1R identified from random peptide libraries

R11	WWTDDGLW
S14	DWDQFGLWRGAA
NU1	RWDDNGLWVVVL
CYC1	CWSMHGLWLC
T12	GGRWDQAGLWVA
MC1	KLWSEQGIWMGE
IL1	DWDTRGLWVY
IL7	QWDTRGLWVA
IL9	SWDTRGLWVE
IL12,17	DWDTRGLWVA
IL13	SWGRDGLWIE

had no effect on binding of ^{125}I-labeled IL-1α to the Type I IL-1R (at concentrations up to 1 mM) and it had no effect on a number of IL-1 mediated cellular responses. Thus, it appears that we have identified a family of peptides that bind the Type I IL-1R in a manner that is non-competitive with that of IL-1.

Two methods were used to block this non-competitive site during the phage selection process in an attempt to identify new peptide sequences which compete with IL-1 for binding to the Type I IL-1R. Since most of the "GLW" family peptides contain tryptophan at positions 2 and 8, we constructed a random 12-mer library which lacked tryptophan at these positions by using NNW (where W equals A or T) at positions 2 and 8 and NNK at the other positions. We also screened some of the phage libraries in Table 1 in the presence of 250 μM peptide RB16 to block the non-competitive site. Using these methods, additional peptides were obtained, as

Table 3 - IL-1 blocking peptides identified from phage libraries

Name	Sequence	IC$_{50}$ (μM)
T6	RLVYWQPYSVQR	59
CW13	WEQPYALPLE	45
CW11	REYEQPYALW	140
AF11475	DNSSWYDSFLL	71
PG42	IMWFCQPGGACYSV	230

shown in Table 3. These peptides were synthesized and tested for their ability to block the binding of ^{125}I-labeled IL-1α to the Type I IL-1R. They were found to block IL-1 binding with IC$_{50}$ values in the range of 60–250 μM (Tab. 3).

Affinity maturation process

Additional phage libraries were designed based on the sequences of T6 and AF11475. These libraries represented 3 different approaches towards obtaining peptides with a higher affinity for the Type I IL-1R. Libraries were generated using either the T6 or AF11475 sequence in which the peptide coding region was mutagenized with a 70-10-10-10 approach (i.e. 70% of the correct nucleotide triphosphate at each position and 10% each of the other nucleotide triphosphates). Several libraries were constructed in which half of the sequence was fixed and the remainder was replaced with random sequences or the peptide sequence was extended by putting additional residues on either side of the core sequence. These libraries were screened against immobilized IL-1RtI as described above and a large number of IL-1RtI binding peptides were identified. More than 130 of these were synthesized and tested for inhibition of ^{125}I IL-1α binding to the Type I IL-1R. The most potent of these are shown in Table 4.

While these peptides were significantly more potent than the initial sequences, the screening process that was utilized did not permit affinity-based selection. To enrich for phage expressing peptides with high affinity for the Type I IL-1R, we modified the selection procedure to include a 15 min ligand-mediated dissociation step. After a 2-h incubation of phage with immobilized receptor, unbound phage were removed by washing and buffer containing 3 μM IL-1α was added to the wells. After incubation for 15 min at 4°C to permit dissociation of phage bearing low affinity peptides, bound phage were eluted with acid as before and the process was repeated. The phage from the third and fourth cycles of this process were used to infect *E. coli* and plated on agarose. After incubation overnight at 37°C, colonies

Table 4 - IL-1RtI binding peptides recovered from mutagenesis and extension libraries

Name	Sequence	IC_{50} (μM)
3H4	TFVYWQPYALPL	5
806-1	EYEWYQPYALPL	0.76
AF11788	DNTAWYENFLL	1.5
AF11789	DNTAWYESFLA	3.5

Table 5 - IL-1RtI binding peptides identified by use of colony lifts

Name	Sequence	IC_{50} (nM)
AF10847	ETPFTWEESNAYYWQPYALPL	2.6
AF10961	TANVSSFEWTPGYWQPYALPL	2.6
AF11308	DGYDRWRQSGERYWQPYALPL	2.1
AF12233	QIDNTAWYERFLLQYNA	7.0
AF12311	TYTYDNTAWYERFLMSY	16
AF12235	HIDNTAWYENFLLTYTP	30

were transferred to nitrocellulose and probed using either radiolabeled IL-1RtI (labeled with ^{33}P using PKA) or a bivalent radiolabeled IL-1R-Fc fusion [13].

Thus, the use of ligand-mediated dissociation to enrich for phage expressing high affinity peptides coupled with the colony lift technique to identify high affinity sequences resulted in the identification of peptides with low nanomolar affinity for the IL-1RtI. However, to obtain this increase in potency, additional residues were added, resulting in going from 10–12 residue peptides to 17–21-mers (Tab. 5). AF10847, AF10961 and AF11308 were obtained from libraries in which the YWQPYALPL was fixed and an additional 12 random residues were placed at the N-terminus. AF12233 and AF12235 were obtained from a library based on AF11789 with two random residues on the N-terminus, four random residues at the C-terminus and a 70-10-10-10 mutagenesis of the core sequence. AF12311 was obtained from a library based on AF11789 with four random residues at the N-terminus, two random residues at the C-terminus and 70-10-10-10 mutagenesis of the core sequence. Comparison of these sequences reveals that there appear to be numerous ways to obtain high affinity binding to the Type I IL-1R, as the residues outside of the core regions are quite different among the high affinity peptides.

Table 6 - Truncations and analogs of high affinity IL-1 antagonists

Name	Sequence	IC_{50} (nM)
AF10961	TANVSSFEWTPGYWQPYALPL	2.6
AF11377	FEWTPGYWQPYALPL	1.9
AF11490	FEWTPGYWQPY-NH$_2$	30
AF11486	FEWTPGYWQJY-NH$_2$	8.1
AF11485	EWTPGYWQPY-NH$_2$	2900
AF10847	ETPFTWEESNAYYWQPYALPL	2.6
AF11170	FTWEESNAYYWQPYALPL	9.9
AF11171	FTWEESNAYYWQPY-NH$_2$	120
AF11303	FTWEESNAYYWQJY-NH$_2$	14
AF11308	DGYDRWRQSGERYWQPYALPL	2.1
AF11440	WRQSGERYWQPYALPL	100
AF12233	QIDNTAWYERFLLQYNA	7.0
AF12407	DNTAWYERFLLQYNA-NH$_2$	15
AF12431	QIDNTAWYERFLLQY-NH$_2$	17
AF12411	DNTAWYERFLLQY-NH$_2$	50

While it is clear that the sequences in Table 5 can be grouped into two families, they are related. The core sequence in the AF10847 family contains two aromatic residues followed by QPY and two hydrophobic residues (AL). Similarly, the AF12233 family contains two aromatic residues followed by ERF or ENF and two hydrophobic residues (LL or LM).

To determine the minimal sequence requirement for high affinity IL-1RtI binding, a series of truncations were performed (Tab. 6). Up to six residues could be removed from the amino-terminus of AF10961 without significant loss of affinity. Truncation from the C-terminus of this series revealed that the ALPL could be substituted with an amide without dramatic loss of affinity. Replacement of the central proline with azetidine (designated "J") resulted in about a four-fold increase in potency, with the resulting compound being an 11-mer with 8 nM affinity for IL-1RtI. Only three residues could be removed from the N-terminus of AF10847 without dramatic loss of affinity. Removal of the C-terminal ALPL in AF11170 resulted in greater than ten-fold loss in affinity, which could be mostly regained by the azetidine for proline substitution (AF11303). With AF12233, two residues could be removed from the N-terminus with only a two-fold drop in potency. Similarly, the two C-terminal residues could be replaced with an amide with only a two-fold drop in potency. However, truncation of both N- and C-termini resulted in a seven-fold drop in potency.

Species selectivity of IL-1RtI binding peptides

The activity of the peptides above was determined by inhibition of ^{125}I IL-1α binding to an antibody immobilized extracellular domain of the IL-1RtI. These peptides had similar activity with respect to inhibition of ^{125}I IL-1β binding to immobilized IL-1RtI extracellular domain (11–15 nM). They inhibited IL-1α binding to the full length IL-1 receptor on the surface of normal human dermal fibroblast cells (IC$_{50}$ of 5.6 nM). However, AF10847 did not inhibit binding of ^{125}I IL-1α or ^{125}I IL-1β to mouse EL4 cells at concentrations up to 12 μM. This peptide was also unable to inhibit IL-1 induced IL-6 expression in murine 3T3 cells. Thus, AF10847 does not appear to bind to the murine IL-1 receptor. AF11377 was tested for its ability to block IL-1 induced EGF receptor down-regulation on the Rhesus monkey cell line CL160. AF11377 blocked this response with an IC$_{50}$ of 35 nM, indicating that this peptide binds with high affinity to the monkey IL-1 receptor.

In vitro and *in vivo* biological characterization of AF-12198

We further explored the structure-activity relationship of peptides related to AF11377. Substitution of an unnatural amino acid l-azetidine-z-carboxylic acid (J) for proline in the core QPY motif increased binding affinity (AF11869) two-fold (Tab. 7). Deletion of the four C-terminal residues (ALPL) from AF11869 resulted in a 3–4-fold loss of affinity (AF11486). Despite the amidation of the C-terminus of AF11486, this peptide only had an *in vitro* human plasma t$_{1/2}$ of 0.5 h. Acetylation of the N-terminus of AF11486 improved stability in human plasma greater than four-fold (2.7 h) accompanied by a two-fold increase in affinity (AF11805). However, there was a loss of functional activity (less than two-fold) as measured by the ability of the peptide to antagonize IL-1β (50 pg/ml) to induce IL-8 production, determined by ELISA, using human dermal fibroblasts. IL-1RA had an IC$_{50}$ value of 24 pM in this assay. Inversion of Trp-7 and Tyr-8 (AF11567) in the protected peptide again diminished binding affinity; but returned the functional antagonist activity, IL-8 inhibition, to the levels of the non-acetylated AF11486. The re-introduction of the ALPL residues to the C-terminus of the protected peptide (AF12198) resulted in a 15-mer with the best overall combination of binding activity (IC$_{50}$ = 0.55 nM), functional activity (IC$_{50}$ = 25 nM) and stability (t$_{1/2}$ = 2.6 h).

AF12198 was further characterized for *in vitro* and *in vivo* antagonism of IL-1 biological activity. Human umbilical vein endothelial cells (HUVEC) normally express relatively low levels of cellular adhesion molecules such as ICAM-1 and E-selectin on their surface. However, in response to IL-1 both ICAM-1 and E-selectin are induced to much higher levels of surface expression. Utilizing fluorescein conjugated mab to ICAM-1 or E-selectin, followed by FACS analysis, the ability of AF12198 to inhibit IL-1 upregulation of these adhesion molecules was assessed.

Table 7 - Biological activity and stability of high affinity IL-1 antagonist

Name	Sequence	Binding IC_{50} (nm)	IL-8 inhibition IC_{50} (nm)	*In vitro* plasma $t_{1/2}$ (h)
AF11377	FEWTPGYWQPYALPL	1.9	N.D.	N.D.
AF11869	FEWTPGYWQJYALPL	0.99	N.D.	N.D.
AF11486	FEWTPGYWQJY-NH$_2$	3.6	85	0.5
AF11805	Ac-FEWTPGYWQJY-NH$_2$	1.5	130	2.7
AF11567	Ac-FEWTPGWYQJY-NH$_2$	3.2	74	2.3
AF12198	Ac-FEWTPGWYQJYALPL-NH$_2$	0.55	25	2.6

AF12198 inhibited IL-1β induction of ICAM-1 and E-selectin expression on HUVEC with IC_{50} values of 9 nM and 24 nM, respectively. AF12198 alone did not demonstrate any agonist activity. IL-1RA inhibited the induction of these adhesion molecules with an IC_{50} of less than 20 pm.

As mentioned previously, peptides from this family do not bind the murine IL-1R or inhibit IL-1 mediated biological activity in murine cells. This made further biological characterization of AF12198 more difficult, since many of the existing preclinical inflammatory and autoimmune rodent models, where IL-1 has been shown to be critical, could not be utilized. Fortunately, as mentioned above, this family of peptides, including AF12198, were found to bind monkey IL-1RtI with similar affinity to the human receptor. Therefore, we went on to characterize the ability of AF12198 to inhibit the IL-1 driven induction of IL-6 in cynomolgus monkeys [14]. Initially, AF12198 was evaluated *in vitro* utilizing heparinized whole blood from monkeys and humans. IL-1β was used at a final concentration of 3 ng/ml or 6 ng/ml for human or monkey samples, respectively. IL-6 analysis was performed by ELISA. AF12198 inhibited IL-1 induced IL-6 production in monkey and human whole blood with IC_{50} values of 17 μM and 15 μM, respectively. IL-1RA inhibited IL-6 induction in monkey and human whole blood with IC_{50} values of 30 nM and 2 nM, respectively. AF12198 alone did not induce any detectable IL-6 in blood from monkeys or humans. *In vivo*, the i.v. bolus administration of IL-1β (0.3 mg/kg) gave extremely variable levels of plasma IL-6 concentrations (1.9 to 42.5 ng/ml) peaking at 3 h post infusion. However, in those animals with a strong inducible IL-6 response (> 15 ng/ml), AF12198 (16 mg/kg/h), infused (i.v.) over a 90 min period (–30 min to +60 min), was very effective in inhibiting IL-1 induced IL-6 (> 90%). IL-1RA (0.3 mg/kg) was also very effective in reducing IL-1 induced IL-6 (> 98%) in all animals tested. Due to the variable IL-6 induction in IL-1 treated animals, an *ex vivo* protocol was established to further assess the activity of AF12198. AF12198 was given as an infusion at 128 mg/kg for 15 min, blood was drawn and stimulated with IL-1 (6 ng/ml). Under this protocol, AF12198 completely blocked (100%) *ex vivo* IL-1 induction of IL-6 with a peptide plasma concentration of 78 nmol/ml at 15 min. IL-1RA (30 mg/kg) achieved 98% inhibition with a plasma concentration of 8.7 pmol/ml at 15 min. Two major metabolites of AF12198 were observed, an 11-mer, Ac-FEWTPGWYQJY-OH and a 6-mer, Ac-FEWTPG-OH. Both metabolites were inactive. These combined results demonstrate that AF12198 is effective at blocking IL-1 driven IL-6 induction.

Crystallographic studies on IL-1 antagonism

Crystallographic studies on IL-1R antagonism started with the crystal structure of the IL-1RA molecule alone. The IL-1RA crystallized over a wide range of pH'S (from 6–8) in the presence of PEG and organic salts. Two different crystal forms were obtained: triclinic and tetragonal. Whereas the triclinic crystals diffracted only out to 2.75 Å resolution, the tetragonal crystals diffracted much better up to about 2.0 Å and allowed a detailed analysis of the IL-1RA crystal structure. IL-1RA crystal structures were described by three independent groups in three papers which appeared in 1994 and 1995 [24–26]. In all cases, the asymmetric unit contained two independent IL-1RA molecules, raising the possibility that IL-1RA dimerizes in solution under suitable conditions (e.g. during crystallization).

IL-1RA has the same fold as IL-1α and IL-1β, consisting of a six-stranded β-barrel, closed at one side by three β-hairpin loops (Fig. 1). This fold has been named Kunitz, or IL-1 fold, and is shared by a large family of protein molecules. Interestingly, none of its members has enzymatic activity. They are all involved in protein-protein interactions, either as protease inhibitors or as receptor ligands, suggesting that this fold is particularly well suited for protein-protein interactions.

Comparison of the structures of IL-1RA, IL-1α and IL-1β revealed that the six stranded β-barrel core is well preserved with root-mean-square differences in Cα positions of less than 1.0 Å, while some of the connecting loops are quite different (Fig. 1). Surprisingly, the loops which were identified by mutagenesis studies to be the most important for receptor interaction (the N-terminus and loops D and G) [27], are exactly the loops which differ most between the three molecules. This means that the interaction of these molecules with the receptor must be different, which opens the possibility of fine-tuning the affinity of IL-1α, IL-1β and IL-1RA towards the type-I, type-II and soluble receptors.

However, inferring receptor interaction from the structure of the ligand alone remains speculative, a situation which was remedied by the back-to-back publication of the structure of IL-1R in complex with IL-1RA [15] or IL-1β [28].

The IL-1R crystal structures, shown in Figure 2, revealed that the extra-cellular portion of the IL-1R consists of three immunoglobulin-like domains which completely surround the ligand and bury about 30% of the solvent accessible surface of

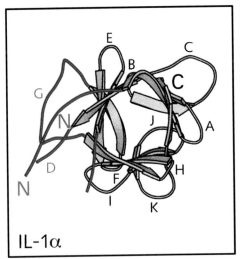
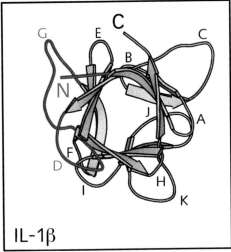
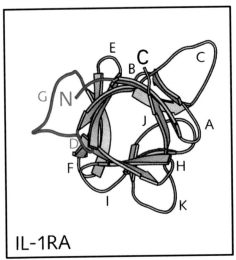

Figure 1
Folding the three IL-1 molecules. The N-terminal region and loops D and G are indicated in red. These loops are important for receptor interaction, but are very different in the three molecules (see text). This figure has been produced with Molscript [31].

the ligand. Figure 3 shows the topology of the IL-1R. The third domain is of the standard telokin- or I-type topology, but the topology of domains 1 and 2 differs significantly from the canonical I-set and may represent a new class of immunoglobulin folds. The most striking feature of this fold is that one of the two β-sheets, which

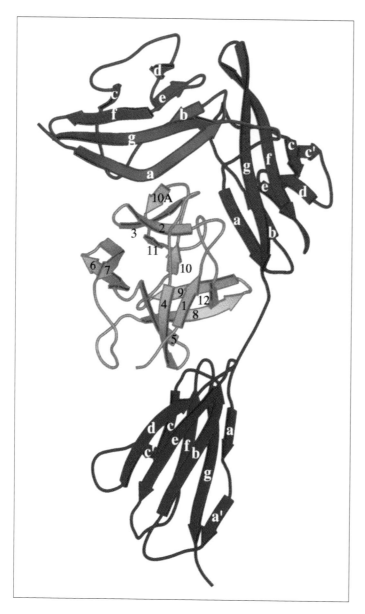

Figure 2

Ribbon diagram [31] of the IL-1R-IL1RA complex. The agonist is yellow and the receptor domains 1, 2 and 3 are red, green and blue, respectively. In the full length receptor, the C terminus of domain 3 (blue) is connected to the membrane-spanning domain. This means that in the natural situation, the membrane will be near the bottom of the figure.

Reprinted with permission from Nature 386: 196 © 1997, Macmillan Magazines Ltd. [15].

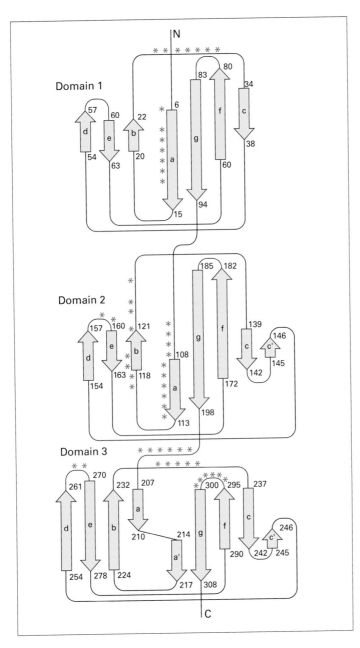

Figure 3
Topology of the IL-1R, β-strands are depicted by arrows. Residues which interact with the
IL-1RA are indicated with a star.
Reprinted with permission from Nature 386: 196. © 1997, Macmillan Magazines Ltd.

build the immunoglobulin β-sandwich, is extremely short with strands of only 3–4 residues. This is caused by the presence of a Pro residue immediately after the disulfide bond which connects the two sheets of the sandwich. The presence of such as CP motif in the sequence of immunoglobulin domains points to this type of fold.

Receptor domains 1 and 2 are tightly linked with strands g and f of domain 2 lying on top of domain 1 precluding any hinge movement between the two domains. In contrast, domain 3 is connected with a long and flexible linker to domain 2 and is able to move freely with respect to domains 1 and 2, allowing the receptor to open so that the ligand can enter the pocket between the three domains.

There are two major interaction sites between IL-1R and its ligands. The first one is around the cleft between domains 1 and 2. The second interaction site is with domain 3. The most important interactions of IL-1RA with the receptor are in the first region, with the edges of the a strands of domains 1 and 2 (Figs. 2 and 3). In particular, the side chains of G1n20 and G1n36 of IL1RA make multiple hydrogen bonds with the backbone of the receptor (Fig. 4), fully exploiting the complementarity of the side chain amide and the peptide amide. These interactions are conserved in the IL-1β complex where G1n14 and G1n32 are equivalent to G1n20 and G1n36 in IL-1RA. Other IL-1RA residues important for receptor interactions are Trp16, Tyr34 and Tyr147 [27]. These residues are also situated near the cleft between domains 1 and 2. The side chain of Tyr34 is tightly fixed by a hydrogen bond to the IL-1RA main chain and faces a hydrophobic area on the receptor surface. Trp16 and Tyr146 are next to each other on adjacent β-strands. The side chain of Trp16 makes a hydrogen bond with the receptor main-chain and has hydrophobic interactions with Met114 of the receptor. Tyr147 interacts with a hydrogen-bonding network involving some bound water molecules on top of domain 2. The IL-1RA residues interacting with domain 3 do not seem to contribute much to the receptor binding. Interestingly, only five residues out of the 18 residues which directly contact the receptor contribute to binding. Apparently the loss of entropy due to the fixation of flexible side chains in the complex appears to offset the binding energy gained. Indeed, the residues which do contribute to the binding are already fixed in unbound IL-1RA.

Agonist versus antagonist activity

When we solved the IL-1R/IL1-RA complex [15], the structure of IL-1β was superimposed onto the IL-1RA in the receptor complex to get a preliminary model of the IL-1R/IL-1β complex. In this model, we noticed a strongly positively charged region on IL-1β, involving Arg4, Lys92, Lys93 and Lys94 (the so called receptor trigger site), facing a negatively charged region on domain 3 of the receptor consisting of three aspartates and two glutamates (Fig. 4). We postulated that binding of IL-1β to the receptor would trigger a rotation of domain 3, which would bring the two

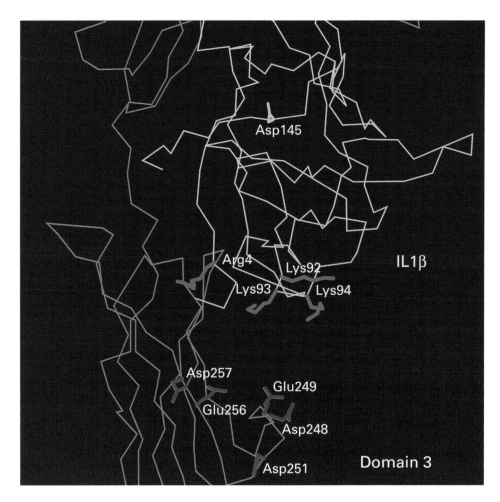

Figure 4
Model obtained after superimposing IL-1β onto IL-1RA in the IL-1R-IL-1RA complex, show-ing the positively charged receptor trigger site (Arg4, Lys92, Lys93 and Lys94) and a nega-tively charged region on the IL-1R domain 3 (Asp248, Glu249, Asp251, Glu256 and Asp257). In the actual IL-1β complex [15], the two regions interact, causing a rotation of receptor domain 3 of –20° with respect to the the IL-1RA complex [28].
Reprinted with permission from Nature 388: 196. © 1997, Macmillan Magazines Ltd. [15].

patches together. Indeed, the crystal structure of the IL-1R/IL-1β complex showed exactly the predicted rotation of ~20° (Fig. 5). The absence of such a conforma-tional change in the IL-1RA complex could be a reason why IL-1RA does not acti-vate the receptor.

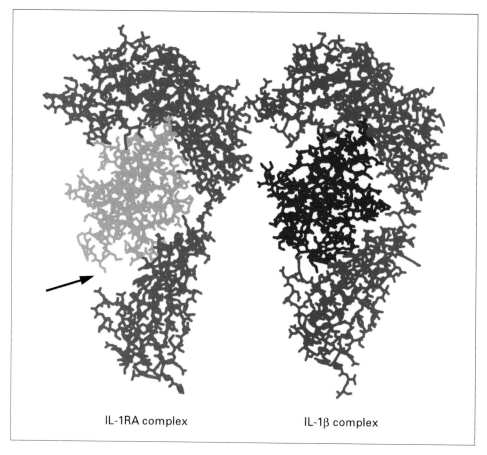

IL-1RA complex   IL-1β complex

Figure 5
Comparison of the IL-1R complexes with IL-1RA and IL-1β. The IL-1R is indicated in green and cyan, IL-1RA in yellow and Il-1β in dark-blue. The arrow indicates the cleft between domain 3 of the receptor and IL-1RA, which is not present in the IL-1β complex, due to the interaction of the "receptor trigger site" of IL-1β with the receptor.

During the structure determination of the IL-1R complexes, an IL-1R-like protein, the IL-1R accessory protein was discovered [29] and it is believed that association of the IL-1R with the IL-1R accessory protein triggers the receptor response. The accessory protein does not bind to either the receptor alone or to an agonist alone. Therefore, it needs either the conformational change in the receptor, induced by IL-1β, or interaction sites on both the receptor and the agonist, or both, in order to associate with the IL-1R. Hints that the accessory protein binds to IL-1β in the IL-1R/IL-1β complex, come from mutagenesis studies, which showed that changing

Asp145 in IL-1β to Lys creates an antagonist, while changing Lys145 in IL-1RA to Asp creates an agonist [30]. Asp145 is at the surface of IL-1β and does not interact with the IL-1R at all (Fig. 5), suggesting that this residue might bind to the accessory protein.

Summary

Despite extensive screening efforts and numerous attempts to use peptide fragments derived from IL-1 ligands by many in the pharmaceutical industry, until our efforts, no one had identified a low molecular weight IL-1 antagonist. The tremendous molecular diversity that was achieved by screening large recombinant peptide libraries was necessary for us to succeed where so many others had failed. Furthermore, our crystallographic studies confirm and identify structurally the same critical residues (Tyr, Trp, G1n) present in the consensus sequence (YWQPYA) identified by screening and fully explaining previous site-directed mutagenesis studies [27].

References

1   Dinarello CA (1994) The interleukin-1 family: 10 years of discovery. *FASEB J* 15: 1314–1325

2   Dinarello CA (1993) Modalities for reducing interleukin-1 activity in disease. *Immunol Today* 14: 260–264

3   Dinarello CA (1992) The role of interleukin-1 in host responses to infectious diseases. *Infect Agents Dis* 1: 227–236

4   March CJ, Mosely B, Larsen A, Cerretti DP, Braedt G, Price V, Gillis S, Henney CS, Kronheim SR, Grabstein K et al (1985) Cloning, sequence and expression of two distinct human interleukin-1 complementary DNAs. *Nature* 315: 641–647

5   Eisenberg SP, Arend WP, Verderber E, Brewer MT, Hannm CH, Thompson RC (1990) Primary structure and functional expression from complementary DNA of a human interleukin-1 receptor antagonist. *Nature* 343: 341–346

6   Hannum CH, Wilcox CJ, Arend WP, Joslin FG, Dripps DJ, Heimdal PL, Armes LG, Sommer A, Eisenberg SP, Thompson RC (1990) Interleukin-1 receptor antagonist activity of a human interleukin-1 inhibitor. *Nature* 343: 336–340

7   Sims JE, Acres RB, Grubin CE, McMahan CJ, Wignall JM, March CJ, Dowr SK (1989) *Proc Natl Acad Sci* 86: 8946–8950

8   McMahan CJ, Slack JL, Mosely B, Cosman D, Lupton SD, Brunton LL, Grubin CE, Wignall JM, Jenkins NH et al (1991) A novel IL-1 receptor, cloned from B cells by mammalian expression, is expressed in many cell types. *Embo J* 10: 2821–2832

9   Sims JE, Gayle MA, Slack JL, Alderson MR, Bird TA, Giri JG, Colotta F, Re F, Manto-

vani A, Shanebeck K, Grabstein KH, Dower SK (1993) Interleukin 1 signaling occurs exclusively via the type I receptor. *Proc Natl Acad Sci USA* 90: 6155–6159

10   Colotta F, Re F, Muzio M, Bertini R, Polentarutti N, Sironi M, Giri JG, Dower SK, Sims JE, Mantovani A (1993) Interleukin-1 type II receptor: a decoy target for IL-1 that is regulated by IL-4. *Science* 26: 472–475

11   Symons JA, Duff GW (1990) A soluble form of the interleukin-1 receptor produced by a human B cell line. *FEBS Lett* 272: 133–136

12   Arend WP, Malyak M, Guthridge CJ, Gabay C (1998) Interleukin-1 receptor antagonist: role in biology. *Annu Rev Immunol (US)* 16: 27–55

13   Yanofsky SD, Baldwin DN, Butler JH, Holden FR, Jacobs JW, Balasubramanian P, Chinn JP, Cwirla SE, Peters-Bhatt E, Whitehorn A et al (1996) High affinity type I interleukin 1 receptor antagonists discovered by screening recombinant peptide libraries. *Proc Natl Acad Sci USA* 93: 7381–7386

14   Akeson AL, Woods CW, Hsieh LC, Bohnke RA, Ackermann BL, Chan KY, Robinson JL, Yanofsky SD, Jacobs JW, Barrett RW, Bowlin TL (1996) AF12198, a novel low molecular weight antagonist, selectively binds the human type I interleukin (IL)-1 receptor and blocks *in vivo* responses to IL-1. *J Biol Chem* 271: 30517–30523

15   Schreuder HA, Tardif C, Trump-Kallmeyer S, Soffientini A, Sarubbi E, Akeson A, Bowlin TL, Yanofsky S, Barrett RW (1997) A new cytokine-receptor binding mode revealed by the crystal structure of the IL-1 receptor with an antagonist. *Nature (London)* 386: 194–200

16   Whitehorn EA, Tate E, Yanofsky SD, Kochersperger L, Davis A, Mortensen RB, Yonkovich S, Bell K, Dower WJ, Barrett RW (1995) A generic method for expression and use of "tagged" soluble versions of cell surface receptors. *Biotechnol* 13: 1215–1219

17   Li BL, Langer JA, Schwartz B, Petska S (1989) Creation of phosphorylation sites in proteins: Construction of a phosphorylatable human interferon alpha. *Proc Natl Acad Sci USA* 86: 558–562

18   Martens CL, Cwirla SE, Lee RY, Whitehorn E, Chen EY, Bakker A, Martin EL, Wagstrom C, Gopalan P, Smith CW (1995) Peptides which bind to E-selectin and block neutrophil adhesion. *J Biol Chem* 270: 21129–21136

19   Cwirla SE, Balasubramanian P, Duffin DJ, Wagstrom CR, Gates CM, Singer SC, Davis AM, Tansik RL, Mattheakis LC, Boytos CM et al (1997) Peptide agonist of the thrombopoietin receptor as potent as the natural cytokine. *Science* 276: 1696–1699

20   Wrighton NC, Farrell X, Chang R, Kasyhap AK, Barbone FP, Mulcahy LS, Johnson DL, Barrett RW, Jolliffe LK, Dower WJ (1996) Small peptides as potent mimetics of the protein hormone erythropoietin. *Science* 273: 458–444

21   Cwirla SE, Peters EA, Barrett RW, Dower WJ (1990) Peptides on phage: A vast library of peptides for identifying ligands. *Proc Natl Acad Sci USA* 87: 6378–6382

22   Cull MG, Miller JF, Schatz PJ (1992) Screening for receptor ligands using large libraries of peptides linked to the C terminus of the lac repressor. *Proc Natl Acad Sci USA* 89: 1865–1869

23 Barrett RW, Cwirla SE, Ackerman MS, Olson AM, Peters EA, Dower WJ (1992) Selective enrichment and characterization of high affinity ligands from collections of random peptides on filamentous phage. *Anal Biochem* 204: 357–364

24 Clancy LL, Finzel BC, Yem AW, Deibel MR jr, Strakalaitis NA, Einspahr HM (1994) Initial chrystallographic analysis of a recombinant human interleukin-1 receptor antagonist protein. *Acta Crystallogr* D50: 197–201

25 Vigers GPA, Caffes P, Evans RJ, Thompson RC, Eisenberg SP, Brandhuber BJ (1994) X-ray structure of interleukin-1 receptor antagonist at 2.0-Å resolution. *J Biol Chem* 269: 12874–12879

26 Schreuder HA, Rondeau JM, Tardif C, Soffientini A, Sarubbi E, Akeson A, Bowlin TL, Yanofsky S, Barrett RW (1995) Refined crystal structure of the interleukin-1 receptor antagonist. Presence of a disulfide link and a cis-proline. *Eur J BioChem* 227: 838–847

27 Evans RJ, Bray J, Childs JD, Vigers PA, Brandhuber BJ, Skalicky JJ, Thompson RC, Eisenberg SP (1995) Mapping receptor binding sites in interleukin (IL)-1 receptor antagonist and IL-1 beta by site-directed mutagenesis. Identification of a single site in IL-1RA and two sites in IL-1 beta. *J Biol Chem* 270: 11477–11483

28 Vigers PA, Anderson LJ, Caffes P, Brandhuber B (1997) Crystal structure of the type-I interleukin-1 receptor complexed with interleukin-1 beta. *Nature (London)* 386: 190–194

29 Greenfeder SA, Nunes P, Kwee L, Labow M, Chizzonite RA, Ju G (1995) Molecular cloning and characterization of a second subunit of the interleukin-1 receptor complex. *J Biol Chem* 270: 13757–13765

30 Ju G, Labriola-Tompkins E, Campen CA, Benjamin WR, Karas J, Plocinski J, Biondi D, Kaffka KL, Kilian PL, Eisenberg SP, Evans RJ (1991) Conversion of the interleukin 1 receptor antagonist into an agonist by site-specific mutagenesis. *Proc Natl Acad Sci USA* 88: 2658–2662

31 Kraulis P (1991) Molscript: A program to produce both detailed and schematic plots of protein structures. *J Appl Crystallogr* 24: 946–950

Phosphodiesterase inhibitors for respiratory diseases

Mark A. Giembycz

Thoracic Medicine, Imperial College of School of Medicine at the National Heart & Lung Institute, Dovehouse Street, London SW3 6LY, UK

Introduction

Asthma and chronic obstructive pulmonary disease (COPD) impose a large financial burden on health services worldwide and it is predicted that this will continue to grow well into the 21st century. Recent epidemiological studies indicate that the prevalence and severity of allergic asthma is increasing [1] together with the number of reported cases of fatal asthma [2, 3]. These statistics are of concern given the marked increase in the prescribing of various anti-asthma therapies [4, 5]. Similarly, it is projected that by the year 2020 the world ranking of COPD relative to the most important causes of death will rise to three, below ischaemic heart and cerebrovascular diseases, with an associated increase in mortality [6].

Asthma and COPD are inflammatory disorders to a greater or lesser extent but differ fundamentally in their cellular basis. Thus, whereas asthmatic inflammation is often allergic involving eosinophils and T lymphocytes, the inflammation seen in COPD has no allergic component and it is believed to be attributable to the recruitment and activation of neutrophils within lung and airways. Although the last decade has seen significant advances in our understanding of the pathogenesis of asthma essentially nothing is known about COPD. Since the incidence of asthma and COPD is already pandemic, it is only too clear that drugs that can prevent the overt and covert manifestations of these diseases could have a profound clinical and global economic impact. While glucocorticosteroids are considered the most effective anti-inflammatory drugs currently available for asthma they are non-selective in action and not without adverse effects. Moreover, patients with COPD do not respond to steroids [7–9] and no alternative therapies are available. Thus, new drugs with enhanced selectivity and improved side-effect profiles are clearly required. One group of drugs that, from a theoretical perspective, may exhibit powerful anti-inflammatory and immunomodulatory activity is inhibitors of the cyclic AMP phosphodiesterase (PDE) isoenzyme families, more commonly known as PDE3 and PDE4 inhibitors [10–21]. Theoretically, these drugs should possess many of the desirable activities of steroids without the associated side effects. This article reviews

High Throughput Screening for Novel Anti-Inflammatories, edited by M. Kahn the progress of anti-inflammatory PDE inhibitors, identifies problems that have been encountered by the pharmaceutical industry in their clinical development and what strategies are being considered to overcome them.

PDE3: definition and multiplicity

PDE3 is a cyclic AMP PDE that is selectively inhibited by micromolar concentrations of cyclic GMP and, for that reason, was originally classified as the cyclic GMP-inhibited, cyclic AMP PDE. Selective inhibitors of the PDE3 isoenzyme family were developed primarily for the treatment of congestive heart failure with the hope that a greater therapeutic index could be achieved over cardiac glycosides [22]. Latterly, their potential utility as bronchodilators and anti-inflammatory agents was explored (see below) given that a PDE3 is present in a number of cells and tissues relevant to airway inflammation (Tab. 1).

Two genes (PDE3A, PDE3B) have thus far been identified that encode PDE3 isoenzymes [23]. PDE3A was originally cloned from a human heart cDNA library and had a predicted molecular weight (125 kDa), similar to the partially purified PDE3 from human cardiac sarcoplasmic reticulum [24]. Transcripts for at least two different forms of human PDE3A have been described that are transcribed from different start codons. One form encodes a membrane-bound protein of 125 kDa for which cyclic GMP has high affinity, while the other is considerably smaller (80 kDa) since it lacks a large portion at the N-terminus. This truncated enzyme is soluble and cyclic GMP has relatively lower affinity [25]. In addition, two distinct, but related, PDE3 cDNAs also have been cloned from rat adipose tissue cDNA libraries [26]. One of these, RcGIP2 (rat cyclic GMP-inhibited phosphodiesterase 2), is highly homologous to the human heart PDE3 and probably is derived from vascular elements within adipose tissue. The other isoenzyme, RcGIP1, is the hormone-stimulated adipocyte PDE3 and is transcribed from a distinct gene, PDE3B [26]. Neither RcGIP1 nor RcGIP2 cDNA's strongly hybridise to total RNA extracted from rat liver, which may indicate the presence of the third PDE3 isoform.

PDE4: definition and multiplicity

PDE4 is a generic term used to describe a large family of enzymes that share several common characteristics. Without apparent exception, PDE4 isoenzymes are acidic proteins that exclusively hydrolyse cyclic AMP [27, 28]. Moreover, the activity of PDE4 is suppressed by nanomolar concentrations of rolipram, an archetypal inhibitor of this enzyme family. Four mammalian cDNA homologues [29–32] of the *Drosophila melanogaster* "dunce" cyclic AMP PDE [33] have been identified and cloned establishing a molecular basis for the observed heterogeneity of gene prod-

Table 1 - *Human cells and tissues implicated in the pathogenesis of asthma and COPD and the distribution of PDE enzymes families*

Cell/Tissue	PDE families identified
T lymphocytes	3, 4, 7*
B lymphocytes	3, 4, 7
Eosinophils	4, 7*
Basophils	3, 4, 5
Mast cells	3, 4
Monocytes	3, 4, 7*, 8*
Macrophages	1, 3, 4, 5
Neutrophils	4
Airways smooth muscle	1, 2, 3, 4, 5, 7*, 8*
Epithelial cells	1, 2, 3, 4, 5, 7*
Endothelial cells	3, 4,
Platelet	1, 2, 3, 5
Nerves	1**, 3, 4, 5

*Identified at the mRNA level by RT-PCR; **Represents >90% of the total PDE activity in guinea-pig de-sheathed vagus nerve which contains parasympathetic and sensory fibres.*

ucts within this PDE family. These clones, originally denoted ratPDEs 1–4, represent transcripts of four different genes and have been reclassified such that ratPDE1, PDE2, PDE3 and PDE4 are now known as RNPDE4C, RNPDE4A, RNPDE4D and RNPDE4B respectively where RN refers to the species *Rattus norvegicus*. Evidence was recently provided for the existence of at least four human genes that encode PDE4 isoenzymes [28, 34–40]. Like their rat counterparts there is a restricted localisation of mRNA transcripts between tissues [34, 35].

An astonishing finding that emerged from the molecular cloning of PDE4 isoenzymes is the presence of mRNA transcripts of different sizes for each of the four variants that are differentially expressed between tissues [28, 41, 42]. An example of this multiplicity is exemplified in human T lymphocytes where at least three different mRNA transcripts derived from the PDE4D gene have been identified [43]. Furthermore, mRNA transcripts show a distinct tissue distribution. Thus, PDE4A mRNA transcripts are present in brain, heart and testis of rats but not in liver or kidney whereas mRNA for PDE4C is localised to the liver and testis only [44]. The basis for this profound heterogeneity of PDE4 isoenzymes is attributable to alternative mRNA splicing and the finding that the genes encoding PDE4 express multiple promoter regions providing several potential start codons for translation of protein [45].

Table 2 - PDE4 subtypes identified in human airways smooth muscle and pro-inflammatory cells by RT-PCR

Cell/Tissue	Phosphodiesterase isogene expression			
	HSPDE4A	HSPDE4B	HSPDE4C	HSPDE4D
T lymphocytes	+	+	–	+
B lymphocytes	+	+	–	+
Eosinophil	+	+	–	+
Neutrophil	+	+	–	+
Monocyte	+	+	–	+
Epithelial cell	+	–	+	+
Trachea	+	+	+	+

+ mRNA present; – mRNA absent

Although PDE4 is present in essentially all cell types that have been implicated in allergic disease (Tab. 1), it is perhaps surprising, given recent molecular biological data, that PDE4 isogene products are not expressed differentially across cells and tissues of the immune system (Tab. 2).

Rationale for the development of PDE4 inhibitors for inflammatory diseases

The prototype PDE inhibitors that have been used in the treatment of asthma for many years are the alkylxanthines of which theophylline is the most widely prescribed. The main beneficial activity of theophylline was originally attributed to its weak bronchodilator action. However, evidence accumulated in the early 1990s points to an anti-inflammatory action of this compound at sub-bronchodilator doses [46–48], which has provoked a remarkable resurgence of interest in theophylline and, so called, "second generation" PDE inhibitors not only as smooth muscle relaxants but as potential anti-allergic and/or anti-inflammatory agents [10, 14, 15, 17–21].

The rationale for developing new PDE inhibitors has stemmed primarily from the realisation that PDEs represent a highly heterogeneous group of enzymes (nine families have thus far been identified) that are differentially expressed between different cell types and presumably regulate specific functional responses. Accordingly, it was rapidly appreciated that selective inhibition of a particular PDE isoenzyme may result in a discrete functional alteration of cells that express that PDE variant and, theoretically, specific functional responses within the same cell. In this respect, almost every cell type that has been implicated in the pathogenesis of asthma expresses representatives of the PDE4 isoenzyme family (Tab. 1). Conceptually, PDE4 inhibitors should show a pleiotropic profile of activity on many cells types involved in asthmatic inflammation and so differ from classical mediator antagonists whose importance in disease progression might vary between asthma sufferers and so have limited usefulness. Torphy [21] recently emphasised this point by reference to the eosinophil. Thus, inhibition of PDE4 can attenuate the elaboration of eosinophil chemotaxins from several cell types, the adherence of eosinophils to the post capillary microvascular endothelium and the secretion of survival-enhancing cytokines such as IL-5 and GM-CSF. In addition, PDE4 inhibitors exert direct effects on the eosinophil and can suppress degranulation, activation of the NADPH oxidase and the generation of lipid mediators. A further prediction is that inhibiting PDE4 should potentiate the effects of endogenous anti-inflammatory agents that stimulate adenylyl cyclase through Gs-coupled receptors such as catecholamines, prostaglandin E_2 and prostacyclin [21, 49]. Taken together, the pharmacology of these compounds provides an exciting rational basis for the development of novel anti-inflammatory pharmaceuticals.

Current pre-clinical status

The results from extensive *in vitro* experiments and *in vivo* studies in laboratory animals have provided much optimism for the development of "second generation" PDE inhibitors. Almost without exception, drugs that inhibit the activity of PDE4 suppress a diverse range of functional responses across many cell types (including all of those indicated in Tab. 1) implicated in the pathogenesis of asthma and COPD [50–93]. Significantly, these agents negatively regulate the secretion not only of acute inflammatory mediators, such as histamine and cysteinyl leukotrienes, but also of other factors that are believed significant to disease progression and chronicity. The more important of these are the cytokines and chemokines including GM-CSF, IL-4, IL-5, IL-8 and eotaxin. Additionally, PDE4 inhibitors block adhesion of a variety of leukocytes to vascular endothelial cells, chemotaxis and the generation of oxygen-derived free radicals. From these data, it is clear that PDE4 inhibitors act at multiple sites and, thus, would be expected to have a general suppressive action on many indices of the inflammatory response. For a detailed description of the *in vitro* pharmacology of PDE4 inhibitors interested readers should consult references [20, 21].

Generally, studies designed to assess if the *in vitro* results described above are predictive of the behaviour of PDE4 inhibitors *in vivo* are borne out in a number of species including the mouse, rat, guinea-pig, dog and monkey. Given that asthmatic inflammation is believed to be eosinophil-driven, it is noteworthy that PDE4 inhibitors suppress IL-5-, PAF-, LTD_4- and, above all, antigen-induced eosinophilia in sensitized animals together with airway hyper-reactivity, the late phase response, microvascular leakage and cytokine generation [94–117]. Of particular significance are the results obtained in cynomolgous monkeys sensitized to *Ascaris suum* with rolipram [100] and the PDE4 inhibitor, CP-80,633 [101]. Given subcutaneously, rolipram significantly suppressed antigen-induced pulmonary neutrophil and eosinophil accumulation and the associated increase in IL-8 and TNFα in the bronchoalveolar lavage fluid (BAL) at a dose (10 mg/kg) that increased the cAMP content of BAL fluid leukocytes. Rolipram also reduced pulmonary eosinophilia and airways hyper-responsiveness to methacholine that occurred over a seven-day period in response to multiple antigen challenges [100]. PDE4 inhibitors also are active after antigen challenge [107, 109] indicating that stabilisation of mast cells cannot account totally for these activities. Indeed, the finding that PDE4 inhibitors suppress pulmonary eosinophil recruitment by agents that are selective eosinophil chemotaxins, including IL-5 [111], suggests multiple sites of action including a general suppressive action of those mechanisms that govern the emigration of eosinophils from the circulation to the airways [21].

No satisfactory animal models have been described for COPD. Nevertheless, in models of adult respiratory distress syndrome, inhibitors of PDE4 (rolipram, zardaverine) effectively antagonise neutrophilia following a non-allergic challenge with high dose lipopolysaccharide given systemically [118–120]. In rats, the effect is impressive where zardaverine blunts neutrophil accumulation in the lungs and the associated oedema and elevated level of elastase [119], which has direct relevance to COPD.

Clinical experience

Asthma

Despite extensive *in vitro* and *in vivo* data in laboratory animals, clinical trials with cyclic AMP PDE inhibitors are relatively limited. However, a number of studies have emerged over the last five years with equivocal results. Oral administration of the selective PDE3 inhibitor, cilostazol, produced a bronchodilator and anti-spasmolytic effect in normal human volunteers [121]. More recently, the effect of the PDE3 inhibitor, MKS 492 (40 mg), was examined in 18 atopic asthmatic subjects where it abolished allergen-induced bronchoconstriction (assessed by the measurement of FEV_1) and significantly attenuated the late phase response [122]. The reduction of the late phase response by MKS 492 is almost certainly due to functional antagonism since PDE3 inhibitors are effective smooth muscle relaxants but have limited anti-inflammatory activity. Unfortunately, the desirable actions of these compounds are accompanied by side effects that result from the inhibition of PDE3 in the cardiovascular system [123]. Tachycardia, hypotension, often with coincident headache, and arrhythmias, which reflected ventricular extrasystole in one patient, are the most serious deleterious effects [121–124]. One strategy aimed at reducing these cardiovascular limitations of PDE3 inhibitors has been the synthesis of compounds that inhibit PDE3 and PDE4 in the hope that lower doses will be clinically effective than a PDE3 inhibitor alone. However, thus far, this approach has yielded inconclusive results. Foster and colleagues [125] reported that benafentrine given by inhalation produced bronchodilatation in normal volunteers but was inactive when administered by the oral or intravenous routes. Another structurally dissimilar PDE3/PDE4 inhibitor, zardaverine, demonstrated modest bronchodilator activity in subjects with asthma when given by inhalation [126]. The hybrid PDE3/PDE4 inhibitor, tolafentrine similarly was inactive in a group of subjects with mild asthma [127]. Inhalation of 500 μg tolafentrine did not significantly affect airways responsiveness to histamine or adenosine monophosphate, which is thought to release histamine from mast cells and so promote bronchoconstriction indirectly. The level of exhaled nitric oxide, a surrogate marker of airways inflammation, also was unchanged by tolafentrine [127].

The appreciation that many side effects of PDE inhibitors reflect an extension of their pharmacology has persuaded the pharmaceutical industry to concentrate on selective inhibitors of PDE4 despite their limited direct effect on airway smooth muscle tone. Israel and co-workers with tibenalast [128] reported the earliest clinical study of the effect of a PDE4 inhibitor in asthma. Although this compound increased FEV_1 in a group of asthmatic patients the effect did not reach statistical significance [128]. The second-generation PDE4 inhibitor, piclamilast (RP 73401), also is without effect in individuals with moderate asthma [129]. Indeed, inhalation of piclamilast (1.2 mg for 15 min) failed to attenuate allergen-induced bronchoconstriction in 11 subjects [129] despite the nanomolar potency of this compound as an inhibitor of PDE4 [59]. However, given that mast cell-derived mediators are primarily responsible for allergen-induced early phase responses, these data are not necessarily surprising as selective PDE4 inhibitors generally are poorly active at stabilising mast cells [53]. More disappointing is that piclamilast (50 and 100 μg inhaled b.i.d. for six weeks) did not improve FEV_1, airway responsiveness to methacholine or the level of exhaled nitric oxide [129, 130]. Nevertheless, some encouragement can be derived from the results obtained with CDP 840, a potent and selective PDE4 inhibitor [131]. Studies with 54 asthmatic subjects in doubled-blind, placebo controlled trials indicated that 9.5 days treatment with 30 mg/day CDP 840 had no effect on the early response elicited by allergen (cf. piclamilast) but attenuated the late phase response by ~30% implying that the inflammatory response *per se* was being modified [132]. Indeed, that conclusion is concordant with the inability of single doses of CDP 840 (15 and 30 mg) to promote bronchodilatation in asthmatic subjects [132]. Unexpectedly, CDP 840 had no effect on airways responsiveness to histamine although the authors argue that the treatment period may have been too short since at least two weeks are required before changes in reactivity are seen in response to steroids [132]. Further positive clinical data have been published for another PDE4 inhibitor, SB 207499, recently named Ariflo [77]. At a press conference in London last year it was reported that SB 207499 produced a greater effect on FEV_1 than salmeterol and that it suppressed the early and late phase responses to allergen in asthmatic subjects (see [133]). Nieman and colleagues [134] also found that in 27 patients with exercise-induced asthma, SB 207499 (10 mg b.i.d.) produced significant improvements in lung function after 7 days of treatment.

COPD

Studies of PDE inhibitors in COPD are sparse and inconclusive. The PDE3 inhibitor, enoximone, given by the intravenous route, has been shown to improve lung function in patients with COPD [124] although another trial with the PDE3/PDE4 inhibitor, zardaverine, was inactive [135]. Perhaps the most exciting clinical data thus far reported has been from a trial of SB 207499. At a conference held in London in September 1998, it was reported that in a group of patients with moderate COPD (mean FEV_1 = 47% of predicted), SB 207499 (15 mg b.i.d.) improved FEV_1 by 130 ml (13% of their initial FEV_1) over a six week treatment period [136]. Studies are now underway to establish if PDE4D is functionally the most important isoform in neutrophils (with respect to degranulation, the NADPH oxidase and cytokine generation), which might explain, at least in part, its apparent efficacy in this disease. These data thus provide new optimism that PDE4 inhibitors do, indeed, have potential as anti-inflammatory agents.

Why have PDE4 inhibitors not demonstrated clinical efficacy in asthma?

Despite the animal and clinical results described above, experience with several structurally dissimilar "second generation" PDE4 inhibitors in the clinic has, thus far, been disappointing. While beneficial effects on airways smooth muscle tone have been documented, little evidence is available to support an anti-inflammatory action of these compounds. A number of factors could account for the lack of efficacy reported by many investigators that are not mutually exclusive. Some of these are described below.

Pharmacokinetics and drug metabolism

A major difficulty in selecting PDE4 inhibitors for asthma has been extrapolating drug metabolism and pharmacokinetic properties of promising compounds across species. This is illustrated with rolipram where oral administration of 50 mg/kg to the rhesus and cynomolgous monkeys, the rat, rabbit and humans results in complete absorption and an approximately equivalent half life (1–3 h) but with bio-availabilities of 0.1%, 0.37%, 3.6%, 3.7% and 75% respectively [137]. Reasons for the poor efficacy of CDP 840 in clinical trials, despite its potency as an inhibitor of PDE4, is provided in patent applications from Celltech which cite low bioavailability and short half-life probably due to extensive first pass metabolism [138, 139]. An assessment of biological activity in whole blood can provide invaluable information on the behaviour of PDE4 inhibitors *in vivo*. For example, CP 293,121 has reduced emetic potential but is extensively protein bound and, therefore, is not bio-available [133, 136]. However, poor bioavailability is not an insurmountable problem. Using piclamilast as an example, which is only 1% bioavailable in humans, as it was designed for the inhaled route, several changes to the central benzimide moiety has profound effects. Thus, replacement of the cyclopentyl and phenyl rings with tetrahydrofuran and pyridine N-oxide respectively, and oxidation of the pyridine ring to pyridine N-oxide produces a compound (RPR 114597) that is 77% bio-available in humans [140].

Difficulties in evaluating measures of efficacy and toxicity

Perhaps the single most confounding approach in the selection of PDE4 inhibitors for clinical development has been the evaluation of efficacy and toxicity in different species. The emetic potential of drugs is invariably examined in dogs or ferrets, whereas measures of biological activity almost always involve *in vivo* studies in rats, guinea-pigs and monkeys and *in vitro* experiments in human blood leukocytes. From these very different test systems the efficacious and toxic effects can be separated through the calculation of therapeutic concentration/dose ratios. A tempting but incorrect assumption is that these ratios always hold in humans regardless of the test systems employed for the analyses. Thus, it is vital to select the correct models of efficacy and toxicity for the evaluation of PDE4 inhibitors [141]. Clearly, a model where indices of clinical efficacy and toxicity could be measured in the same species is an ideal solution to some of these limitations although this can be technically challenging.

Dose-limiting side effects

Another explanation for the lack of efficacy of PDE4 inhibitors in asthma is that the level of drug ingested is too low to inhibit PDE4 in target cells and tissues. This invariably is because of dose-limiting side effects, nausea and vomiting, which are believed to represent an extension of the pharmacology of these compounds [142]. It would seem to be important in clinical evaluations of PDE4 inhibitors to establish that the amount of drug given inhibits PDE4 *in vivo*. While this is difficult to accomplish directly, several surrogate markers of PDE activity can be used such as the *ex vivo* measurement of cyclic AMP in bronchoalveolar lavage leukocytes, akin to the experiments performed in non-human primates [100], or more indirect measurements such as *ex vivo* cytokine production from peripheral blood leukocytes.

Strategies to minimize side effects

If it is accepted that dose-limiting side effects account, in large part, for the poor clinical activity of PDE4 inhibitors in human asthma, then what strategies could be adopted to increase the therapeutic ratio? Several possibilities have been considered.

The PDE4 isogene family

Molecular genetics has established that PDE4 is a generic term that refers to a family of closely related proteins. Thus, one approach to minimise side effects while retaining beneficial activity might be to develop "third generation" inhibitors selective for a particular PDE4 gene product [143, 144]. Currently, there is little information in the literature that addresses this issue and the functional significance of a particular PDE4 gene product in pro-inflammatory and immune cells is unknown. However, evidence is available that subtype-selective compounds can be synthesised. Indeed, the "second generation" PDE4 inhibitors SB 207499 and V11294A are 10- and 30-fold selective for PDE4D over the other enzyme families respectively [136]. In this respect it is intriguing that V11294A is non-emetic in ferrets at 30 mg/kg despite being >70% bioavailable and achieving a plasma concentration (>1 μM) that is sufficient to significantly inhibit PDE4 *in vitro* [136, 145, 146]. The lack of emesis also has been observed in humans in Phase I clinical trials at doses up to 300 mg. These findings are significant as V11294A is similarly bio-available (~50%) with a half-life of ~7 h [136, 145, 146]. However, a note of caution is merited here. While conceptually this approach seems logical, it pre-supposes that all dose-limiting side effects are, indeed, attributable to PDE4 inhibition. Moreover, the deliberate targeting of a PDE4 subtype also assumes that deleterious actions of PDE4 inhibitors are associated with a specific gene product(s) that is distinct from those that regulate cyclic AMP levels in pro-inflammatory and immune cells. This latter assumption seems unlikely. Even if supporting evidence is ultimately provided, it is difficult to envisage how this strategy could be exploited given that almost all peripheral cells and tissues contain representatives of the A, B and D gene families (Tab. 2). Indeed, human T lymphocytes express at least 5 proteins that are derived from these three genes [43]. The same is true for other cells including human eosinophils, neutrophils, monocytes and macrophages [147, 148]. It is also probable that there is significant PDE4 redundancy such that inhibition of a specific subtype will have little long-lasting impact due to the induction of an alternative isoenzyme. Perhaps the best family to target is PDE4C [38]. These enzymes are not present in inflammatory cells, but are abundantly expressed in the CNS [149] where PDE4 inhibitors are believed to promote many of their adverse effects. However, whether this is through inhibition of PDE4C is unknown.

Conformational states of PDE4

An alternative approach (patented by SmithKline Beecham) is based on the ability of certain PDE4 isoforms to adopt at least two non-interconvertible, or slowly interconvertible, conformations, $PDE4_H$ and $PDE4_L$, for which rolipram has high and low affinity respectively [150–152]. Significantly, the rank order of potency of a variety of compounds to inhibit $PDE4_H$ and $PDE4_L$ is distinct enabling a specific conformational state of PDE4 to be selectively targeted. The additional finding that the relative amounts of each conformer vary considerably between cells and tissues and that inhibition of $PDE4_L$ and $PDE4_H$ are associated with a number of anti-inflammatory and adverse responses respectively, has provided a rational basis for designing new compounds with a high $PDE4_H/PDE4_L$ ratio [150–152]. *In vitro* and *in vivo* studies have established that inhibition of $PDE4_L$ is linked to the suppression of the NADPH oxidase in eosinophils [153], IL-2 release from splenocytes [154] and TNFα generation from monocytes [76, 155]. Conversely, emesis [142], perhaps the major dose-limiting side effect of these drugs, and gastric acid secretion [156] are believed to result exclusively from inhibition of $PDE4_H$. It is noteworthy that certain functional responses, that might be considered desirable, are evoked following inhibition of $PDE4_H$ such as bronchodilatation [157] and degranulation of human neutrophils [76]. In addition, other effects that are not apparently related to inhibition of either $PDE4_H$ or $PDE4_L$ have been described suggesting that additional conformations of PDE4 might exist. These findings notwithstanding, compounds have been synthesised that have a considerably increased $PDE4_H/PDE4_L$ ratio when compared to rolipram (H/L = 0.01 to 0.001) such as CDP 840 (H/L = 0.27) [152], RP 73401 (H/L = 3) [59, 150] and Ariflo (H/L = 1.1) [77, 158] with the hope of retaining anti-inflammatory activity while reducing side effects. Indeed, SB 207499 was selected for clinical development based on a markedly improved $PDE4_H/PDE4_L$ ratio and its negative charge at physiological pH, which should reduce penetration across the blood brain barrier and, so, lower the potential for side effects. However, Phase IIb clinical trials have established that although apparently free of cardiovascular effects, SB 207499 (15 mg orally) was emetic. Interestingly, this adverse reaction was produced with only the first and second doses suggesting that the mechanisms governing emesis desensitise rapidly [159]. Based upon these clinical data it would appear that $PDE4_H/PDE4_L$ ratios considerably greater than 1 may be necessary to provide an acceptable therapeutic index. Ironically, it has seemingly been difficult to synthesise compounds with this property although Pfizer [160, 161] and Rhône-Poulenc Rorer [162] now have reported some success with novel series of oxindoles, catechol benzimidazoles and quaternary substituted γ-lactams. For example, CP 146,523 inhibits PDE4 with an IC_{50} of ~400 nM but is poorly able to displace [^{3}H]rolipram from rat brain cortex, a tissue rich in $PDE4_H$. Similarly, CP 293,121 has reduced emetic potential due to its high $PDE4_H/PDE4_L$ ratio [133, 136].

Pharmacokinetic strategies and alternative routes of administration

A primary objective of the pharmaceutical industry is to synthesise orally active PDE4 inhibitors that display *in vivo* efficacy in humans with an acceptable therapeutic ratio. Current experience with PDE4 inhibitors suggests that this goal can prove difficult to achieve when adverse effects simply are an extension of the pharmacology of these compounds. However, side effects may be limited by identifying methods of delivery that improve the pharmacokinetic behaviour of existing PDE4 inhibitors. One possibility is to administer the drug of choice as a slow-release formulation such that the peak concentration achieved in the plasma is lowered relative to overall systemic exposure [163]. This approach has been successfully adopted for pentoxifylline, a non-selective PDE inhibitor, which allows for the administration of higher doses before side effects become manifest [164]. Alternatively, direct application of PDE4 inhibitors to the airways as an inhaled formulation might be the preferred route of administration. Indeed, preliminary data suggest that this approach should retain the desired therapeutic activity while minimising side effects [165–167].

Development of combined PDE3/PDE4 inhibitors

In many "up-stream" immune and pro-inflammatory cells such as T lymphocytes and macrophages, which drive eosinophilic inflammation, PDE3 is widely expressed. However, inhibitors of this isoenzyme family generally are inactive or poorly active *in vitro* and in *in vivo* models of allergic inflammation but reproducibly potentiate the effect of inhibitors of PDE4 [20, 21]. This has been demonstrated in many cell types including human T lymphocytes where mitogen-induced IL-2 production was studied [53, 80]. Based on these findings it has been proposed that compounds that inhibit both PDE3 and PDE4 should be less prone to produce side effects than selective PDE4 inhibitors since activity would be expected at lower doses [168]. While this approach certainly appears attractive from a superficial perspective, it is not without potential problems when the clinical pharmacology of PDE3 inhibitors is considered. Indeed, these drugs originally were developed for the therapy of congestive heart failure and, therefore, certain predications can be made regarding their side effect profile. Of particular concern is their potential arrhythmogenic and vasodilator activities together with their ability to produce positive inotropism and chronotropism in the heart [169, 170]. Although this approach has not been rigorously tested in human volunteers, many researchers are of the opinion that the cardiovascular complications of PDE3 inhibitors preclude the development of hybrid inhibitors for asthma. Furthermore, logic dictates that if inhibitors PDE3 and PDE4 act synergistically in the resolution of inflammation, they could also synergise in the production of side effects. Nevertheless, the knowledge that the PDE3 in cardiac muscle (PDE3A) is different to isoform (PDE3B) detected in inflammatory cells such as T lymphocytes [43] does provide an opportunity to engineer molecules that have reduced activity against PDE3A. Although opposite of the desired selectivity, the PDE3 inhibitor, vesnarinone, is 10- to 50-fold more potent against PDE3A than PDE3B [171]. This is the first evidence that individual members of the PDE3 isoenzyme family can be distinguished pharmacologically.

Development of inhibitors of PDE7 and PDE8

An additional concern over the development of selective PDE4 inhibitors is the report that rats given rolipram repeatedly for two weeks displayed a profile of side effects similar to the toxicology of PDE3 inhibitors [172]. In particular, rolipram produced cardiac fibrosis, degeneration and epicarditis similar to the histopathology effected by milrinone and ICI 153,110 [173, 174]. Other effects produced by rolipram normally associated with the administration of PDE3 inhibitors were arteritis of the abdominal vasculature [172]. Although these lesions are believed to occur only in rodents, the recent discovery of new PDE families that are expressed in cells and tissues relevant to the pathogenesis of asthma provide alternative targets for increasing cyclic AMP with potential therapeutic opportunity. In addition to PDE3 and PDE4, two other isoenzyme families have been discovered that regulate the cyclic AMP content in a number of cells and tissues. In 1993, a gene isolated from a human glioblastoma cDNA library was expressed in a cyclic AMP PDE-deficient strain of the yeast, *Saccharomyces cerevisiae* [175]. This gene, originally named HCP-1 (high affinity, cyclic AMP-specific phosphodiesterase 1) encodes a cyclic AMP-specific PDE which is insensitive to cyclic GMP and inhibitors of the PDE3 and PDE4 isoenzyme families and does not hydrolyse cyclic GMP. Furthermore, HCP-1 does not share extensive homology to the *Drosophila* dunce cyclic AMP PDE (i.e. PDE4) and, therefore, represents a member of a novel PDE family that has been designated PDE7 [175]. PDE7 is believed to be encoded by a single gene, although at least two splice variants (PDE7A1, PDE7A2) have been reported [176, 177].

Northern blot analyses have identified an abundance of PDE7 mRNA in human skeletal muscle. In addition, transcripts of identical size are present in human heart and kidney [175]. In the context of allergic diseases, Bloom and Beavo [178], in 1994, identified high levels of PDE7 mRNA in the human T cell line, HUT 78 and, more recently, evidence has emerged that PDE7 mRNA and protein are ubiquitously expressed throughout mammalian tissues including human peripheral blood CD4[+] and CD8[+] T lymphocytes [80, 176], epithelial cells [179, 180], human monocytes, neutrophils, eosinophils and airways smooth muscle (unpublished observations). Selective inhibitors of PDE7 have not yet been described and so the functional role of these enzymes is undefined. However, recent antisense studies indicate that PDE7 regulates T-cell proliferation in response to ligation of CD3/CD28 [181]. Inevitably, the discovery of compounds that selectively inhibit PDE7 will provoke a considerable research effort to determine whether PDE7 represents a viable therapeutic target.

The other novel PDE family was discovered in 1998 by expressed sequence tag data base searching and was denoted PDE8 to distinguish it from PDE3, 4 and 7 [182, 183]. Two genes have so far been identified [182–184], PDE8A and PDE8B, that have a discrete tissue distribution; at the mRNA level PDE8A is abundantly expressed in the human testis, ileum, colon and ovary with lower levels in the heart, brain, kidney and pancreas [183]. In contrast, PDE8B mRNA is enriched in the thyroid gland [184]. Although pro-inflammatory and immune cells have not been systematically screened, PDE8 mRNA is present in human monocytes and airways smooth muscle (unpublished observations). The functions that these novel PDE isoenzymes subserve has to await the discovery of selective inhibitors, but the possibility that these proteins could be exploited therapeutically is one that, almost certainly, will be examined.

A re-examination of theophylline

Until relatively recently, the therapeutic efficacy of theophylline in asthma was attributed to its weak bronchodilator activity resulting from the inhibition of cyclic nucleotide PDEs in airways smooth muscle cells. However, there is now increasing evidence that theophylline exerts an immunomodulatory action at plasma concentrations that do not effect airways smooth muscle tone [185, 186]. Several lines of investigation have lead to this conclusion. In essentially all studies that have been conducted, theophylline protects against the late asthmatic response following allergen provocation implying that the emigration of pro-inflammatory and immunocompetent cells from the circulation in to the lung and/or their subsequent activation is suppressed. In a study of Ward et al., [46] theophylline, at a mean plasma concentration of 7.8 µg/ml, inhibited the late phase reaction in asthmatic subjects in response to allergen and the typical increase in CD4[+] and CD8[+] T lymphocytes.

Similarly, it has been reported that the number of CD8+ T lymphocytes in the peripheral blood of asthmatic children is suppressed compared to normal individuals and that the degree to which this occurs correlates with the severity of the disease [187, 188]. Significantly, treatment of those children for one month with theophylline restored the T cell count to the level found in the control group. Further support for an immunomodulatory effect of theophylline has been derived from studies examining the clinical effects of controlled withdrawal in patients on high dose inhaled steroids [189, 190]. Such intervention is associated with a deterioration in symptoms and lung function, a reduction in activated CD4+ and CD8+ T lymphocytes in the peripheral blood and a commensurate increase in the number of these cells in the lung as evidenced from bronchial biopsies [189, 190]. Recently, it was reported that in patients with moderate asthma and persistent symptoms, theophylline, at a dose below the recommended therapeutic range, in combination with low-dose budesonide, produced clinical benefits equivalent to high-dose budesonide given as a monotherapy [191]. Thus, in addition to the economic implications of reducing steroid usage, these data would suggest that theophylline is steroid sparing [185].

In addition to T lymphocytes, theophylline also modulates other pro-inflammatory and immune cells. In asthmatic children treated chronically for 10 days with theophylline both neutrophil and macrophage activity (chemotaxis, superoxide anion generation, bacterial killing) assessed *ex vivo* is suppressed, the degree of which correlates positively with the concentration of theophylline measured in the BAL fluid [192, 193]. Similar experiments have demonstrated that the number of EG2+ (activated) eosinophils and CD4+ T cells are reduced in allergic subjects given low dose theophylline (mean plasma concentration 6.6 μg/ml) for six weeks [47, 194] and that this might relate to the ability of theophylline to promote eosinophil apoptosis [195]. At the mediator level, oral administration of theophylline (mean level 10.9 μg/ml) to moderately severe atopic asthmatics has been shown to reduce the number of cells (mostly mast cells) staining for IL-4 and IL-5 implying that theophylline may repress transcription of the IL-4 and IL-5 genes [48, 196]. Moreover, Mascali and colleagues [197] reported an increase in the elaboration of the anti-inflammatory cytokine IL-10 from peripheral blood mononuclear cells harvested from 24 asthmatic subjects.

The molecular mechanism(s) underlying the immunomodulatory actions of theophylline is far from clear, but several activities have been considered that could act in concert. The most attractive of these is through the inhibition of cyclic AMP PDEs. However, the concentration of theophylline in the blood necessary to produce anti-inflammatory effects generally is less than 10 μg/ml, which has a negligible effect on cyclic AMP hydrolysis and, accordingly, has resurrected the proposal of a cyclic AMP-independent mechanism of action. Although several possibilities have been advanced including adenosine receptor antagonism, the inhibition of Ca^{2+} influx into target cells and the elaboration of catecholamines, none satisfactorily account for the results described above. It is of considerable interest that theophylline was recently shown to inhibit the activation of the transcription factor, nuclear factor κB (NF-κB), in human mast cells at concentrations (6 to 18 μg/ml–30 to 100 μM) achieved therapeutically [198]. Potentially, this is a significant finding as many pro-inflammatory genes relevant to asthma pathogenesis are regulated by NF-κB including TNFα, IL-1β, GM-CSF and RANTES [199]. If theophylline does, indeed, owe its therapeutic activity to a mechanism other that PDE inhibition, then a dedicated chemistry effort around the alkylxanthine structure could result in compounds with enhanced therapeutic activity and reduced side effects [200] that, paradoxically, might be achieved by reducing the ability of such compounds to inhibit PDE. In this respect, the xanthine derivative, arofylline (LAS 31025), has now entered Phase III clinical trials for the treatment of asthma based on encouraging Phase II studies in which a dose of 20 mg significantly improved FEV_1 after oral administration [201, 202]. Arofylline is a relatively weak inhibitor of PDE4 but, nevertheless, displays an anti-inflammatory profile in animal models of asthma similar to rolipram. It has been reported that arofylline is free of cardiovascular and CNS side effects in animals and is considerably less emetic in dogs than rolipram with a 10-times greater therapeutic index (see [133]). Results from further clinical trials are eagerly awaited.

What is the future of PDE4 inhibitors as anti-inflammatory agents?

Despite an extensive research effort, "proof of concept" studies in human volunteers designed to assess if PDE4 inhibition exerts an anti-inflammatory influence in clinical asthma are still not available. In the absence of this critical information what are the ways forward? Assuming that the concept is correct, then the identification of PDE4 inhibitors with markedly improved therapeutic indices clearly is desirable if these drugs are to be used as a mono-therapy in asthma. However, in light of the success in combining a β_2-adrenoceptor agonist (salmeterol) with a steroid (fluticasone) as a single formulation (Seretide) it is tempting to ask if similar benefit would be derived in combining low dose PDE4 inhibitors with existing therapies. Indeed, synergy might be predicted at the level of cyclic AMP accumulation with a combination of a β_2-adrenoceptor agonist and a PDE4 inhibitor that, theoretically, could be more efficacious than either drug alone. The idea of combining a PDE4 inhibitor with a steroid also is attractive since this could be steroid sparing.

If the inflammation that underlies asthma ultimately is shown not to respond adequately to PDE4 inhibitors it is important to appreciate that other diseases such as rheumatoid arthritis [163], atopic dermatitis [203] and COPD [136, 204, 205] which have a different inflammatory basis, may well be sensitive to intervention with these drugs. Indeed, recent trials of SB 207499 in COPD tend to endorse this possibility.

238

Acknowledgements
The author gratefully acknowledges the Medical Research Council (UK), the National Asthma Campaign (UK), the British Lung Foundation (BLF) and Glaxo-Wellcome Research & Development for financial support.

References

1   Flemming DM, Crombie DL (1987) Prevalence of asthma and hay fever in England and Wales. *Br Med J* 294: 279–283

2   Sly RM (1984) Increases in death from asthma. *Ann Allergy* 53: 2–25

3   Barnes PJ, Chung KF, Page CP (1988) Platelet activating factor as a mediator of allergic disease. *J Allergy Clin Immunol* 81: 919–934

4   Keating G, Mitchell EA, Jackson R, Beaglehole R, Rea H (1983) Trends in the sales of drugs for asthma in New Zealand, Australia and the United Kingdom. *Br Med J* 289: 348–351

5   Hay IFC, Higgenbotham TW (1987) Has the management of asthma improved? *Lancet* ii: 609–611

6   Murray CJL, Lopez AL (1997) Alternative projections of mortality and disability by cause 1990–2020: global burden of disease study. *Lancet* 349: 1498–1504

7   McEvoy CE, Niewoehner DE (1997) Adverse effects of corticosteroid therapy for COPD. A critical review. *Chest* 111: 732–743

8   Renkema TE, Schouten JP, Koeter GH, Postma DS (1996) Effects of long term treatment with corticosteroids in COPD. *Chest* 109: 1156–1161

9   Pauwels RA, Lofdahl CG, Pride NB, Postma DS, Laitinen LA, Ohlsson SV (1992) European Respiratory Society study on chronic obstructive pulmonary disease (EUROSCOP): hypothesis and design. *Eur Respir J* 5: 1254–1261

10   Torphy TJ, Undem BJ (1991) Phosphodiesterase inhibitors: new opportunities for the treatment of asthma. *Thorax* 46: 512–523

11   Giembycz MA (1992) Could isoenzyme-selective phosphodiesterase inhibitors render bronchodilator therapy redundant in the treatment of bronchial asthma? *Biochem Pharmacol* 43: 2041–2051

12   Giembycz MA, Dent G (1992) Prospects for selective cyclic nucleotide phosphodiesterase inhibitors in the treatment of bronchial asthma. *Clin Exp Allergy* 22: 337–344

13   Raeburn D, Souness JE, Tomkinson A, Karlsson J-A (1993) Isoenzyme-selective cyclic nucleotide phosphodiesterase inhibitors: biochemistry, pharmacology and therapeutic potential in asthma. *Prog Drug Res* 40: 9–31

14   Nicholson CD, Shahid M (1994) Inhibitors of cyclic nucleotide phosphodiesterase isoenzymes – their potential utility in the therapy of asthma. *Pulmon Pharmacol* 7: 1–17

15   Torphy TJ, Murray KJ, Arch JRS (1994) Selective phosphodiesterase isoenzyme inhibitors. In: CP Page, WJ Metzger (eds): *Drugs and the lung*, Raven Press, New York, 397–477

16 Torphy TJ, Barnette MS, Hay DW, Underwood DC (1994) Phosphodiesterase IV inhibitors as therapy for eosinophil-induced lung injury in asthma. *Environ Health Perspect* 102 (10): 79–84

17 Dent G, Giembycz MA (1996) Phosphodiesterase inhibitors: Lily the Pink's medicinal compound for asthma? *Thorax* 51: 647–649

18 Dent G, Giembycz MA (1996) Interaction of PDE4 inhibitors with enzymes and cell functions. In: C Schudt, G Dent, KF Rabe (eds): *Handbook of immunopharmacology: Phosphodiesterase inhibitors*, Academic Press, London, 111–126

19 Giembycz MA, Souness JE (1996) Phosphodiesterase IV inhibitors as potential therapeutic agents in allergic disease. In: RG Townley, DK Agarwal (eds): *Immunopharmacology of allergic disease*, Marcel-Dekker, New York, 523–559

20 Giembycz MA, Dent G, Souness JE (1997) Theophylline and isoenzyme-selective phosphodiesterase inhibitors. In: AB Kay (ed): *Allergy and allergic diseases*, Blackwell Scientific, Oxford, 531–567

21 Torphy TJ (1998) Phosphodiesterase isozymes: molecular targets for novel antiasthma agents. *Am J Respir Crit Care Med* 157: 351–370

22 Fischer TA, Erbel R, Treese N (1992) Current status of phosphodiesterase inhibitors in the treatment of congestive heart failure. *Drugs* 44: 928–945

23 Degerman E, Belfrage P, Manganiello VC (1997) Structure, localization, and regulation of cGMP-inhibited phosphodiesterase (PDE3). *J Biol Chem* 272: 6823–6826

24 Meacci E, Taira M, Moos M, Jr., Smith CJ, Movsesian MA, Degerman E, Belfrage P, Manganiello V (1992) Molecular cloning and expression of human myocardial cGMP-inhibited cAMP phosphodiesterase. *Proc Natl Acad Sci USA* 89: 3721–3725

25 Kasuya J, Goko H, Fujita-Yamaguchi Y (1995) Multiple transcripts for the human cardiac form of the cGMP-inhibited cAMP phosphodiesterase. *J Biol Chem* 270: 14305–14312

26 Taira M, Hockman SC, Calvo JC, Belfrage P, Manganiello VC (1993) Molecular cloning of the rat adipocyte hormone-sensitive cyclic GMP-inhibited cyclic nucleotide phosphodiesterase. *J Biol Chem* 268: 18573–18579

27 Conti M, Swinnen JV (1990) Structure and function of the rolipram-sensitive, low Km cyclic AMP phosphodiesterase: a family of highly related proteins. In: MD Houslay, J Beavo (eds): *Molecular pharmacology of cell regulation: Cyclic nucleotide phosphodiesterase structure and drug action*, Wiley, New York, 243–66

28 Bolger G, Michaeli T, Martins T, St.John T, Steiner B, Rodgers L, Riggs M, Wigler M, Ferguson K (1993) A family of human phosphodiesterases homologous to the dunce learning and memory gene product of Drosophila melanogaster are potential targets for antidepressant drugs. *Mol Cell Biol* 13: 6558–6571

29 Colicelli J, Birchmeier C, Michaeli T, O'Neill K, Riggs M, Wigler M (1989) Isolation and characterization of a mammalian gene encoding a high-affinity cAMP phosphodiesterase. *Proc Natl Acad Sci USA* 86: 3599–3603

30 Davis RL, Takayasu H, Eberwine M, Myres J (1989) Cloning and characterization of

mammalian homologs of the *Drosophila* dunce⁺ gene. *Proc Natl Acad Sci USA* 86: 3604–3608

31 Swinnen JV, Joseph DR, Conti M (1989) The mRNA encoding a high-affinity cAMP phosphodiesterase is regulated by hormones and cAMP. *Proc Natl Acad Sci USA* 86: 8197–8201

32 Swinnen JV, Joseph DR, Conti M (1989) Molecular cloning of rat homologues of the *Drosophila melanogaster* dunce cAMP phosphodiesterase: evidence for a family of genes. *Proc Natl Acad Sci USA* 86: 5325–5329

33 Chen CN, Denome S, Davis RL (1986) Molecular analysis of cDNA clones and the corresponding genomic coding sequences of the *Drosophila* dunce⁺ gene, the structural gene for cAMP phosphodiesterase. *Proc Natl Acad Sci USA* 83: 9313–9317

34 Livi GP, Kmetz P, McHale MM, Cieslinski LB, Sathe GM, Taylor DP, Davis RL, Torphy TJ, Balcarek JM (1990) Cloning and expression of cDNA for a human low-Km, rolipram-sensitive cyclic AMP phosphodiesterase. *Mol Cell Biol* 10: 2678–2686

35 McLaughlin MM, Cieslinski LB, Burman M, Torphy TJ, Livi GP (1993) A low-Km, rolipram-sensitive, cAMP-specific phosphodiesterase from human brain. Cloning and expression of cDNA, biochemical characterization of recombinant protein, and tissue distribution of mRNA. *J Biol Chem* 268: 6470–6476

36 Obernolte R, Bhakta S, Alvarez R, Bach C, Zuppan P, Mulkins M, Jarnagin K, Shelton ER (1993) The cDNA of a human lymphocyte cyclic-AMP phosphodiesterase (PDE IV) reveals a multigene family. *Gene* 129: 239–247

37 Sullivan M, Egerton M, Shakur Y, Marquardsen A, Houslay MD (1994) Molecular cloning and expression, in both COS-1 cells and *S. cerevisiae*, of a human cytosolic type-IVA, cyclic AMP specific phosphodiesterase (hPDE-IVA-h6.1). *Cell Signal* 6: 793–812

38 Obernolte R, Ratzliff J, Baecker PA, Daniels DV, Zuppan P, Jarnagin K, Shelton ER (1997) Multiple splice variants of phosphodiesterase PDE4C cloned from human lung and testis. *Biochim Biophys Acta* 1353: 287–297

39 Baecker PA, Obernolte R, Bach C, Yee C, Shelton ER (1994) Isolation of a cDNA encoding a human rolipram-sensitive cyclic AMP phosphodiesterase (PDE IVD). *Gene* 138: 253–256

40 Engels P, Sullivan M, Muller T, Lubbert H (1995) Molecular cloning and functional expression in yeast of a human cAMP-specific phosphodiesterase subtype (PDE IV-C). *FEBS Lett* 358: 305–310

41 Conti M, Nemoz G, Sette C, Vicini E (1995) Recent progress in understanding the hormonal regulation of phosphodiesterases. *Endocrine Rev* 16: 370–389

42 Houslay MD, Sullivan M, Bolger GB (1998) The multienzyme PDE4 cyclic adenosine monophosphate-specific phosphodiesterase family: intracellular targeting, regulation, and selective inhibition by compounds exerting anti-inflammatory and antidepressant actions. *Adv Pharmacol* 44: 225–342

43 Seybold J, Newton R, Wright L, Finney PA, Suttorp N, Barnes PJ, Adcock IM, Giembycz MA (1998) Induction of phosphodiesterases 3B, 4A4, 4D1, 4D2, and 4D3 in Jurkat T-cells and in human peripheral blood T-lymphocytes by 8-bromo-cAMP and Gs-

coupled receptor agonists. Potential role in β_2-adrenoreceptor desensitization. *J Biol Chem* 273: 20575–20588

44   Conti M, Swinnen JV, Tsikalas KE, Jin SL (1992) Structure and regulation of the rat high-affinity cyclic AMP phosphodiesterases. A family of closely related enzymes. *Adv Second Messenger Phosphoprotein Res* 25: 87–99

45   Monaco L, Vicini E, Conti M (1994) Structure of two rat genes coding for closely related rolipram-sensitive cAMP phosphodiesterases. Multiple mRNA variants originate from alternative splicing and multiple start sites. *J Biol Chem* 269: 347–357

46   Ward AJM, McKenniff M, Evans JM, Page CP, Costello JF (1993) Theophylline – an immunomodulatory role in asthma. *Am Rev Respir Dis* 147: 518–523

47   Sullivan PJ, Bekir S, Jaffar Z, Page CP, Costello JF (1994) The effect of low dose theophylline on the bronchial wall infiltrate after antigen challenge. *Lancet* 343: 1006–1008

48   Djukanovic R, Finnerty JP, Lee C, Wilson S, Madden J, Holgate ST (1995) The effect of theophylline on mucosal inflammation in asthmatic airways: biopsy results. *Eur Resp J* 8: 831–833

49   Kuehl FA, Zanetti ME, Soderman DD, Miller DK, Ham EA (1987) Cyclic AMP-dependent regulation of lipid mediators in white cells: a unifying concept for explaining the efficacy of theophylline in asthma. *Am Rev Respir Dis* 136: 210–213

50   Au BT, Teixeira MM, Collins PD, Williams TJ (1998) Effect of PDE4 inhibitors on zymosan-induced IL-8 release from human neutrophils: synergism with prostanoids and salbutamol. *Br J Pharmacol* 123: 1260–1266

51   Louis R, Bury T, Corhay JL, Radermecker M (1992) LY186655, a phosphodiesterase inhibitor, inhibits histamine release from human basophils, lung and skin fragments. *Int J Immunopharmacol* 14: 191–194

52   Peachell PT, Undem BJ, Schleimer RP, MacGlashan DW, Jr., Lichtenstein LM, Cieslinski LB, Torphy TJ (1992) Preliminary identification and role of phosphodiesterase isozymes in human basophils. *J Immunol* 148: 2503–2510

53   Weston MC, Anderson N, Peachell PT (1997) Effects of phosphodiesterase inhibitors on immunological release of histamine and on lung contraction. *Br J Pharmacol* 73: 287–295

54   Cooper KD, Kang K, Chan SC (1985) Phosphodiesterase inhibition by Ro 20–1724 reduces hyper-IgE synthesis by atopic dermatitis *in vitro*. *J Invest Dermatol* 84: 477–482

55   Dent G, Giembycz MA, Rabe KF, Barnes PJ (1991) Inhibition of eosinophil cyclic nucleotide PDE activity and opsonised zymosan-stimulated respiratory burst by 'type IV'-selective PDE inhibitors. *Br J Pharmacol* 103: 1339–1346

56   Dent G, Giembycz MA, Evans PM, Rabe KF, Barnes PJ (1994) Suppression of human eosinophil respiratory burst and cyclic AMP hydrolysis by inhibitors of type IV phosphodiesterase: interaction with the beta adrenoceptor agonist albuterol. *J Pharmacol Exp Ther* 271: 1167–1174

57   Souness JE, Carter CM, Diocee BK, Hassall GA, Wood LJ, Turner NC (1991) Characterization of guinea-pig eosinophil phosphodiesterase activity. Assessment of its involvement in regulating superoxide generation. *Biochem Pharmacol* 42: 937–945

58   Souness JE, Villamil ME, Scott LC, Tomkinson A, Giembycz MA, Raeburn D (1994) Possible role of cyclic AMP phosphodiesterases in the actions of ibudilast on eosinophil thromboxane generation and airways smooth muscle tone. *Br J Pharmacol* 111: 1081–1088

59   Souness JE, Maslen C, Webber S, Foster M, Raeburn D, Palfreyman MN, Ashton MJ, Karlsson JA (1995) Suppression of eosinophil function by RP 73401, a potent and selective inhibitor of cyclic AMP-specific phosphodiesterase: comparison with rolipram. *Br J Pharmacol* 115: 39–46

60   Hatzelmann A, Tenor H, Schudt C (1995) Differential effects of non-selective and selective phosphodiesterase inhibitors on human eosinophil functions. *Br J Pharmacol* 114: 821–831

61   Berends C, Dijkhuizen B, Demonchy JGR, Dubois AEJ, Gerritsen J, Kauffman HF (1997) Inhibition of PAF-induced expression of CD11b and shedding of L-selectin on human neutrophils and eosinophils by the type IV selective PDE inhibitor, rolipram. *Eur Respir J* 10: 1000–1007

62   Kaneko T, Alvarez R, Ueki IF, Nadel JA (1995) Elevated intracellular cyclic AMP inhibits chemotaxis in human eosinophils. *Cell Signalling* 7: 527–534

63   Tenor H, Hatzelmann A, Church MK, Schudt C, Shute JK (1996) Effects of theophylline and rolipram on leukotriene C_4 (LTC_4) synthesis and chemotaxis of human eosinophils from normal and atopic subjects. *Br J Pharmacol* 118: 1727–1735

64   Schudt C, Tenor H, Hatzelmann A (1995) PDE isoenzymes as targets for anti-asthma drugs. *Eur Respir J* 8: 1179–1183

65   Seldon PM, Barnes PJ, Meja K, Giembycz MA (1995) Suppression of lipopolysaccharide-induced tumor necrosis factor-α generation from human peripheral blood monocytes by inhibitors of phosphodiesterase 4: interaction with stimulants of adenylyl cyclase. *Mol Pharmacol* 48: 747–757

66   Semmler J, Wachtel H, Endres S (1993) The specific type IV phosphodiesterase inhibitor rolipram suppresses tumor necrosis factor-α production by human mononuclear cells. *Int J Immunopharmacol* 15: 409–413

67   Molnar Kimber K, Yonno L, Heaslip R, Weichman B (1993) Modulation of TNFα and IL-1β from endotoxin-stimulated monocytes by selective PDE isozyme inhibitors. *Agents Actions* 39: C77–C79

68   Prabhakar U, Lipshutz D, Bartus JO, Slivjak MJ, Smith EF-3, Lee JC, Esser KM (1994) Characterization of cAMP-dependent inhibition of LPS-induced TNFα production by rolipram, a specific phosphodiesterase IV (PDE IV) inhibitor. *Int J Immunopharmacol* 16: 805–816

69   Griswold DE, Webb EF, Breton J, White JR, Marshall PJ, Torphy TJ (1993) Effect of selective phosphodiesterase type IV inhibitor, rolipram, on fluid and cellular phases of inflammatory responses. *Inflammation* 17: 333–344

70   Derian CK, Santulli RJ, Rao PE, Soloman HF, Barrett JA (1995) Inhibition of chemotactic peptide-induced neutrophil adhesion to vascular endothelium by cAMP modulators. *J Immunol* 154: 308–317

71 Wright CD, Kuipers PJ, Lobylarz-Singer D, Devall LJ, Klinkefus BA, Weishaar RE (1990) Differential inhibition of human neutrophil functions. Role of cyclic AMP-specific and cyclic GMP-insensitive phosphodiesterase. *Biochem Pharmacol* 40: 699–707

72 Schudt C, Winder S, Forderkunz S, Hatzelmann A, Ullrich V (1991) Influence of selective phosphodiesterase inhibitors on human neutrophil functions and levels of cAMP and Ca_i. *Naunyn-Schmiedeberg's Arch Pharmacol* 344: 682–690

73 Ottonello L, Morone MP, Dapino P, Dallegri F (1995) Cyclic AMP-elevating agents down-regulate the oxidative burst induced by granulocyte/macrophage colony-stimulating factor (GM-CSF) in adherent neutrophils. *Clin Exp Immunol* 101: 502–506

74 Ottonello L, Marone G, Dapino G, Dallegri F (1995) Tumour necrosis factor α-induced oxidative burst in neutrophils adherent to fibronectin: effects of cyclic AMP-elevating agents. *Br J Haematol* 91: 566–570

75 Nourshargh S, Hoult JRS (1986) Inhibition of human neutrophil degranulation by forskolin in the presence of phosphodiesterase inhibitors. *Eur J Pharmacol* 122: 205–212

76 Barnette MS, Bartus JO, Burman M, Christensen SB, Cieslinski LB, Esser KM, Prabhakar US, Rush JA, Torphy TJ (1996) Association of the anti-inflammatory activity of phosphodiesterase 4 (PDE4) inhibitors with either inhibition of PDE4 catalytic activity or competition for [^{3}H]rolipram binding. *Biochem Pharmacol* 51: 949–956

77 Barnette MS, Christensen SB, Essayan DM, Grous M, Prabhakar U, Rush JA, Kagey Sobotka A, Torphy TJ (1998) SB 207499 (Ariflo), a potent and selective second-generation phosphodiesterase 4 inhibitor: *in vitro* anti-inflammatory actions. *J Pharmacol Exp Ther* 284: 420–426

78 Nielson CP, Vestal RE, Sturm RJ, Heaslip RJ (1990) Effects of selective phosphodiesterase inhibitors on the polymorphonuclear leukocyte respiratory burst. *J Allergy Clin Immunol* 86: 801–808

79 Fonteh AN, Winkler JD, Torphy TJ, Heravi J, Undem BJ, Chilton FH (1993) Influence of isoproterenol and phosphodiesterase inhibitors on platelet-activating factor biosynthesis in the human neutrophil. *J Immunol* 151: 339–350

80 Giembycz MA, Corrigan CJ, Seybold J, Newton R, Barnes PJ (1996) Identification of cyclic AMP phosphodiesterases 3, 4 and 7 in human CD4$^+$ and CD8$^+$ T-lymphocytes: role in regulating proliferation and the biosynthesis of interleukin-2. *Br J Pharmacol* 118: 1945–1958

81 Essayan DM, Huang S, Undem BJ, Kagey Sobotka A, Lichtenstein LM (1994) Modulation of antigen- and mitogen-induced proliferative responses of peripheral blood mononuclear cells by non-selective and isozyme-selective cyclic nucleotide phosphodiesterase inhibitors. *J Immunol* 153: 3408–3413

82 Essayan DM, Huang S, Kagey Sobotka A, Lichtenstein LM (1995) Effects of non-selective and isozyme selective cyclic nucleotide phosphodiesterase inhibitors on antigen-induced cytokine gene expression in peripheral blood mononuclear cells. *Am J Respir Cell Mol Biol* 13: 692–702

83 Banner KH, Roberts NM, Page CP (1995) Differential effect of phosphodiesterase 4

inhibitors on the proliferation of human peripheral blood mononuclear cells from normals and subjects with atopic dermatitis. *Br J Pharmacol* 116: 3169–3174

84   Van Wauwe J, Aerts F, Walter H, De Boer M (1995) Cytokine production by phytohemagglutinin-stimulated human blood cells: effect of corticosteroids, T-cell immunosuppressants and phosphodiesterase IV inhibitors. *Inflamm Res* 44: 400–405

85   Anastassiou ED, Paliogianni F, Balow JP, Yamada H, Boumpas DT (1992) Prostaglandin E2 and other cyclic AMP-elevating agents modulate IL-2 and IL-2α gene expression at multiple levels. *J Immunol* 148: 2845–2852

86   Chan SC, Li SH, Hanifin JM (1993) Increased interleukin-4 production by atopic mononuclear leukocytes correlates with increased cyclic adenosine monophosphate-phosphodiesterase activity and is reversible by phosphodiesterase inhibition. *J Invest Dermatol* 100: 681–684

87   Crocker IC, Townley RG, Khan MM (1996) Phosphodiesterase inhibitors suppress proliferation of peripheral blood mononuclear cells and interleukin-4 and -5 secretion by human T-helper type 2 cells. *Immunopharmacol* 31: 223–235

88   Crocker IC, Ohia SE, Church MK, Townley RG (1998) Phosphodiesterase type 4 inhibitors, but not glucocorticoids, are more potent in suppression of cytokine secretion by mononuclear cells from atopic than nonatopic donors. *J Allergy Clin Immunol* 102: 797–804

89   Essayan DM, Kagey Sobotka A, Lichtenstein LM, Huang SK (1997) Regulation of interleukin-13 by type 4 cyclic nucleotide phosphodiesterase (PDE) inhibitors in allergen-specific human T-lymphocyte clones. *Biochem Pharmacol* 53: 1055–1060

90   Kaminuma O, Mori A, Wada K, Kikkawa H, Ikezawa K, Suko M, Okudaira H (1998) A selective type 4 phosphodiesterase inhibitor, T-440, modulates intracellular cyclic AMP level and interleukin-2 production of Jurkat cells. *Immunopharmacol* 38: 247–252

91   Kaminuma O, Mori A, Suko M, Kikkawa H, Ikezawa K, Okudaira H (1996) Interleukin-5 production by peripheral blood mononuclear cells of asthmatic patients is suppressed by T-440: relation to phosphodiesterase inhibition. *J Pharmacol Exp Ther* 279: 240–246

92   Seldon PM, Barnes PJ, Giembycz MA (1998) Interleukin-10 does not mediate the inhibitory effect of PDE4 inhibitors and other cAMP-elevating drugs on lipopolysaccharide-induced tumor necrosis factor-a generation from human peripheral blood monocytes. *Cell Biochem Biophys* 29: 179–201

93   Blease K, Burke-Gaffney A, Hellewell PG (1998) Modulation of cell adhesion molecule expression and function on human lung microvascular endothelial cells by inhibitors of phosphodiesterases 3 and 4. *Br J Pharmacol* 124: 229–237

94   Howell RE, Sickles BD, Woeppel SL (1993) Pulmonary anti-allergic and bronchodilator effects of isozyme-selective phosphodiesterase inhibitors in guinea-pigs. *J Pharmacol Exp Ther* 264: 609–615

95   Underwood DC, Osborn RR, Novak LB, Matthews JK, Newsholme SJ, Undem BJ, Hand JM, Torphy TJ (1993) Inhibition of antigen-induced bronchoconstriction and

eosinophil infiltration in the guinea pig by the cyclic AMP-specific phosphodiesterase inhibitor, rolipram. *J Pharmacol Exp Ther* 266: 306–313

96   Teixeira MM, Rossi A, Williams TJ, Hellewell PG (1994) Effect of phosphodiesterase isoenzyme inhibitors on cutaneous inflammation in the guinea-pig. *Br J Pharmacol* 112: 332–340

97   Raeburn D, Underwood SL, Lewis SA, Woodman VR, Battram CH, Tomkinson A, Sharma S, Jordan R, Souness JE, Webber SE et al (1994) Anti-inflammatory and bronchodilator properties of RP 73401, a novel and selective phosphodiesterase type IV inhibitor. *Br J Pharmacol* 113: 1423–1431

98   Hughes B, Howat D, Lisle H, Holbrook M, James T, Gozzard N, Blease K, Hughes P, Kingaby R, Warrelow G et al (1996) The inhibition of antigen-induced eosinophilia and bronchoconstriction by CDP 840, a novel stereo-selective inhibitor of phosphodiesterase type 4. *Br J Pharmacol* 118: 1183–1191

99   Gozzard N, Herd CM, Blake AM, Holbrooke M, Hughes B, Higgs GA, Page CP (1996) Effect of theophylline and rolipram on antigen-induced airway responses in neonatally immunised rabbits. *Br J Pharmacol* 117: 1405–1412

100 Turner CR, Andreson CJ, Smith WB, Watson JW (1994) Effects of rolipram on responses to acute and chronic antigen exposure in monkeys. *Am J Respir Crit Care Med* 149: 1153–1159

101 Turner CR, Cohan VL, Cheng JB, Showell HJ, Pazoles CJ, Watson JW (1996) The *in vivo* pharmacology of CP-80,633, a selective inhibitor of phosphodiesterase 4. *J Pharmacol Exp Ther* 278: 1349–1355

102 Nagai H, Takeda H, Iwama T, Yamaguchi S, Mori H (1995) Studies on anti-allergic activity of AH-21-132, a novel isozyme-selective phosphodiesterase inhibitor in airways. *Jap J Pharmacol* 67: 149–156

103 Danahay H, Broadley KJ (1997) Effects of inhibitors of phosphodiesterase, on antigen-induced bronchial hyperreactivity in conscious sensitized guinea-pigs and airway leukocyte infiltration. *Br J Pharmacol* 120: 289–297

104 Danahay H, Broadley KJ (1998) PDE4 inhibition and a corticosteroid in chronically antigen exposed conscious guinea-pigs. *Clin Exp Allergy* 28: 513–522

105 Elwood W, Sun J, Barnes PJ, Giembycz MA, Chung KF (1995) Inhibition of allergen-induced lung eosinophilia by type IV and combined type III- and IV-selective phosphodiesterase inhibitors in Brown Norway rats. *Inflammation Res* 44: 83–86

106 Howell RE, Jenkins LP, Fielding LE, Grimes D (1995) Inhibition of antigen-induced pulmonary eosinophilia and neutrophilia by selective inhibitors of phosphodiesterases types 3 or 4 in Brown Norway rats. *Pulmon Pharmacol* 8: 83–89

107 Sturm RJ, Osborne MC, Heaslip RJ (1990) The effect of phosphodiesterase inhibitors on pulmonary inflammatory cell influx in ovalbumin-sensitized guinea-pigs. *J Cell Biochem* 14: 337

108 Underwood DC, Matthews JK, Osborn RR, Bochnowicz S, Torphy TJ (1997) The influence of endogenous catecholamines on the inhibitory effects of rolipram against early-

and late-phase response to antigen in the guinea pig. *J Pharmacol Exp Ther* 280: 210–219

109 Underwood DC, Bochnowicz S, Osborn RR, Kotzer CJ, Luttmann MA, Hay DW, Gorycki PD, Christensen SB, Torphy TJ (1998) Antiasthmatic activity of the second-generation phosphodiesterase 4 (PDE4) inhibitor SB 207499 (Ariflo) in the guinea pig. *J Pharmacol Exp Ther* 287: 988–995

110 Lagente V, Moodley I, Perrin S, Mottin G, Junien JL (1994) Effects of isozyme-selective phosphodiesterase inhibitors on eosinophil infiltration in the guinea-pig lung. *Eur J Pharmacol* 255: 253–256

111 Lagente V, Pruniaux MP, Junien JL, Moodley I (1995) Modulation of cytokine-induced eosinophil infiltration by phosphodiesterase inhibitors. *Am J Respir Crit Care Med* 151: 1720–1724

112 Santing RE, Olymulder CG, Van der Molen K, Meurs H, Zaagsma J (1995) Phosphodiesterase inhibitors reduce bronchial hyperreactivity and airway inflammation in unrestrained guinea pigs. *Eur J Pharmacol* 275: 75–82

113 Howell RE, Woeppel SL, Howell DE, Rubin EB, Jenkins LP, Golankiewicz JM, Lombardo LJ, Heaslip RJ (1995) Pulmonary antiallergic and antiinflammatory effects of a novel, orally-active phosphodiesterase IV inhibitor (WAY-127093B) in guinea pigs and rats. *Inflamm Res* 44 (2): S172–S173

114 Holbrook M, Gozzard N, James T, Higgs G, Hughes B (1996) Inhibition of bronchospasm and ozone-induced airway hyperresponsiveness in the guinea-pig by CDP840, a novel phosphodiesterase type 4 inhibitor. *Br J Pharmacol* 118: 1192–1200

115 Raeburn D, Karlsson J-A (1993) Effect of isoenzyme-selective inhibitors of cyclic nucleotide phosphodiesterase on microvascular leak in guinea-pig airways *in vivo*. *J Pharmacol Exp Ther* 267: 1147–1152

116 Ortiz J, Cortijo J, Valles JM, Bou J, Morcillo EJ (1993) Rolipram inhibits airway microvascular leakage induced by platelet-activating factor, histamine and bradykinin in guinea-pig. *J Pharmacol* 45: 1090–1092

117 Ortiz JL, Valles JM, Marticabrera M, Cortijo J, Morcillo EJ (1996) Effects of selective phosphodiesterase inhibitors on platelet-activating factor- and antigen-induced airway hyperreactivity, eosinophil accumulation, and microvascular leakage in guinea pigs. *Naunyn-Schmiedeberg's Arch Pharmacol* 353: 200–206

118 Turner CR, Esser KM, Wheeldon ER (1993) Therapeutic intervention in a rat model of ARDS: IV. Phosphodiesterase IV inhibition. *Circ Shock* 39: 237–245

119 Kips JC, Joos GF, Pauwels RA (1993) The effect of zardaverine, an inhibitor of phosphodiesterase isoenzymes III and IV, on endotoxin-induced airway changes in rats. *Clin Exp Allergy* 23: 518–523

120 Rabinovici R, Feuerstein G, Abdullah F, Whiteford M, Borboroglu P, Sheikh E, Phillip DR, Ovadia P, Bobroski L, Bagasra O et al (1996) Locally produced tumor necrosis factor-alpha mediates interleukin-2-induced lung injury. *Circ Res* 78: 329–336

121 Fujimura M, Kamio Y, Saito M, Hashimoto T, Matsuda T (1995) Bronchodilator and

bronchoprotective effects of cilostazol in humans *in vivo*. *Am J Respir Crit Care Med* 151: 222–225

122   Bardin PG, Dorward MA, Lampe FC, Franke B, Holgate ST (1998) Effect of selective phosphodiesterase 3 inhibition on the early and late asthmatic responses to inhaled allergen. *Br J Clin Pharmacol* 45: 387–391

123   Skoyles JR, Sherry KM (1992) Pharmacology, mechanisms of action and uses of selective phosphodiesterase inhibitors. *Br J Anaesth* 68: 293–302

124   Leeman M, Lejeune P, Melot C, Naeije R (1987) Reduction in pulmonary hypertension and in airway resistance by enoximone (MDL 17,043) in decompensated COPD. *Chest* 91: 662–666

125   Foster RW, Rakshi K, Carpenter JR, Small RC (1992) Trials of the bronchodilator activity of the isoenzyme-selective phosphodiesterase inhibitor, AH 21-132 in healthy volunteers during methacholine challenge test. *Br J Clin Pharmacol* 34: 527–534

126   Brunnee T, Engelstatter R, Steinijans VW, Kunkel G (1992) Bronchodilatory effect of inhaled zardaverine, a phosphodiesterase III and IV inhibitor, in patients with asthma. *Eur Respir J* 5: 982–985

127   Evans DJ, Aikman SL, Kharitanov SA, O'Connor BJ (1996) Inhaled tolafentrine, a PDE III/IV inhibitor: acute effect on histamine- and AMP-induced bronchoconstriction and exhaled NO in mild asthma *Am J Respir Crit Care Med* 153: A347

128   Israel EP, Mathur PN, Tashkin D, Drazen JM (1988) LY 186655 prevents bronchospasm in asthma of moderate severity. *Chest* 91: 715–718

129   Jonker GJ, Tijhuis GJ, De Monchy JGR (1996) RP 73401 (A phosphodiesterase IV inhibitor) single dose does not prevent allergen-induced bronchoconstriction during the early phase reaction in asthma *Eur Respir J* 9: 82S

130   McGrath JL, Aikman SL, Cook RM, Kharitonov SA, O'Connor BJ (1997) Six weeks treatment with inhaled RP 73401, a PDE IV inhibitor: effect on airway hyperresponsiveness and exhaled nitric oxide in mild to moderate asthma *Am J Respir Crit Care Med* 155: A660

131   Perry MJ, O'Connell J, Walker C, Crabbe T, Baldock D, Russell A, Lumb S, Huang Z, Howat D, Allen R et al (1998) CDP840: a novel inhibitor of PDE-4. *Cell Biochem Biophys* 29: 113–132

132   Harbinson PL, MacLeod D, Hawksworth R, O'Toole S, Sullivan PJ, Heath P, Kilfeather S, Page CP, Costello JF, Holgate ST et al (1997) The effect of a novel orally active selective PDE4 isoenzyme inhibitor (CDP840) on allergen-induced responses in asthmatic subjects. *Eur Respir J* 10: 1008–1014

133   Norman P (1998) PDE4 Inhibitors 1998. *Exp Opin Ther Patents* 8: 771–784

134   Nieman RB, Fisher BD, Amit O, Dockhorn RJ (1998) SB 207499 (Ariflo™), a second generation, selective oral phosphodiesterase type 4 (PDE4) inhibitor, attenuates exercise-induced bronchoconstriction in patients with asthma *Am J Respir Crit Care Med* 157: A413

135   Ukena D, Rentz K, Reiber C, Sybrecht GW (1995) Effects of the mixed phosphodi-

esterase III/IV inhibitor, zardaverine, on airway function in patients with chronic airflow obstruction. *Respir Med* 89: 441–444

136 Rogers DF, Giembycz MA (1998) Asthma therapy for the 21st century. *Trends Pharmacol Sci* 19: 160–164

137 Krause W, Kuhne G (1988) Pharmacokinetics of rolipram in the rhesus and cynomolgous monkeys, the rat and the rabbit. Studies on species differences. *Xenobiotica* 18: 561–571

138 Celltech Therapeutics Ltd (1997) WO9723460

139 Celltech Therapeutics Ltd (1997) WO9723461

140 Society for Medicines Research (1996) Trends in Medicinal Chemistry Meeting Report, London

141 Escott KJ, Birrell M, Webber SE, Souness JE, Geiger LE, Aldous D, Sargent CA (1998) Efficacy versus toxicity of PDE4 inhibitors *Am J Respir Crit Care Med* 157: A413

142 Duplantier AJ, Biggers MS, Chambers RJ, Cheng JB, Cooper K, Damon DB, Eggler JF, Kraus KG, Marfat A, Masamune H et al (1996) Biarylcarboxylic acids and -amides: inhibition of phosphodiesterase type IV versus [^{3}H]rolipram binding activity and their relationship to emetic behavior in the ferret. *J Med Chem* 39: 120–125

143 Muller T, Engels P, Fozard JR (1996) Subtypes of the type 4 cAMP phosphodiesterases: structure, regulation and selective inhibition. *Trends Pharmacol Sci* 17: 294–298

144 Bushnik T, Conti M (1996) Role of multiple cAMP-specific phosphodiesterase variants. *Biochem Soc Trans* 24: 1014–1019

145 Cavalla D, Gale DD, Spina D, Seeds E, Banner K, Page CP, Wong RH, Jordan S, Burch RM, Chasin M (1997) Activity of V11294A, a novel phosphodiesterase 4 (PDE4) inhibitor, in cellular and animal models of asthma. *Am Rev Respir Crit Care Med* 155: A660

146 Cavalla D, Gale D (1997) A case history in successful virtual research. *Drugs News Perspect* 10: 470–476

147 Engels P, Fichtel K, Lubbert H (1994) Expression and regulation of human and rat phosphodiesterase type IV isogenes. *FEBS Lett* 350: 291–295

148 Verghese MW, McConnell RT, Lenhard JM, Hamacher L, Jin SL (1995) Regulation of distinct cyclic AMP-specific phosphodiesterase (phosphodiesterase type 4) isozymes in human monocytic cells. *Mol Pharmacol* 47: 1164–1171

149 Engels P, Abdel'Al S, Hulley P, Lubbert H (1995) Brain distribution of four rat homologues of the *Drosophila* dunce cAMP phosphodiesterase. *J Neurosci Res* 41: 169–178

150 Souness JE, Rao S (1997) Proposal for pharmacologically distinct conformers of PDE4 cyclic AMP phosphodiesterases. *Cell Signalling* 9: 227–236

151 Barnette MS, Christensen SB, Underwood DC, Torphy TJ (1997) Phosphodiesterase 4: biological underpinnings of the design of improved inhibitors. *Pharmacol Rev Commun* 8: 65–73

152 Hughes B, Owens R, Perry M, Werrellow G, Allen R (1997) PDE4 inhibitors: the use of molecular cloning in the design and development of novel drugs. *Drug Disc Today* 2: 89–101

153 Barnette MS, Manning CD, Cieslinski LB, Burman M, Christensen SB, Torphy TJ (1995) The ability of phosphodiesterase IV inhibitors to suppress superoxide production in guinea pig eosinophils is correlated with inhibition of phosphodiesterase IV catalytic activity. *J Pharmacol Exp Ther* 273: 674–679

154 Souness JE, Houghton C, Sardar N, Withnall MT (1997) Evidence that cyclic AMP phosphodiesterase inhibitors suppress interleukin-2 release from murine splenocytes by interacting with a "low affinity" phosphodiesterase 4 conformer. *Br J Pharmacol* 121: 743–750

155 Souness JE, Griffin M, Maslen C, Ebsworth K, Scott LC, Pollock K, Palfreyman MN, Karlsson JA (1996) Evidence that cyclic AMP phosphodiesterase inhibitors suppress TNFα generation from human monocytes by interacting with a 'low-affinity' phosphodiesterase 4 conformer. *Br J Pharmacol* 118: 649–658

156 Barnette MS, Grous M, Cieslinski LB, Burman M, Christensen SB, Torphy TJ (1995) Inhibitors of phosphodiesterase IV (PDE IV) increase acid secretion in rabbit isolated gastric glands: correlation between function and interaction with a high-affinity rolipram binding site. *J Pharmacol Exp Ther* 273: 1396–1402

157 Harris AL, Connell MJ, Ferguson EW, Wallace AM, Gordon RJ, Pagani ED, Silver PJ (1989) Role of low Km cyclic AMP phosphodiesterase inhibition in tracheal relaxation and bronchodilation in the guinea pig. *J Pharmacol Exp Ther* 251: 199–206

158 Christensen SB, Guider A, Forster CJ, Gleason JG, Bender PE, Karpinski JM, DeWolf WE, Jr., Barnette MS, Underwood DC, Griswold DE et al (1998) 1,4-Cyclohexanecarboxylates: potent and selective inhibitors of phosphodiesterase 4 for the treatment of asthma. *J Med Chem* 41: 821–835

159 Murdoch RD, Cowley H, Upward J, Webber D, Wyld P (1998) The safety and tolerability of ArifloTM (SB 207499), a novel and selective phosphodiesterase 4 inhibitor, in healthy male volunteers *Am J Respir Crit Care Med* 157: A409

160 Masamune H, Cheng JB, Cooper K, Eggler JF, Marfat A, Marshall SC, Shirley JT, Tickner JE, Umland JP, Vazquez E (1995) Discovery of micromolar PDE IV inhibitors that exhibit much reduced affinity for the [^{3}H] rolipram binding site; 3-Norboryl-4-methoxyphenylmethylene oxindoles. *Bioorganic Med Chem Letts* 5: 1965–1968

161 Cheng JB, Cooper K, Duplantier AJ, Eggler JF, Kraus KG, Marshall SC, Marfat A, Masamune H, Shirley JT, Tickner JE et al (1995) Synthesis and *in vitro* profile of a novel series of catechol benzimidazoles. The discovery of potent, selective phosphodiesterase type IV inhibitors with greatly attenuated affinity for the [3H] rolipram binding site. *Bioorganic Med Chem Letts* 5: 1969–1972

162 Hulme C, Moriarty K, Huang FC, Mason J, McGarry D, Labaudiniere R, Souness J, Djuric S (1998) Quaternary substituted PDE IV inhibitors II: the synthesis and *in vitro* evaluation of a novel series of g-lactams. *Bioorg Med Chem Letts* 8: 399–404

163 Souness JE, Foster M (1998) Potential of phosphodiesterase type 4 inhibitors in the treatment of rheumatoid arthritis. *Curr Res Rheum Arthr* 2: 255–268

164 Ward A, Clissold SP (1987) Pentoxifylline: A review of its pharmacokinetic properties, and its therapeutic efficacy. *Drugs* 34: 50–97

165 Kamijo S, Imai J (1989) Eur. Pat. 3200032

166 Kamijo S, Imai J, Kodaira H (1989) Eur. Pat. 319902

167 Masakatsu K, Ohashi M (1990) Eur. Pat. 350913

168 Hatzelmann A, Engelstatter R, Morley J, Mazzoni L (1996) Enzymatic and functional aspects of dual-selective PDE3/4 inhibitors. In: C Schudt, G Dent, KF Rabe (eds): *Handbook of immunopharmacology: Phosphodiesterase inhibitors*, London, Academic Press, 21–40

169 Wood MA, Hess ML (1989) Long term therapy of congestive heart failure with phosphodiesterase inhibitors. *J Am Med Sci* 297: 105–113

170 Naccarelli GV, Goldstein RA (1989) Electrophysiology of phosphodiesterase inhibitors. *Am J Cardiol* 63: 35A–40A

171 Masuoka H, Ito M, Sugioka M, Kozeki H, Konishi T, Tanaka T, Nakano T (1993) Two isoforms of cGMP-inhibited cyclic nucleotide phosphodiesterases in human tissues distinguished by their responses to vesnarinone, a new cardiotonic agent. *Biochem Biophys Res Commun* 190: 412–417

172 Larson JL, Pino MV, Geiger LE, Simeone CR (1996) The toxicity of repeated exposures to rolipram, a type IV phosphodiesterase inhibitor, in rats. *Pharmacol Toxicol* 78: 44–49

173 Alousi A, Fabian RJ, Baker JF, Stroshane RM (1985) Milrinone. In: A Scriabine (ed) *New drugs annual: Cardiovascular drugs*, Raven Press, New York, 245–83

174 Westwood FR, Iswaran TJ, Greaves P (1990) Pathologic changes in blood vessels following administration of an inotropic vasodilator (ICI 153,110) to the rat. *Fund Appl Toxicol* 14: 797–809

175 Michaeli T, Bloom TJ, Martins T, Loughney K, Ferguson K, Riggs M, Rodgers L, Beavo JA, Wigler M (1993) Isolation and characterization of a previously undetected human cAMP phosphodiesterase by complementation of cAMP phosphodiesterase-deficient Saccharomyces cerevisiae. *J Biol Chem* 268: 12925–12932

176 Bloom TJ, Beavo JA (1996) Identification and tissue-specific expression of PDE7 phosphodiesterase splice variants. *Proc Natl Acad Sci USA* 93: 14188–14192

177 Han P, Zhu X, Michaeli T (1997) Alternative splicing of the high affinity cAMP-specific phosphodiesterase (PDE7A) mRNA in human skeletal muscle and heart. *J Biol Chem* 272: 16152–16157

178 Bloom TJ, Beavo JA (1994) Identification of PDE VII in HUT78 T-lymphocyte cells *FASEB J* 8: A372

179 Wright LC, Seybold J, Robichaud A, Adcock IM, Barnes PJ (1998) Phosphodiesterase expression in human epithelial cells. *Am J Physiol* 275: L694–L700

180 Fuhrmann M, Jahn HU, Seybold J, Neurohr C, Barnes PJ, Hippenstiel S, Kraemer HJ, Suttorp N (1999) Identification and function of cyclic nucleotide phosphodiesterase isoenzymes in airway epithelial cells. *Am J Respir Cell Mol Biol* 20: 292–302

181 Li L, Yee C, Beavo JA (1999) CD3- and CD28-dependent induction of PDE7 required for T cell activation. *Science* 283: 848–851

182 Soderling SH, Bayuga SJ, Beavo JA (1998) Cloning and characterization of a cAMP-specific cyclic nucleotide phosphodiesterase. *Proc Natl Acad Sci USA* 95: 8991–8996

183 Fisher DA, Smith JF, Pillar JS, St Denis SH, Cheng JB (1998) Isolation and characterization of PDE8A, a novel human cAMP-specific phosphodiesterase. *Biochem Biophys Res Commun* 246: 570–577

184 Hayashi M, Matsushima K, Ohashi H, Tsunoda H, Murase S, Kawarada Y, Tanaka T (1998) Molecular cloning and characterization of human PDE8B, a novel thyroid-specific isozyme of 3',5'-cyclic nucleotide phosphodiesterase. *Biochem Biophys Res Commun* 250: 751–756

185 Markham A, Faulds D (1998) Theophylline. A review of its potential steroid sparing effects in asthma. *Drugs* 56: 1081–1091

186 Chung KF (1996) Theophylline in chronic asthma – evidence for disease-modifying properties. *Clin Exp Allergy* 26 (2): 22–27

187 LaHat N, Nir E, Horenstein L, Colin AA (1985) Effect of theophylline on the proportion and function of T-suppressor cells in asthmatic children. *Allergy* 40: 453–457

188 Shohat B, Volovitz B, Varsano I (1983) Induction of suppressor T-cells in asthmatic children by theophylline treatment. *Clin Allergy* 13: 487–493

189 Brenner M, Berkowitz R, Marshall N, Strunk RC (1988) Need for theophylline in severe steroid-requiring asthmatics. *Clin Allergy* 18: 143–150

190 Kidney JC, Dominguez M, Taylar P, Rose M, Chung KF, Barnes PJ (1995) Immunomodulation by theophylline: demonstration by withdrawal of therapy. *Am J Respir Crit Care Med* 151: 1907–1914

191 Evans DJ, Taylor DA, Zetterstrom O, Chung KF, O'Connor BJ, Barnes PJ (1997) A comparison of low-dose inhaled budesonide plus theophylline and high-dose inhaled budesonide for moderate asthma. *New Engl J Med* 337: 1412–1418

192 O'Neill SJ, Sitar DS, Klass DJ, Taraska VA, Kepron W, Mitenko PA (1986) The pulmonary disposition of theophylline and its influence on human macrophage bactericidal function. *Am Rev Respir Dis* 134: 1225–1228

193 Condino-Neto A, Vilela MM, Cambiucci EC, Ribeiro JD, Guglielmi AA, Magna LA, De Nucci G (1991) Theophylline therapy inhibits neutrophil and mononuclear cell chemotaxis from chronic asthmatic children. *Br J Clin Pharmacol* 32: 557–561

194 Jaffar Z, Sullivan P, Page C, Costello J (1996) Low-dose theophylline modulates T-lymphocyte activation in allergen-challenged asthmatics. *Eur Respir J* 9: 456–462

195 Ohta K, Sawamoto S, Nakajima M, Kubota S, Tanaka Y, Miyasaka T, Nagai A, Hirai K, Mano K, Miyashita H (1996) The prolonged survival of human eosinophils with interleukin-5 and its inhibition by theophylline via apoptosis. *Clin Exp Allergy* 26: 10–15

196 Finnerty JP, Lee C, Wilson S, Madden J, Djukanovic R, Holgate ST (1996) Effects of theophylline on inflammatory cells and cytokines in asthmatic subjects: a placebo-controlled parallel group study. *Eur Respir J* 9: 1672–1677

197 Mascali JJ, Cvietusa P, Negri J, Borish L (1996) Anti-inflammatory effects of theophylline: modulation of cytokine production. *Ann Allergy Asthma Immunol* 77: 34–38

198 Coward WR, Sagara H, Church MK (1998) Asthma, adenosine, mast cells and theophylline. *Clin Exp Allergy* 28 (3): 42–46

199 Blackwell TS, Christman JW (1997) The role of nuclear factor-kB in cytokine gene reg-
     ulation. *Am J Respir Cell Mol Biol* 17: 3–9
200 Montana JG, Cooper N, Dyke HJ, Gowers L, Gregory JP, Hellewell PG, Miotla J, Mor-
     ris K, Naylor R, Tuladhar B et al (1998) PDE4 inhibitors: new xanthine analogues.
     Bioorg Med Chem Letts 8: 2925–2930
201 LAS 31025 (1997) *Clin Trials Monitor* 69: 25–26
202 Ferrer P, Dihn-Xuan T, Chanal I, Lockhart A, Bousquet J, Luria X (1997) Bronchodila-
     tor activity of LAS 31025, a new selective phosphodiesterase inhibitor *Am J Respir Crit
     Care Med* 155: A660
203 Hanifin JM, Chan SC, Cheng JB, Tofte SJ, Henderson WR, Kirby DS, Weiner ES (1996)
     Type 4 phosphodiesterase inhibitors have clinical and *in vitro* anti-inflammatory effects
     in atopic dermatitis. *J Invest Dermatol* 107: 51–56
204 Barnes PJ (1998) Chronic obstructive pulmonary disease: new opportunities for drug
     development. *Trends Pharmacol Sci* 19: 415–423
205 Barnes PJ (1998) New therapies for chronic obstructive pulmonary disease. *Thorax* 53:
     137–147

Index